Neuroendocrinology

Neuroendocrinology
An Integrated Approach

DAVID A. LOVEJOY

Associate Professor of Zoology
University of Toronto
Toronto, Canada

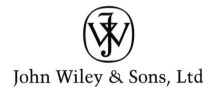

John Wiley & Sons, Ltd

Copyright © 2005   John Wiley & Sons Ltd, The Atrium, Southern Gate, Chichester,
West Sussex PO19 8SQ, England

Telephone   (+44) 1243 779777

Email (for orders and customer service enquiries): cs-books@wiley.co.uk
Visit our Home Page on www.wiley.com

Other Wiley Editorial Offices

John Wiley & Sons Inc., 111 River Street, Hoboken, NJ 07030, USA

Jossey-Bass, 989 Market Street, San Francisco, CA 94103-1741, USA

Wiley-VCH Verlag GmbH, Boschstr. 12, D-69469 Weinheim, Germany

John Wiley & Sons Australia Ltd, 33 Park Road, Milton, Queensland 4064, Australia

John Wiley & Sons (Asia) Pte Ltd, 2 Clementi Loop #02-01, Jin Xing Distripark, Singapore 129809

John Wiley & Sons Canada Ltd, 22 Worcester Road, Etobicoke, Ontario, Canada M9W 1L1

Wiley also publishes its books in a variety of electronic formats. Some content that appears in print may not
be available in electronic books.

British Library Cataloguing in Publication Data

A catalogue record for this book is available from the British Library

ISBN 0-470-84431-0 (HB)
ISBN 0-470-84432-9 (PB)

Typeset in 10/12pt Times by Integra Software Services Pvt. Ltd, Pondicherry, India
Printed and bound in Great Britain by Antony Rowe Ltd, Chippenham, Wiltshire.
This book is printed on acid-free paper responsibly manufactured from sustainable forestry
in which at least two trees are planted for each one used for paper production.

For my teachers

Nancy M. Sherwood

Richard E. Peter

Wylie W. Vale

Contents

Preface   xi

Acknowledgments   xiii

1 History of Neuroendocrinology and Neurohormones   1
Introduction   1
Early history of physiology   2
Renaissance and the growth of western science   12
Scientific revolution   20
The 19th-century physiology and medicine   25
Neurosecretion and the hypothalamus–pituitary regulation   31
Chapter summary   34

2 Origin of Life and the First Signalling Molecules   37
Introduction   37
Theories of the evolution of the first cells   38
The first cells   47
The first true signalling molecules   57
Chapter summary   60

3 Rise of Metazoans and the Elaboration of Signalling Systems   61
Introduction   61
Colonialism and multicellularity   62
The elaboration of hormone pathways   67
Nervous systems and rudimentary neuroendocrine systems   78
Increase in genetic complexity and the rise of triploblastic organisms   82
Chapter summary   83

4 Elaboration of Neuroendocrine Systems   85
Introduction   85
Elaboration of nervous system and development of organismal
   complexity   86
Nervous and neuroendocrine systems in phylogenetically
   younger invertebrates   91
Nervous and neuroendocrine systems in the deuterostomes   95

Peripheral and autonomic nervous systems — 99
Blood–brain barriers — 100
Cerebrospinal fluid and the choroid plexus — 103
Neurohaemal and circumventricular organs: Neurovascular interfaces — 104
Hypothalamus–pituitary gland complex — 106
Chapter summary — 115

5   Neurohormones and Receptors: Structure, Function and Co-evolution — 119
Introduction — 119
Orthology and paralogy — 120
Structural description of non-peptide ligands — 122
Peptide and polypeptide signalling molecules — 131
Structure and classes of receptors — 137
Receptor–ligand interactions — 145
Receptor–ligand co-evolution — 146
Chapter summary — 148

6   Osmoregulation, Metabolism and Energy Production — 149
Introduction — 149
Osmoregulation — 150
Role of prolactin — 161
Feeding and appetite regulation — 166
Neural circuitry associated with feeding — 173
Chapter summary — 183

7   Growth and Development — 189
Introduction — 189
Growth and the growth hormone, prolactin, somatolactin superfamily — 190
Metamorphosis and development — 198
Sexual differentiation — 205
Mechanisms of ageing — 208
Chapter summary — 211

8   Biological Rhythms — 215
Introduction — 215
Origin of biological clocks — 216
Circadian rhythms — 217
Infradian rhythms — 220
Clock circuitry in vertebrates — 224
The role of melatonin — 228
Chapter summary — 239

9   Stress, Arousal and Homeostatic Challenge — 243
Introduction — 243
Physiology and behaviour associated with stress — 244
Components of the stress-response system — 246

Corticotrophin-releasing factor superfamily of peptides   254
Proopiomelanocortin and adrenocorticotrophic hormone   261
Integration of HPA/I components with other systems   262
Complementary neuroendocrine circuits associated
   with stress   265
Chapter summary   272

10   Reproduction   275
Introduction   275
Selection of sexual reproduction   276
Regulation of reproduction   276
Gonadotrophin-releasing hormone   282
Gonadotrophins and their regulation   288
Neuroendocrine regulation of the HPG axis   295
Pregnancy, parturition and lactation   298
Seasonal reproduction   300
Reproduction and stress   301
Chapter summary   305

11   Behaviour, Learning and Memory   307
Introduction   307
Basic behavioural circuits   307
Memory   310
Motivation: Reward and fear   310
Stress and the modulation of learning
   and behaviour   314
Hormonal facilitation of behaviour   316
Galanin modulation of neurological circuits   323
An integrated approach to behavioural modulation   324
Neurodegeneration and trauma   325
Chapter summary   327

12   Pheromones and Chemo-attractants   329
Introduction   329
Evolution of pheromones   330
Classification of pheromones   332
Pheromones in invertebrates   332
Pheromones in vertebrates   337
Physiological actions of vertebrate pheromones   340
Pheromones in mammals   342
Chapter summary   344

13   Xenobiotics and Hormone Mimics   345
Introduction   345
Types of xenobiotics   345
Vertebrate toxins and defences   348
Toxins and xenobiotics in invertebrates   353

Toxins and hormone mimics in plants   357
Hormone mimics from anthropogenic sources   362
Chapter summary   363

Glossary   **365**
References   **367**
Index   **389**

Preface

Although the conservation of mass and energy and the transduction of one to the other has been explored in relatively great detail in science, the qualities of information flow has only been investigated until relatively recently. This has perhaps been stimulated with the vast quantities of information humans have begun accumulating. The disciplines of information technology and bioinformatics have helped stimulate new philosophies of understanding information flow.

Neuroendocrinology might be considered as the science that transduces information from both the environment (external milieu) and the organism (internal milieu) via sensory systems into a form that can be processed by the cells, tissues and organs of an organism to develop an 'informed' and integrated response to a particular stimulus. In practice, neuroendocrinology involves four basic areas of study. These include the actions of the nervous system on the functions of the endocrine processes, the reciprocal actions of hormones on nervous functions and behaviour, and the neurosecretions by the brain into the blood stream, and more recently, the function of neuromodulators and neurotransmitters inside the brain that ultimately act to direct actions outside of the brain.

Although neuroendocrinology is a relatively new science, it has expanded exponentially over the last 50 years. This book is intended to be used at the undergraduate level to introduce students to neuroendocrinology from an evolutionary and comparative point of view. Clearly, it is not possible to discuss every neurohormone system and its role in every physiological system; however, the major concepts of neurohormonal regulation, origin and evolution can be introduced. Thus this book is unique in the sense that we begin the study of neuroendocrinology with the origin of life to investigate where the first hormones came from. The development of neural signalling systems is traced from the first multicellular organisms to the most complex living organisms living today. Finally we end the book with how the neuroendocrine system integrates the organism with its environment, whether it is a human in a shopping mall or an insect in its ecosystem.

David A. Lovejoy

Acknowledgments

Completion of this book would not have been possible without the monumental efforts of my editor, Nicky McGirr, and Lizzy Kingston and the production staff at John Wiley and Sons in Chichester. It was through their hard work, encouragement and support that this book became a reality. I am indebted to the work of Sowmya Balaraman and her team at Integra Software Services Pvt. Ltd in India for transforming this work into a published format.

An author can never take sole credit for the writing of a book of science, particularly when the field is changing literally on a daily basis. Many of the sections and topics in the book were selected as a result of discussions with colleagues and associates from all aspects of neuroendocrinology.

I would like to thank my colleagues from the University of Manchester, and the University of Toronto for numerous helpful discussions. In particular I would like to thank Profs Stephen Tobe, Denise Belsham, John Yeomans and Nicholas Mrozovsky of the University of Toronto, Dr Hugh Piggins at the University of Manchester, Dr Susan Rotzinger at the Centre for Addiction and Mental Health in Toronto, and my wife, Dr Dalia Baršyte-Lovejoy at the Ontario Cancer Institute. I am particularly appreciative of the effort of my friend and colleague at the University of Manchester, Prof. Richard Balment, who critically examined an early draft of this book.

My warmest thanks to my colleagues with whom I have had the honour and privilege of interacting with, and who have kindly contributed profiles on their work: Howard Bern (University of California, Berkeley); Jackson Bittencourt (University of Sao Paulo); Imogen Coe (York University); Bob Denver (University of Michigan); Bob Dores (University of Denver); Matt Edwards (University of Toronto); Frank Horodyski (Ohio University College of Osteopathic Medicine); Wendi Neckameyer (St Louis University); Hugh Piggins (University of Manchester); Martin Ralph (University of Toronto); Nancy Sherwood (University of Victoria) and Hubert Vaudry (University of Rouen). Their contributions helped make this book an international and integrative work!

Special thanks goes to Roy Pearson and Matt Edwards at the Gerstein Library at the University of Toronto, who introduced me to a number of research papers and manuscripts I would not have found on my own. I also thank the Thomas Fisher Rare Book Library at the University of Toronto, for the digital reproductions from the older texts.

Much credit is due to the efforts and research of my present and past graduate students, Arij Al Chawaf, Xianjuan Qian, Yasmin Mohammad and David Tellam, my friend and colleague, Dr Liqun Wang, and some very talented undergraduate assistants, Jason Wasserman, Stacy Kyritsis, Cassandra Yau and Laura Tan who prepared some of the material used in this book. I must thank the students of my Zoo325 'Endocrine Physiology' course at the University of Toronto, who allowed me to 'field test' much of the material in this book, and my students at the University of Manchester where the concept of this book originated.

Finally I would like to thank my wife, Dalia, and my daughter, Sabine, for their help, understanding, patience and support while I endeavoured to complete this book.

David A. Lovejoy

1

History of neuroendocrinology and neurohormones

Introduction

Neuroendocrinology, as a separate discipline, did not emerge until the latter half of the 20th century. Neuroendocrinology found its roots once physiology, chemistry and biology coalesced out of the ancestral fields of medicine, alchemy and natural philosophy. The theory behind neuroendocrinology emerged only when cross-communication of ideas from these disparate disciplines could occur. Often information flow between these disciplines was stemmed because of lack of understanding, politics and wars, ego and religion. Advances in neuroendocrinology were accelerated once the ability to make the necessary observations on the most appropriate animal species developed. However, this was possible only after the concepts of evolution and animal phylogeny were consolidated. Like so many extinct species, many ideas were lost, after dominating the science for extended periods. Although it is easy to criticize incorrect ideas in retrospect, many such ideas needed to be fully examined before being discarded. Controversial ideas, even though they may eventually be shown to be incorrect, can stimulate research and experimentation in an area, which eventually lead to the discovery of new facts that would not ordinarily have happened. This chapter is not meant to be an all-encompassing summary of the history of neuroendocrinology, but rather represents an attempt to identify some of the major trends that led eventually to the formation of the field. If it can be said we are remembered for our successes, then this chapter represents

Neuroendocrinology: An Integrated Approach   David A. Lovejoy
© 2005 John Wiley & Sons, Ltd

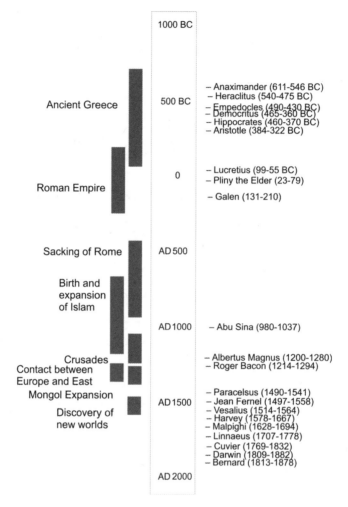

Figure 1.1   *Schematic representation of some of the birth and death dates of key historical figures who played a role in the development of neuroendocrinology.*

a celebration of the intellectual progress that led eventually to the science of neuro-endocrinology (Fig. 1.1).

Early history of physiology

In the earliest societies, physiological knowledge came from observing natural processes such as childbirth, injury, disease and death. Pharmacological knowledge of the medicinal uses of plants sprang from the knowledge of food and nutrition. Once language was developed and acted to consolidate these thoughts, then eventually a cause and effect was placed upon these events. We can only guess the level of understanding that the societies of prehistory possessed as no real historical documents survive. One of the earliest recorded human civilizations flourished in the city state of Babylon. Translated texts give reference to both human and animal anatomies, and medicine. Large collections of animals were kept in zoos, and early veterinarians were trained to keep these collections healthy. We might assume, therefore, that the Babylonians understood many of the similarities and differences among species, although physiological processes were not understood. Egyptian texts, on the other hand, made reference to the metamorphosis of the frog and scarab beetle. Biological and medical knowledge was obtained when it promised a potential solution for situations arising within these societies. Thus, while many facts were obtained by some of the earliest cultures, a philosophical framework upon which to organize this knowledge did not exist.

The science of ancient Greece acted as a catalyst to create a philosophical foundation of the natural and medical sciences. Many of the ideas driving modern science and biomedicine have their roots in Greek science, although one must sort through a number of incorrect notions in order to find them. Ancient Greece did not achieve political unity. It consisted of a series of city states each with a set of local gods and distinct religious customs. Some historians have argued that free thought may have flourished as the religions remained relatively primitive and disorganized. Unlike ancient Greece, science in Babylon, Egypt and India tended to be associated with a relatively powerful priesthood that kept the knowledge in the hands of a comparatively few number of individuals in the society. In addition, Greek influence extended over a large territory around the Mediterranean thereby facilitating the permeation of common ideologies throughout the cultures of the region. This commonality, by improving information flow among the societies, increased cultural and scientific interaction that ultimately fostered a rapid increase in the knowledge and the methods by which to procure knowledge.

Philosophers, such as Heraclitus (540–475 BC), Empedocles (490–430 BC) (Fig. 1.2), Hippocrates (460–370 BC), Aristotle (384–322 BC) (Fig. 1.3) and Epicurus (341–270 BC) (Fig. 1.4), to name a few, endeavoured to extricate the concept of disease from the limitations imposed by observable cause and effect. The pervading Grecian philosophy at this time embodied the concept that all biological systems continually sought to balance various influential factors that were either opposed or allied to one another. This balance was achieved through an interaction of the four humours: black bile, yellow bile, phlegm and blood. These humours combined the characteristics of the four elements – earth, air, fire and water – and reflected a harmony between the environment and the body. Those elements or qualities that fostered this balance, and consequently promoted harmony, were viewed as an essential part of health and survival. We might consider this interaction of the four humours to be a simple physiology. More importantly, however, it introduced the concept of 'dynamic equilibrium' – a chaotic interaction that we use today to characterize complex interactions of matter. Homeostasis, as will be described in later chapters, may also be described as a balance between internal and external conditions.

The ancient Greeks inherited this philosophy of health from older civilizations. The Ayurvedic writings of ancient India make reference to *vayu* (air), *pitta* (bile) and *kapha* (phlegm). These elements combined with other nutrients to form the seven basic tissues. The notion of quantification may also have been passed to the Greek culture from this culture as mathematics was also highly developed in the early Hindu cultures. The

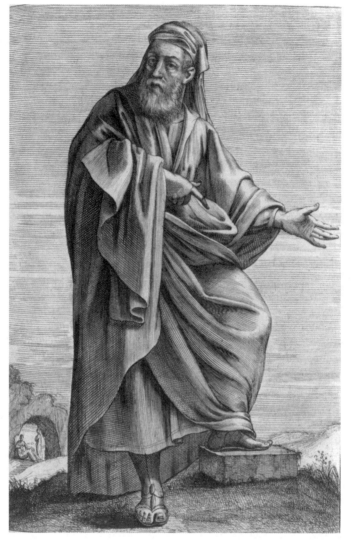

Figure 1.2 *Empedocles (490–430 BC). Reproduced by permission of the Thomas Fisher Library of Rare Books, University of Toronto.*

infusion of these methodological approaches likely had a bearing on the intellectualization and logical rationalization that characterized the Platonic school of thought that dominated much of Greek thinking.

The Greeks and a number of later cultures utilized the practice of 'pseudographia' where the writing of one author would be credited to another. This was considered a form of respect whereby junior philosophers and physicians would align with a more established school of thought. It is sometimes difficult to ascertain who actually penned a particular manuscript. Manuscripts bearing Hippocrates' name were written

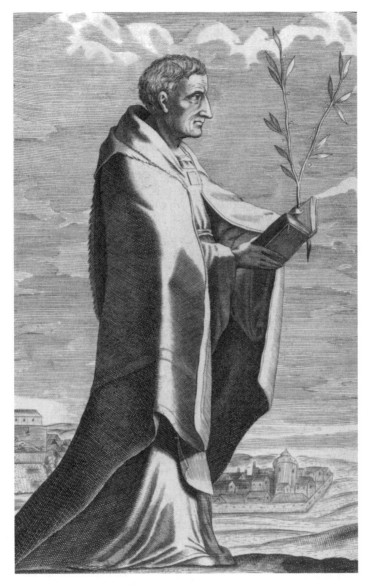

Figure 1.3 *Aristotle (384–322 BC). Reproduced by permission of the Thomas Fisher Library of Rare Books, University of Toronto.*

by a number of different authors. Despite this interaction, there was little understanding of endocrine functions in the various Hippocratean writings. The lymphatic glands were comparatively well described, for example, but there was little knowledge of endocrine glands such as pancreas. Moreover, there was a tendency to confuse nerves with veins. Although the word 'hormone' is derived from the Greek word 'hormonta' meaning to arouse or excite, the term was used by Hippocrates and later writers to

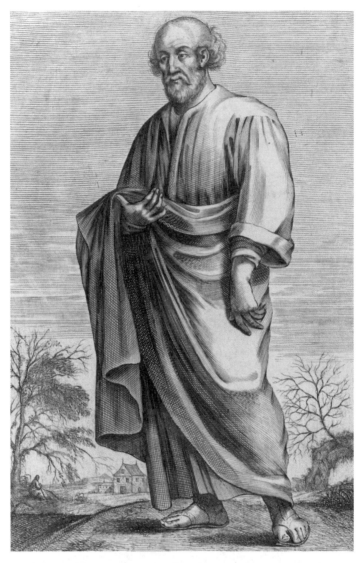

Figure 1.4 *Epicurus (341–270 BC). Reproduced by permission of the Thomas Fisher Library of Rare Books, University of Toronto.*

describe the life force. It did not obtain its modern definition until two millennia later when it was used by Bayliss and Starling in 1902 when they announced their discovery of secretin.

Physiological understanding of the brain was mired in competing theories. Among the first of the philosophers to reflect upon the function of the brain, Alcmaeon (ca.500 BC), suggested that mental processes resided in the brain. Empedocles, on the other hand, located mental processes in the heart, whereas Plato (430–347 BC) (Fig. 1.5) argued that

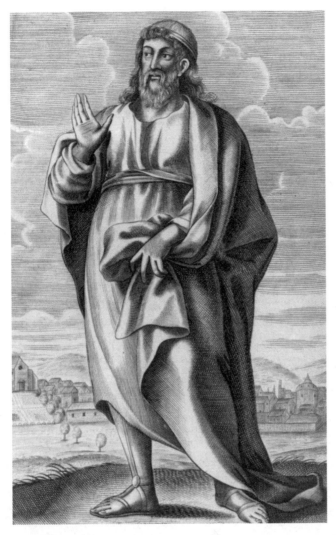

Figure 1.5   *Plato (430–347 BC). Reproduced by permission of the Thomas Fisher Library of Rare Books, University of Toronto.*

rational part of the soul occurred in the brain as it was the closest to the heavens. Aristotle rejected his teacher's beliefs and suggested that the brain only acted to cool the blood. He too believed that thought and rationality occurred in the heart. Democritus (465–360) (Fig. 1.6) also argued that the brain might be the organ of thought. This latter concept was eventually incorporated into some of the Hippocratean writings where emotion and feelings were described as being part of the brain function. With considerable insight, Democritus had forwarded the notion that matter was composed of small particles not visible to the naked eye. Lucretius (99–55 BC) applied this theory of 'atomism' to the

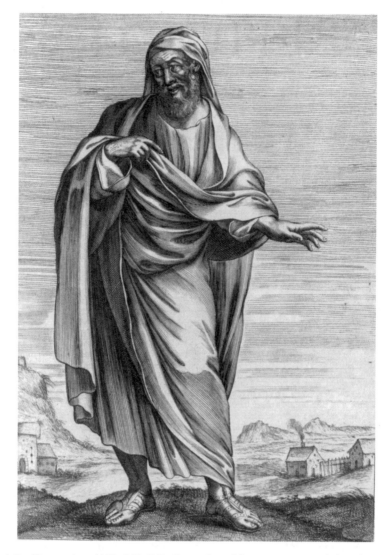

Figure 1.6 *Democritus (465–360 BC). Reproduced by permission of the Thomas Fisher Library of Rare Books, University of Toronto.*

senses. He argued that sense perception occurs when small particles are given off which impinge upon the eyes, tongue and nose. Different particles were responsible for different sensory perceptions. Lucretius' writings helped atomism to survive throughout the middle ages, although it did not really begin to flourish as a theory until the 19th century.

Observations of the animal world had the potential to add much to the understanding of medicine. Anaximander (611–546 BC) may have been the first to introduce the concept of an evolutionary process to explain the related animal forms. Whilst the pattern by which one form changed to another was incorrect, he introduced the notion of the transition of one morphological form to another. Later, Aristotle, drawing upon these ideas along with the concepts of Plato, developed the first systemic classification of animals incorporating comparative principles. Unfortunately, because human were considered to have divine origins to a certain degree, many of the zoological observations were not incorporated into an understanding of human physiology at least until a few hundred more years.

With the knowledge of hindsight, we might wring our hands in anguish and think how close the Greeks were to bring together a modern understanding of physiology, yet they missed the opportunity. Experimentation as a way of procuring knowledge had yet to become entrenched in the psyche of the natural philosophers, and thus they were limited by what was observable. Frequently, it was impossible to differentiate among a number of competing theories. Human dissection was generally banned in the Greek states, thus observations of disease, injury and battlefield wounds provided the primary observations of anatomy and the underlying physiological processes.

As Greek culture waned in influence, Alexandria in Egypt enjoyed a brief heyday before the cultural torch was passed to Rome. The Alexandria Medical School introduced the notion that the level of understanding was dependent upon the detail of the observation. About 300 BC, dissection of the human body was legalized in the Alexandrian school where the bodies of condemned criminals were used for this purpose. Human dissections were practiced with exquisite skill for the time allowing accurate observations to supplant earlier observations based on animal dissections. Galen (AD 131–210), born of Greek parents in the region that is now Turkey, was influenced by the teachings of Alexandria and Greek schools of thought. He later moved to Rome where he developed a considerable following. Galen wrote over five hundred medical treatises of which over one hundred have survived into modern times (Fig. 1.7). Much of our understanding of Roman medicine comes from these sources and, therefore, we have a skewed view of what Roman medicine actually was. Galen understood the physiological processes as food being consumed and transformed in the liver into blood. There, it is passed to the lung to combine with air where it flowed outwards to all organs. He added considerable detail to the morphology of the brain and described motor and sensory nerves. Galen did perform a number of experiments and dissections on animals to determine the significance of various organ systems but continued to utilize the Greek four-humour concept. He refuted Aristotle's theory on the function of the brain by arguing that nerves from the sense organs went to the brain, not the heart.

The Romans added little to the Greek understanding of the zoological world. In the 1st century AD, Pliny the Elder (AD 23–79) wrote the 37-volume 'Natural History'. This book was a mixture of fact and fantasy about European, African and Asian animals. Pliny did little, if any, of his own observation, but rather tended to record and compile the observations of others. Pliny, however, unlike previous writers, quoted his sources in his texts, a practice that was reintroduced in modern times. This influence of this text lasted into the Renaissance times with little attempt to modify or correct the text until about the 15th century.

By the 4th century AD, as a result of inept leadership, high taxes and increased pressure by external societies, the political locus of influence moved from Rome to Constantinople in the East once again shifting the intellectual and scientific focus. The Western Roman Empire eventually collapsed and was replaced by a series of unstable

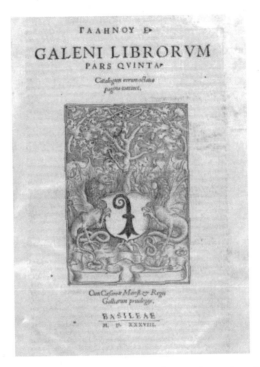

Figure 1.7   *A Renaissance version on Galenic medicine. Reproduced by permission of the Thomas Fisher Library of Rare Books, University of Toronto.*

political and economic states over the next 500 years. Much of the material property and intellectual culture was lost. The Byzantine Empire, arising from the Eastern Roman Empire, inherited much of the Roman approach to science and medicine. However, the Byzantinians took a practical approach to medicine and acquired what information they could find, then combined the elements of natural observation with mysticism and 'magic' in an attempt to solve medical problems. Byzantium overlapped historically with the emergence of Islam, and in the early stages of Islamic growth, the Byzantium knowledge of medicine passed to Islam. Later, much of this was transferred back to Byzantium, albeit in a much expanded and developed state.

Whilst much of Europe laboured under a relatively austere feudal society, the emergence of Islam in the east introduced numerous tribes and cultures to a common ideology. Islam eventually grew into a large cultural and intellectual society that surpassed the knowledge and ability of the western states. The growth of Arabic science was a direct descendent of Greek science. As Islam united the ancient lands of Syria, Babylon, Persia and Egypt, they also acquired the Greek texts scattered throughout the region. The texts of Aristotle and Galen were among the first to be translated into Arabic. Abu Sina (980–1037), one of the early Arabic writers, wrote the *Canon of Medicine* that was built upon the ideas of Galen and Aristotle.

The concept of experimental science was utilized by Muslim scientists centuries before it became widely used in the west. By the 10th century, al-Razi (850–932) described the function of veins and valves, and during the 13th century, Ibn al-Nafs and Ibn al Quff described the circulation of blood and the role of the heart. Opium derivatives were used as anaesthetics; sulphur- and mercury-based compounds were used as anti-microbial agents. Most importantly, however, was the discovery and utilization of drug-like compounds and herbal extracts to treat various conditions. The protosciences of chemistry, botany and pharmacology were all intrinsically linked with Arabic science. The Arabs introduced experimental science particularly in the form of chemistry that was essentially born from the use and understanding of herbal-type concoctions of the ancients. By the 14th century, Ibn Baytar described the use of over 1000 different naturally derived agents. The science of pharmacology, which acted as a foundation for modern endocrine theory, was comparatively well developed in Islam. The word 'drug' is derived from Arabic.

The rise of Islam had a number of effects on information flow in the West, which ultimately affected the direction of western science. Byzantium found itself in the awkward position of having Islam to the east, barbaric peoples to the north and an unstable Europe to the west. Intercultural contacts were frequent although Byzantinian society was maintained by a combination of both diplomatic and armed contacts with each of these groups. During Islamic rule, large parts of their culture came under the rule of a single person, Caliph, and foreigners could travel throughout Muslim countries without hindrance. However, Byzantium and western Europe, being primarily Christian, were restricted from travelling through Islam thereby separating Europe from cultures that lay to the east of Islam, notably India and China. The perceived Muslim threat on Byzantium acted also to increase communication between Constantinople and Rome once western society began to stabilize. Because of the limited interaction between Islam and the west, knowledge of Muslim discoveries eventually made its way to the west via Byzantium. In addition, a number of Arabic writings were introduced to western Europe by the Arab occupation of Spain and Sicily.

By the late 10th century, Christian pilgrimages to the Holy Land were organized into a series of crusades that lasted until the mid-13th century. These crusades that initially began as unruly mobs of poverty stricken and desperate individuals eventually opened Jerusalem back to the west. This coincided with the sweep of the Mongolian Tartars through Islam in the early 13th century and opened a passage for westerners to travel to the east. This overland route to the east lasted for about a century until the Tartar administration of the region began to crumble and Islam coalesced again effectively shutting down this passage.

In the west, science through much of the middle ages was constrained by the doctrines of the Catholic Church. However, many concepts held by the Church were not inconsistent with some of the prevailing scientific views. St Augustine (353–430), for example, had suggested that in the beginning the earth was endowed with the ability to produce plants and animals, and one must not necessarily assume that all creation formed at once. This view was supported, as late as the 13th century, by St Thomas Aquinas (1225–1275).

In the 12th century, the formation of the university occurred. This led to concentrated loci of study that later through inter-university competition acted to drive scientific research. Now for the first time, hundreds or thousands of students could be educated together instead of the few individuals that could be educated in the past. This increased the level of learnedness in society. Ironically, the formation of the universities that were generally formed to be higher learning centres of religious doctrine allowed free thought to flourish in various pockets of society. Roger Bacon (1214–1294) studied at Oxford and Paris, and achieved a position of eminence in the Franciscan order. He was an avid experimentalist and pushed the view that science should be based on the experience gained through observing natural phenomena. Unfortunately, his liberal views landed him in prison. Despite his controversial beliefs, he and others attracted others to this philosophy. Nevertheless, the universities, an infusion of translated texts, ideas and observations from Islam and from eastern sources, ignited free thought in the west and laid the foundations for the Renaissance.

Renaissance and the growth of western science

The Renaissance was essentially born in Italy, which was never far removed from the science of antiquity. During the Renaissance there became a quest for knowledge for knowledge's sake. Coincident with the rediscovery of the ancient texts came the discovery of new worlds or new routes to the east. The loss of the overland route to India and China inspired Portugal to find a new route around Africa to the east. Their eventual success and dominance of this route induced Spain to investigate a direct route across the Atlantic to the east. There became a new component of society that developed the quest for knowledge. Thus, a new type of scientist emerged, one that became a travelling naturalist or a scientific explorer.

At the dawn of the Renaissance, the search for the classic scientific texts was intense with the resurgence in interest of the ancient scholars. However, despite the recovering of the ancient texts, much of the Greek writing of antiquity were inaccessible to most of the western world due to the lack of scholars who were fluent in ancient Greek. It was not until Manuel Chrysolorus arrived in Italy with the Byzantine Emperor Manuel Paleologus in 1396, and later another Byzantinian, Gemistos Plethon, in 1439. This caused a Greek revival that was to affect all scholarly fields in the 15th century. In 1417, Poggio Bracciolini (1380–1459) discovered the only remaining copy of Lucretius (99–55 BC) *De Rerum Natura* to have survived antiquity. This book became a major stimulus for the revived interest in atomism two centuries later. In 1428, Guarino da Verona (1370–1460) found Celsus' treatise *De Medicina* written in the 2nd century AD.

Coincident with the search of these ancient texts was the development of the printing press and improved methods for reducing pictures such as woodcuts and copper plate engraving. Now, for the first time, information and knowledge could be efficiently disseminated to scholars and laypersons alike. Latin, used as a scientific language, had previously kept the communication of ideas within the scientific community. However, the growing use of vernacular language in the 15th and 16th centuries by medical and natural scientists allowed science to be understood by the public.

Medicine during the Renaissance

Galen's theories continued to dominate physiological thinking until well into the Renaissance. Although, al-Razi had written an entire volume on the shortcomings of

Galen's work, some 500 years earlier, much of this thought was inaccessible to western societies. The concept of endocrinology was dependent upon understanding the physics of circulation. Unfortunately, there remained considerable resistance to ideas that contradicted to those of Galen. The divine element of human consciousness remained to be extricated from medical teachings. Thus, many of the physicians attempted to advance physiological understanding by trying to understand the spiritual origin of vitality. In 1553, the Spanish physician, Michael Servetus, was jailed, then later burned at the stake for describing the modern notion of pulmonary circulation in contradiction to what Galen had postulated nearly 1400 years earlier. Serevetus believed that the blood was the origin of the divine spirit or the soul. In his quest for this understanding, he rejected Galen's notion that blood passed through pores of the septum and argued that blood was diverted to the lungs where it mixed with air, became cleaned and reddened, then returned to the auricle. Unfortunately, he described his theory in his *Christianismi Restitutio*, where it was not understood by the theologians who read the book. They eventually burned all known copies of the book along with the author. However, historians have suspected that one of the surviving copies may have been examined by Realdus Columbus, a professor of anatomy, in Rome. In 1559, he published a theory suspiciously similar to that of Serevetus. The theory remained in academic circles and appears to have made an impression upon William Harvey.

In many ways, much of the understanding of natural science and medicine had to be rediscovered in the west. Medicine and modern physiology were dependent on an accurate understanding of anatomy and its function. Functional comprehension continued to be limited by the lack of experimental methods. This inhibition of anatomical studies occurred, in part, because of a ban on human dissection. Andreas Vesalius (1514–1564) (Fig. 1.8) played a major role in finally overthrowing Galen's dominance of medical teachings. Unlike the majority of other professors of anatomy, Vesalius performed his own dissections during public demonstrations and, therefore, was in a position to directly observe the discrepancies between Galen's work and that of human anatomy (Fig. 1.9). However, Vesalius was already intellectually primed to examine the shortcomings of Galen's work having previously translated a Greek version of the ninth volume of al-Razi. Vesalius published *De Humani Corporis Fabrica* in 1543. It consisted of seven volumes detailing human anatomy. Each was supplemented with high quality illustrations. The first book was devoted to the skeleton and the second included all of the musculature. The third book was devoted to all the veins and arteries, where he described the capillary network of the hepatic portal system that would later be utilized by Harvey in describing circulation, and also later in the 20th century as a model to understand the hypothalamus–pituitary portal system. The fourth book described the nerves and the abdominal organs were described in the fifth book. The thoracic organs were covered in the sixth book whereas the seventh book was devoted entirely to the brain (Fig. 1.10). Vesalius' treatise on human anatomy represented a landmark event in the study of physiology for here was the first real attempt to describe the structure of human anatomy in an integrated manner. Around the same time, Charles Estienne published *De Dissectione Partium Corporis Humani*, a treatise on human anatomy, although the descriptions and the figures were of considerably less quality than that of Vesalius' work (Fig. 1.11). The description of the nerves and blood vessels allowed for

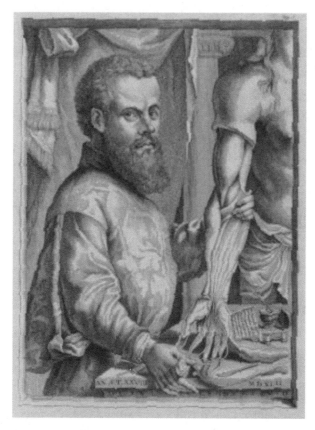

Figure 1.8 *A portrait of Vesalius. Reproduced by permission of the Thomas Fisher Library of Rare Books, University of Toronto.*

deductions of communication between organ systems to be made. Vesalius was initially a follower of Galenic medicine. However, through the course of his dissections, many inaccuracies of Galen's work became apparent and he became an outspoken critic. Unfortunately, the followers of Galen dominated the medical community. Vesalius, not the most diplomatic individual at the best of times, eventually fled, and took a post of physician in the court of Charles V of the united kingdom of Belgium and Spain. Two of Vesalius' contemporaries, Gabriele Fallipio and Bartolomeo Eustachio, and also among his critics, ironically added to the accuracy of human anatomy that Vesalius began. In 1561, Fallipio described the cranial nerves and around the same time, Fallopio, unlike Vesalius left a long legacy of highly regarded former students. One such student, Girolamo Fabrici, or better known as Fabricus ab Aquapendente, became an outstanding teacher, with his students including Harvey and Kasper Bauhim (Fig. 1.12). Eustachio (1520–1574) demonstrated the adrenals and sympathetic ganglia and continued dissections and descriptions of the brain and nervous system. However, much of Eustachio's work remained unpublished and was not rediscovered until the early 1700s (Fig. 1.13).

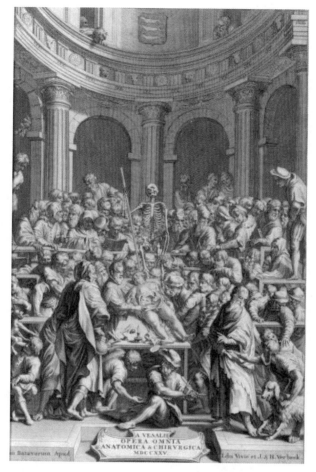

Figure 1.9 *A Renaissance period demonstration theatre. From a 1725 edition of* Opera omnia anatomica and chirurgica, *Vesalius. Reproduced by permission of the Thomas Fisher Library of Rare Books, University of Toronto.*

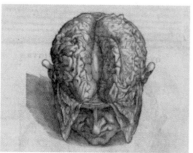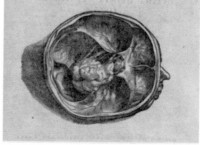

Figure 1.10 *Drawings of the human brain from Vesalius's work* De humani corporis fabrica *(1543). Reproduced by permission of the Thomas Fisher Library of Rare Books, University of Toronto.*

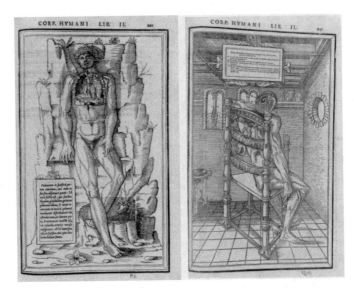

Figure 1.11 *Drawings of human anatomy from Charles Estienne work* De dissectione partium corporis humani *(1545). Reproduced by permission of the Thomas Fisher Library of Rare Books, University of Toronto.*

(a)   (b)

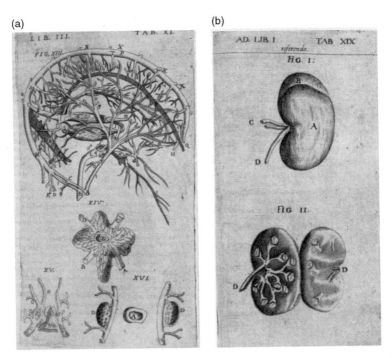

Figure 1.12 *Drawings of (a) blood vessels of the brain and (b) kidney and adrenal gland. From Kaspar Bauhin,* Theatrum anatomicum *(1605). Reproduced by permission of the Thomas Fisher Library of Rare Books, University of Toronto.*

(a)   (b)

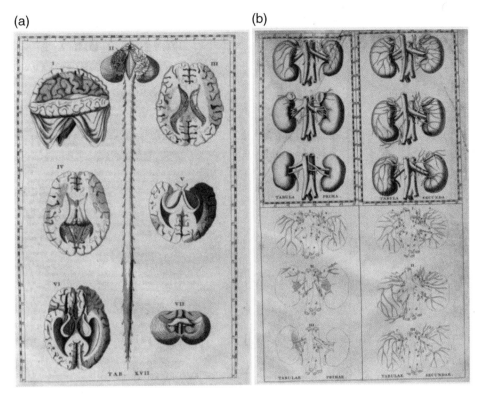

Figure 1.13 *Drawings of (a) brain and spinal cord and (b) kidney and adrenal glands. From Bartolomeo Eustachi,* Explicatio tabularum anatomicarum *(1744). Reproduced by permission of the Thomas Fisher Library of Rare Books, University of Toronto.*

Natural sciences

Pliny the Elder's zoological work continued to be the major comparative work until Ermolao Barbaro (1454–1493) produced *Castigationes Plinanae* in 1492–1493 where he systematically pointed out the errors in the earlier work. However, he did not include any new observations, but rather sought out the ancient sources that Pliny had utilized. This work, however, marked the beginning of several ambitious projects detailing the comparative nature history of animals. Notably among these are the writings of Conrad Gesner (1516–1565) particularly in the five-volume set, *Historiae Animalium* which included all known animals and a description of their habitat, physiology, behaviour and diet, with several new observations (Fig. 1.14). His major contribution was the introduction of illustrations to study biology. The classification was based along Aristotelean lines whereas the description reflected Pliny's general organization. However, the scope and depth of Gesner's work in comparison to earlier works was considerably enriched. Ulisse Androvandi (1522–1605) published three volumes on birds and insects just before his death. Afterwards, his students published an additional eleven volumes based on his notes. Many of these writings included virtually all information that could be obtained. Unfortunately, the tendency to rank fantasy creatures alongside real creatures continued.

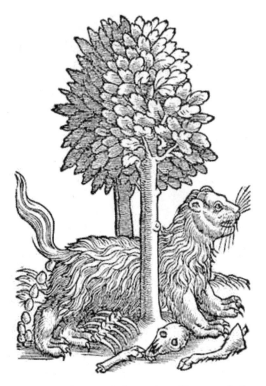

Figure 1.14   *Wolverine (Conrad Gesner). Reproduced by permission of the Thomas Fisher Library of Rare Books, University of Toronto.*

Although the inability to distinguish between fantasy and real animals may have thwarted attempts to organize animals along comparative morphological lines, the lack of physiological understanding of animals likely acted to retain such fantastic notions. In 1474, in the Swiss town of Bale, what was thought to be a rooster laid an egg. With all seriousness and formality the bird was tried for witchcraft, sentenced then burnt at the stake.

By the mid-16th century, descriptive comparative works began to appear. Pierre Belon (1517–1564) toured the near east obtaining information on animals. He subsequently published *La Nature & Diversité des Poissons* in 1551 and *Portraits d'Oyseau, Animaux, Serpens, Herbes, Arbres, Hommes et Femme d'Arabie & Egypte* in Paris in 1557. Whilst this work was notable in that he described the comparative anatomy of humans and birds, drawing attention to homologous structures, many errors and the presence of fantasy animals continued. But by the end of the 17th century, the appearance of more carefully prepared books on comparative anatomy and physiology of animals had appeared, although comparative morphology as a discipline remained in its infancy. Significant among these was Willem Piso's (1611–1678) description of South American animals, and also Jacob Bondt's (1592–1631) work on animals of the East Indies. Many of the descriptions and drawings of the animals in these books bore little similarity to the creatures they were meant to depict. Instead, the emphasis continued to be placed on cataloguing as many species as possible, rather trying to accurately describe the few that were directly observable.

Introduction of chemistry in medicine and natural sciences

The maturation of chemistry into a modern science underwent a particularly long gestation period. Despite the considerable progress of Muslim chemists and physicians, the understanding of chemistry in the west was dominated by the four-element theory of the Greeks until well into the 16th century. There were some notable developments before this, however. For example, Albertus Magnus (1200–1280) was principally a chemist and introduced the term 'affinity' into chemical terminology to denote a chemical relationship.

Paracelsus (1490–1541) (Fig. 1.15) and his followers helped increased awareness in chemistry by their belief that chemistry was the basis for a new understanding of nature. The Paracelsians introduced the concept of creation itself as a chemical unfolding of nature and rejected the humour balance theory of Galenic medicine. They described disease origins as seedlike factors that were introduced to the body through air, food or drink, which became localized in specific organs. Chemistry during Paracelsus time was

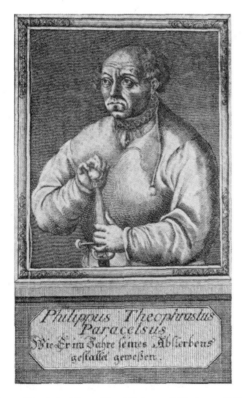

Figure 1.15 *Paracelsus. Reprinted from* The History of Biology, *Erik Nordenskiold (1928). Author's collection.*

essentially alchemy with the focus to transmute one element into another. There was no knowledge of empirical reactions and of the molecular notion of modern chemistry. Paracelsus argued that the goal of alchemy was to prepare medications and not to create gold, for example. The drugs based on Galen's teachings were herbal in origin with no real understanding of dose and response. During Paracelsus time, there was a great expansion of the pharmacopoeias with the increased exploration, a proliferation of medical schools and greater competition among the schools. Paracelsus also introduced the concept of inorganic drugs in medicine. The introduction of medicinal chemistry into the study of health was notable in that it placed more focus on the physical world and less on the divine aspects of human nature. This may have been the inspiration for Jean Fernel (1497–1558) to become the first person to use the word 'physiology' as the study of the body's normal functioning, although he continued to use it in reference to alchemical and spiritual terms. Before Paracelsus, medical teaching was based upon anatomy and botany. Paracelsus and his followers likely had an influence in the addition of chemistry as a branch of medical study. The Paracelsians helped forward the concept that disease state was environmental and not punishment from God *per se*. Physiology in the modern sense was really dependent upon the scientific philosophy of chemistry to develop to a point where it became complementary with the study of medicine.

Scientific revolution

The scientific revolution began in the mid-15th century and continued until the end of the 18th century. By the 17th century came the formation of scientific societies that promoted the science and interaction among scientists thereby facilitating scientific development. These societies reduced some of the constraints of the interacademic, theological and political biases on science. The shifting from a vitalistic view of nature to one of a mechanistic view changed the approach by which scientific investigation was conducted. Renaissance science was based on the Aristotelean vitalistic view of nature and was under considerable attack by the 17th century. However, the 'Aristotelian scientific base' that initially stimulated such critical enquiry had been discredited by the early part of the 17th century. This acted to introduce alternative theories to explain the human condition. Experimentation began to precede conclusion, supplanting the old notions of health and disease with a negative doctrine of objectivity. Thus, during the Renaissance, writers such as Thomas Sydenham (1624–1689) extended the previous philosophical insights to explain how an individual's response to environmental unrest was capable of inducing definable pathological states.

Comparative anatomy

The development of comparative anatomy and physiology was constrained in that researchers of the 15th and 16th centuries did not have a classification system upon which to organize the species. Moreover, there was no real understanding of the evolutionary process. During the Renaissance, with the discovery of the new world and increased exploration, travellers would inaccurately describe creatures they had seen.

This combined with many of the fantasy creatures described in the books of antiquity made it difficult to establish animal phylogeny as a slow transition from one form to another. Thus, the ideas of Charles Darwin and Alfred Russel Wallace on evolution could really only be accepted once most of the fantasy creatures disappeared from popular and scientific literature. This would have to wait until the 19th century. Later in the 17th century, John Ray (1627–1705) (Fig. 1.16) arranged plants and animals into systematic groupings that acted, in part, as a foundation for Carolus Linnaeus (1707–1778) animal classification.

The development of the microscope in the 17th century allowed biologists to extend their observations into the structures of much smaller animals. This allowed researchers the potential to draw homologies among a wider variety of species. Notable among this new breed of comparative anatomist was Marcello Malpighi (1628–1694). He was the first to insist on analogies between organs throughout the animal kingdom. Malpighi made extensive use of simpler animals that could be used in interpreting similar structures in more complex species. Thus in doing so he fostered the development of the model organism that would be so widely utilized in the 20th and 21st centuries. His careful dissections and drawings of insect anatomy and nervous systems, along with his contemporaries Anton van Leeuwenhoek (1632–1723), Jan Swammerdam (1637–1680) and later Pierre Lyonet (1707–1789), ushered in a new standard of biological observation that influenced later comparative anatomists.

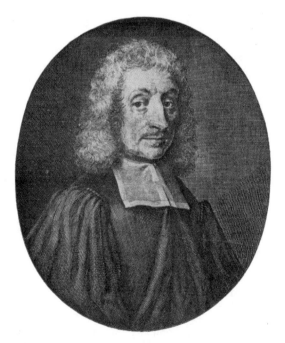

Figure 1.16 *John Ray. Reprinted from* The History of Biology, *Erik Nordenskiold (1928). Author's collection.*

Medicinal chemistry

The need to develop a physical basis to understand chemical principles may have driven the early theories of the atomists back into science simply out of necessity. However, in the 16th century, correct ideas were mixed with fantasy and facts with superstition in chemistry. By the 16th century, the study of medicinal plants was an established branch of medicine. The popularity of illustrated botanical books and the use of herbs in medicine helped to push the proliferation of botanical gardens in universities and institutions. Until the end of the 19th century, most academic botanists tended to be doctors of medicine. By the end of the 16th century, there were thousands of chemists and alchemists who where trying many combinations and chemical reactions therefore having many novel observations. Among these chemists included van Helmont (1577–1644), who, influenced by the Paracelsians, coined the word 'gas' and continued to develop chemistry alongside human physiology. Thomas Sydenham (1624–1689) introduced laudanum, an alcoholic tincture of opium, to which other drugs may be added. This tincture was used for a variety of purposes such as an analgesic, or treatment of some psychological conditions. By 1571, Leaonary Thurniesser advocated the use of quantitative chemical methods such as solubility, crystallography and flame tests to understand novel substances.

Thus, by the 17th century there was considerably momentum in the development of novel concepts in chemistry. Paracelsian philosophy suggested to the physician that poisons rather than vegetable concoctions should be investigated. A poison that caused a disease, they argued, could also become its cure. Logically, this was an extension of their belief that any food or drink, in a great enough concentration, could act as a poison. Here, they anticipated the nutrient–toxin quality of most substances (Chapter 13), suggesting that it was dose rather than the substance itself that cause the problem. This philosophical insight represented a major advancement in the understanding of physiology, although it took a considerable period before this view became ensconced in scientific literature. This concept would later be applied in the fields of molecular pharmacology and endocrinology to understand the mode of action for high- and low-affinity receptors (Chapter 5). However, at the time, the Paracelsian philosophy received a considerable amount of ridicule.

Among the chemical physicians, there was an increasing number who sought to maintain chemistry as the basis of a new philosophy of nature, but rid it of the most mystical and least experimental aspects. Chemistry, they argued, was the proper basis of medicine. Paracelsian physicians described local seats of disease governed by internal archei rather than the imbalance of fluids. Here, we may, perhaps, see the seeds of a concept that was later to mature into Claude Bernards *milieu interieur*. Robert Boyle (1627–1691) was directly influenced by the atomists. He broke away from the mysticism of the alchemists and focused on the breaking up of complex substances into their simplest elements.

Medicine and anatomy

Early in the 17th century, function began to be applied to structure thereby setting the foundation for physiology. Disease eventually came to be associated with organ systems as a knowledge base was built up linking organ conditions with the disease shown during dissection and post-mortem examination. Human dissections, however, were generally considered unacceptable to the public in general, and as a result, restrictions placed on post-mortem examinations slowed the progress of this knowledge.

In 1628, William Harvey (Fig. 1.17) published *On the Motion of the Heart and Blood in Animals* thereby laying down the foundation of circulation. Harvey was a graduate of Padua University in Italy, where much of its curriculum was based on Ibn Sina's and al-Razi's writings. Later that century, the Italian physician Santorio invented a device to count pulses and a thermometer to measure body heat. By this time, chemical processes and explanations were sought to explain fermentation, combustion and decomposition thereby setting the stage for the beginning of a molecular understanding of physiology.

Many of the roots of the modern theories of neurobiology can be traced to this period in history. The theory of atomism was resurrected to varying degrees by René Descartes (1596–1650) and Gottfried Wilhelm Leibniz (1646–1716) to explain soul and consciousness. Descartes attempted to explain sensation and reaction by the existence of small rapidly moving particles that travelled in hollow nerves. Descartes thought that the pineal gland was the locus of the soul. For much of history, it was believed that the soul was resident in the fluids of the ventricles and not the brain tissue *per se*, although this view was refuted by Vesalius who showed that the size of the human brain ventricles and that of other mammals were similar. Descartes had suggested instead that fluids from the ventricles flowed through hollow nerves to effect movement of the muscles. The pineal gland, located near the ventricles of the forebrain,

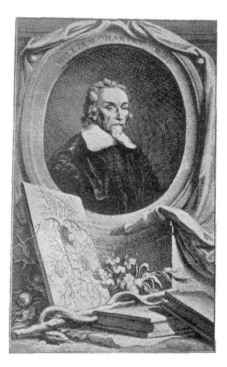

Figure 1.17   *William Harvey. Reprinted from* The History of Biology, *Erik Nordenskiold (1928). Author's collection.*

therefore, could be the actual location of the soul. This theory was notable in that it was the first to suggest that the soul was resident in the actual brain tissues instead of the fluids in and around the brain. Descartes' book *De Homine* is regarded by many as the first European book on physiology, which attempted to explain all physical actions in mechanical terms. Isaac Newton, likely drawing upon van Leeuwenhoek's lack of evidence for hollow nerve fibres, refuted this in 1717 and argued that the nerves were solid.

The first real investigations of glands were reported by Thomas Wharton (1614–1673) in his treatise *Adenographia*. He described, for the first time, the pancreas and also the kidney, testes and thyroid in detail (Fig. 1.18). Wharton rejected Descartes' view of the pineal gland as the origin of the soul and instead described it as an excretory organ to drain waste products, which were subsequently removed by blood vessels. In this description, he stumbled across the concept of neurosecretion, a mechanism that would not be adequately explained until the mid-20th century. Thomas Willis (1621–1675) may be regarded as the first true modern comparative neuroanatomist. He did a detailed investigation of the brain and nervous system. Physiologically, Willis, built upon the

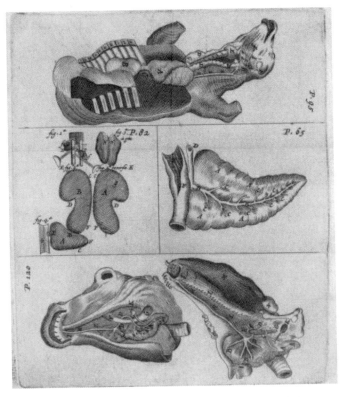

Figure 1.18 *Drawings of glands and organs from a cow. From* Adenographia, *Thomas Wharton (1659). Reproduced by permission of the Thomas Fisher Library of Rare Books, University of Toronto.*

ideas of Descartes, however, placed the seat of thought and ideas in the cerebral cortex. He established the function of the vagus nerve in dogs and established its function in heart and lungs. Glisson (1634–1677) used the term 'irritability' to describe the tendency of living things to respond to an irritating agent by involving muscular contraction. Abrecht von Haller (1708–1777) used the term in a more refined sense to mean the ability of muscle to contract and having noted that irritating nerves caused pain he used the term 'sensitivity' for the property peculiar to nerves conveying sensation. In 1780, Luigi Galvani (1737–1798) showed that an electrical current applied to a frog leg could induce a contraction.

The 19th-century physiology and medicine

At the opening of the 19th century, a scientific philosophy dominated by mechanistic approaches was firmly in place. European science flourished in the 19th century. At the end of the 18th century, Alexander Monro (1733–1817) published a comparative examination of the nervous system (Fig. 1.19). Shortly afterwards, Marc Jean Bougery (1797–1849) produced one of the finest texts on human anatomy, *Traité Complet de l'Anatomie de l'Homme*, with the nerves rendered in exquisite detail (Fig. 1.20). The accurate transmission of comparative morphology was essential to understand the interrelationship of species.

However, at the beginning of the 19th century, theories of evolution remained at the periphery of mainstream science. Up until that time, animal classification was based upon Linnaeus' organization. It was based only on gross morphological similarities among species, and was, therefore, of limited use. Georges Cuvier (1769–1832) (Fig. 1.21) was the first to modify this classification and proposed a grouping based on the knowledge of comparative anatomy. By this time, biologists had already formulated the idea that animals formed a gradient from the simplest to the more complex forms. Despite the organization of species along what might seem to be evolutionary principles, morphological variation was still believed by many biologists to be a function of divine influence. The notion that there existed a natural transition from one form to another was not well accepted. In actuality, the stability of a species became as much of a dogma in science as it did in theology. Lamarck (1744–1829), drawing upon the theories of Erasmus Darwin (1731–1802) and Buffon (1707–1788), began to utilize a branched tree to understand the morphological relationships among species and tried to synthesize a view whereby animals could 'evolve' into different species. Immediately upon the heels of Lamarck came the ideas of Charles Darwin (1809–1882) and Wallace (1809–1882). With the acceptance of Mendel's (1822–1884) theories of inheritance the theory of evolution was firmly established within scientific doctrine by the end of the 19th century. Establishment of the evolutionary process consolidated the concept of linking humans with animals thereby providing a distinct scientific reasoning for engaging in comparative research for the development of model systems upon which to understand certain processes.

Scientific pursuits shaped by the ideologies and cultures of the individual nations effectively reacted a nationalistic competition both among individuals and countries to propel science as a faster pace than had been seen previously. A complex interaction of

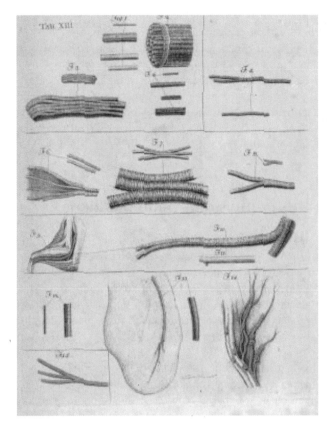

Figure 1.19   *Comparative anatomy of peripheral nerves, from* Observations on the Structure and Functions of the Nervous System, *Alexander Monro (1783). Reproduced by permission of the Thomas Fisher Library of Rare Books, University of Toronto.*

life sciences, chemistry, mixed with the new fields of evolution and physiology acted to mix thought in ways that had not occurred before. The Franco–Prussian War interrupted communication between French and German scientists acting to isolate the scientific communities from each other. Towards the end of the 19th century, Germany devoted a large amount of funding for scientific research and as a result became influential worldwide.

Cells as physiological units

There was a transition of organism to tissue then finally to the cells as the central unit of biological organization in the 19th century. Cells as organisms had been known to biologists for some time before their role as a biological unit was understood and became entrenched in medicine and physiology. Cell theory was limited by the quality of the microscopes. By 1850s, cell theory and the use of the microscope were introduced to the science of pathology. Initially, plants were shown to be composed of cells. Animal tissue was more problematic as it tended to be softer, degraded easier and there were problems

(a)   (b)

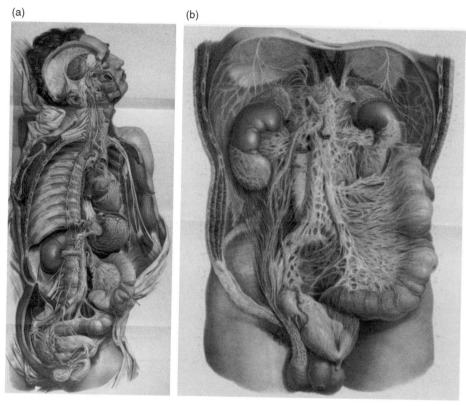

Figure 1.20 *Drawings of (a) autonomic nerves and (b) peripheral nerves of the gut. From* Traité complet de l'anatomie de l'homme *published 1831 to 1854, by Marc Jean Bourgery. Reproduced by permission of the Thomas Fisher Library of Rare Books, University of Toronto.*

with the early microscopes. Cells, at the time, were essentially defined as units of space, but there was little agreement as to what they actually were.

Cell theory defined in the mid-1880s by Matthias Schleiden (1804–1881) and Theodor Schwann (1810–1882) introduced the cell as the fundamental unit of life and its processes, although their concept of how a cell arose was incorrect at the time. By the late 1880s, the cell was recognized as a defined entity possessing a nucleus with chromosomes and a nucleus surrounded by a cytoplasm of complex biochemistry. It was still arguable as to whether the cell possessed a plasma membrane. A number of significant improvements in cytological methods allowed for a clearer resolution of cells in the latter half of the 19th century. As early as 1839, Schwann had argued that cells were the basic unit of the nervous system. About ten years later, van Kolliker established that nerve fibres were linked to the cell body. Drawing upon the methods of Camillo Golgi and Frans Nissl, Santiago Ramon y Cajal exquisitely described a number of nerve cells and argued for the fundamental role of the nerve cell in the brain (Fig. 1.22). By the early 1890s, the term 'neuron' had been coined to describe the brain cell. In the mid-19th century, Fritsch (1838–1929) and Hitzig (1838–1907) showed that the dog neocortex could be electrically

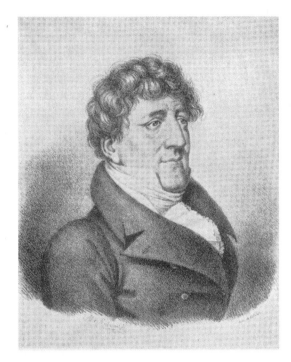

Figure 1.21   *Cuvier. Reprinted from* The History of Biology, *Erik Nordenskiold (1928). Author's collection.*

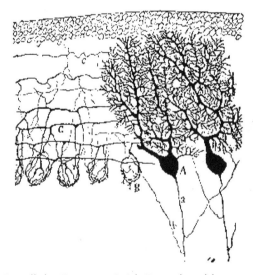

Figure 1.22   *Purkinje cell, by Ramon y Cajal. Reproduced by permission of the Thomas Fisher Library of Rare Books, University of Toronto.*

and selectively excited prompting Bernstein to develop the theory that the membrane of a nerve was polarized and that an action potential was a propagated depolarization of this membrane.

The roots of neuroendocrinology

Physiology as a distinct discipline began to separate from anatomy in the mid-1800s. Experimental physiology was not well received in 19th-century France and many researchers were frequently investigated by the police. This was due in part to the questionable ways in which animals were obtained and sold to physiologists.

The French physiologist, Claude Bernard (Fig. 1.23), had significant impact on the future of modern physiology. Bernard's approach to introduce physics and chemistry into physiology was inherited from his professor Francois Magendie at the Collège de France. Magendie had shown that both sensory and motor nerve fibres travelled together in the whole nerve except near the spinal cord where sensory fibres occupied the dorsal root and the motor fibres were found in the ventral root. Bernard's use of chemical experimentation to solve physiological problems is also believed to have originated from his time as an

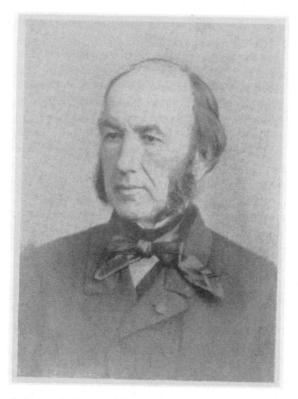

Figure 1.23 *Claude Bernard. Reprinted from* Claude Bernard, Physiologist, *J.M.D. Olmsted (1939). Author's collection.*

assistant to a pharmacist where the first compound entrusted to Bernard was shoe polish. It was the first thing he learned to make. Bernard's chemical approach to physiology was evident in most of his work. In Bernard's Doctor of Medicine dissertation, he showed that gastric juice acting upon cane sugar when injected into the blood of dogs could not be detected in the urine. Cane sugar injected into the blood could be detected. Bernard later began collaborating with the chemist, Barreswill. In 1846, Bernard demonstrated the role of the pancreas in digestion. In 1849, Bernard announced that a slight wound in the floor of the brain near the cerebellum renders an animal temporally diabetic via stimulation of the sympathetic nerve. He had previously shown that cutting the vagus nerves interrupted the secretion of sugar from the liver. Here, Bernard touched upon the essential concepts of neuroendocrinology, although the modern concept of neuroendocrinology was still 100 years into the future. Bernard had a significant influence in experimental physiology and medicine in the UK and the US. John Call Dalton, an American pupil of Bernard, was the first to teach physiology using live material and his textbook in physiology which kept up to date on Bernard's discussions was the most widely used in the US in the 1880s.

Bernard brought experimental approaches to the key physiological processes and helped to entrench an integrative approach of physics and chemistry. In doing so, he helped create the foundation in which to explore and develop molecular neuroendocrinology. Indeed, his demonstration of glycogenesis of liver was a demonstration of that. In the course of trying to understand the course of sugar entering and leaving the liver, he formulated the principles of internal secretions and in doing so he laid the foundation for a new field of study – endocrinology.

Bernard utilized cellular theory in that the cells of the pancreas contained different substances and together they can act upon the emulsification of fats. He also employed a comparative approach to solve endocrine/physiological problems utilizing pancreatic physiology of dog, rabbit and ox to understand the differences and similarities. He explored the developmental issues using the actions of a foetal pancreas on fat digestion. Banting, himself, used this as a starting point to try to extract insulin from the islets of Langerhans at an age when they were not producing trypsin. Bernard differentiated between internal secretions (endocrine) and external secretions (exocrine, e.g. bile). He recognized the thyroid and adrenals as glands using internal secretions. He recognized the concept of homeostasis by comparing the liver to a syringe of sugar that injects its contents little by little into the blood. If injected too quickly, then the symptoms of diabetes occurred.

Bernard's approach to studying peripheral physiological processes, the nervous system and the molecular actions of poison allowed him to make deductions where other individuals focusing on the same problem might not have the same insight. Bernard's work on molecular mechanisms of physiology laid the groundwork for the study of the signalling aspects of endocrinology and chemical signals. During investigations on O_2, CO and CO_2 in blood he recognized the concept of bound and free forms. Hoppe-Seyler coined the term 'haemoglobin' and together with Bernard recognized the role of CO and haemoglobin. Bernard established that curare must enter a wound to be effective and not by the mouth. It attacked the nerves at a point where they enter the muscles. He established that intelligence, sensitivity and will are not touched by the poison but will lose their ability to control muscles. He used curare as an antagonist to disrupt the communication between nerve and muscle and found that the muscle could still respond independently of the nerve. In 1815, Watterton and Brodie in England injected curare into an ass and could keep it alive by artificial respiration with a pair of bellows inserted through an incision in the trachea.

Neurosecretion and the hypothalamus–pituitary regulation

By the late 1800s, the concept of 'ductless' glands being necessary for the normal function of any organism came to be generally accepted by the scientific community. Brown-Sequard, a student of Bernard and later professor of pathology of the nervous system at Harvard, investigated the actions of adrenal glands during 1856–1858. Later in 1889, he announced that his auto-injection of testicular extracts resulted in rejuvenated physical and mental abilities. He anticipated the notion of modern neuroendocrinology and endocrinology, when he wrote that all tissues and cells secrete bioactive substances into the blood that ultimately interact with other cells in other tissues including the brain.

At the turn of the 20th century, Elliot theorized that epinephrine was associated with the nervous system and suggested that it may be a stimulant that is released from a neuron when the appropriate neural impulse is received. Bayliss and Starling reported the identification of the first hormone in 1902. They showed that an intravenous injection of a mucosal extract from the duodenum resulted in the release of bicarbonate and water from the pancreas. They named this hormone 'secretin'. However, it was not until 1961 when the purification of secretin was reported, then finally sequenced and shown to be a 27 amino acid peptide in 1970 by Victor Mutt and his associates. However, it has only been in the last decade when secretin has been found in the brain although its function is not clear.

An understanding of neurosecretion

Early 20th-century science also heralded in the field of comparative endocrinology and neuroendocrinology, although there was a considerable period before such concepts were accepted. By the end of the 19th century, studies indicated that pituitary extracts could elevate blood pressure, stimulate uterine contraction and regulate diuresis; a number of writers were still arguing that the pituitary gland was a vestigial organ with little function. Gaskell, in 1914, demonstrated that leech ganglia possessed pharmacological attributes and Dahlgren described cells in the nervous system of the electric skate that resembled endocrine cells. This was later shown by Spiedel around 1920. Thus, the notion that the brain was capable of secreting bioactive substances and that the appropriate animal model could be used to further our understanding of physiology became well established. Despite the significance of these studies examined in retrospect, their significance was largely ignored by the scientific community at the time. Ernst Scharrer (1905–1965) is generally credited as being the originator of the concept of neurosecretion. In the late 1920s he showed that the preoptic region in the brain (Chapter 10) of the minnow possessed endocrine properties that was associated with pituitary function. Together with his wife, Bertha, the Scharrers engaged in an intense comparative investigation of neurosecretion in other species. They showed the parallel between the corpus cardiacum and corpus allatum intercerebralis system in insects and the hypothalamus–pituitary system of vertebrates (Chapter 4). However, despite the evidence they accumulated on the phylogenetic ubiquity of neurosecretion, the significance of their work was missed by many of the researchers at the time and it was many years before their findings were accepted by mainstream scientists.

By the 1930s the notion that the pituitary gland was the master endocrine gland acting to regulate all, if not most, physiological functions was well accepted. In the late 1930s and early 1940s, Bargmann had shown that a neuronal system ran from the paraventricular nuclei of the hypothalamus (Chapters 6 and 9) to the neural lobe of the pituitary. Bargmann and Scharrer published a paper where they postulated that vasopressin and oxytocin are synthesized in the hypothalamus and are transported to the neural lobe of the pituitary where they are stored until released. Vincent du Vigneaud won the Nobel Prize, for Chemistry in 1955, for isolating vasopressin and oxytocin and showing that these two peptides were responsible for the known effects of the posterior pituitary gland.

Hypothalamus–pituitary interaction

The concept that the hypothalamus exerted control over the anterior lobe of the pituitary gland was gaining acceptance by the 1930s. Around the same time, the work of Walter Cannon and Hans Selye on the concepts of stress and homeostasis complemented each other and this synergism acted to stimulate considerable progress in the field. Earlier studies on the balanced control of biological systems were embellished by Cannon's extension of Bernard's *le milieu interieur* to include psycho-emotional criteria which he termed 'homeostasis'. However, it was not until Hans Selye (1939) (Fig. 1.24) introduced his concept of a *General Adaptation, or Stress Syndrome* that the current paradigm on biological stress was finally founded. Selye's general adaptation syndrome is based upon a three-stage characterization of an organism's biological reactions to severe stress. The first stage, the 'alarm reaction', is characterized by two sub-stages, a 'shock phase' and a 'countershock phase'. During the shock phase the body temperature drops, blood pressure is lowered, there is a loss of fluid from the tissues and muscle tone decreases. During the countershock phase there is an increase in adrenocortical hormones and a general biological defence reaction against the stress begins. The second phase is a 'resistance stage' that continues the recuperative processes begun during the counter-shock. Bodily functions, such as blood pressure and temperature, for example, gradually return to normal, or near normal. However, if the stress is too severe, or prolonged, the third stage 'exhaustion' ensues. Here, the general pattern of the initial shock reappears and ultimately death results. The physiological implications of this were immense and, therefore, the Cannon–Selye concepts ultimately had a significant effect on the direction of neuroendocrine investigations by orienting neuroendocrine research to the hypothalamus–pituitary–adrenal (HPA) axis (Chapter 9).

Although all of the theoretical elements existed in science to understand the neuro-endocrine control of the anterior lobe of the pituitary gland, a working hypothesis was lacking until Geoffrey Harris at Cambridge University put all the pieces in place.

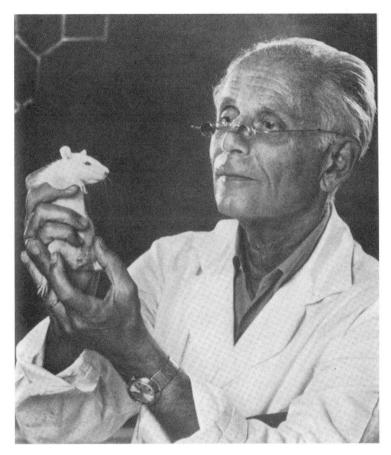

Figure 1.24   *Hans Selye. Reprinted from* The Stress of My Life, *Hans Selye (1939). Author's collection.*

A description of the vascular portal system between the hypothalamus and the pituitary gland had been described by Popa and Fielding in 1930, drawing heavily upon earlier observations. However, a lack of understanding of the direction of blood flow in the portal system limited the theoretical rationale for utilizing the portal system as a vascular means to transport neurosecretory products from the hypothalamus to the pituitary. Depending on the method and the animal model used, studies showed that the blood flow could be either from the pituitary to the hypothalamus or alternatively from the hypothalamus to the pituitary gland. In the 1940s, Harris collaborated with John Green, an anatomist based out of the Wayne University College of Medicine to engage in a comparative examination of the portal system in various species. By 1947, Green showed that the portal blood flow was oriented from the hypothalamus to the pituitary gland. The regulation of the anterior lobe by secretory products from the hypothalamus was summarized and discussed by Harris in 1948.

The competition to be the first to isolate the hypothalamic factors that regulated the anterior pituitary gland was underway by the early 1950s. In 1955, Roger Guillemin, a former post-doctoral fellow of Selye, and Andrew Schally independently reported the isolation of hypothalamic extracts that could release adrenocorticotropic hormone (ACTH) from the anterior pituitary. However, the chemical properties of this corticotrophin-releasing factor (CRF) made it difficult to purify. It was finally purified and the structure determined by 1981 by Wylie Vale, a former post-doctoral fellow of Guillemin, and his colleagues at the Salk Institute in San Diego. Schally and his laboratory succeeded in isolating and characterizing thyrotrophin-releasing factor (TRF) in the 1960s, whereas Guillemin and his associates reported the structure of ovine gonadotropin-releasing hormone (GnRH) in 1971, only six months before the report of porcine GnRH by Schally's group. Jean Rivier and Vale published the structure of growth hormone-releasing hormone (GHRH) in 1983. The development of radioimmunoassays, by Yalow, and autoradiography allowed researchers to determine the presence of cells expressing the hormones and their receptors in the brain. For their efforts, Schally, Guillemin and Yalow were awarded the Nobel Prize for Physiology or Medicine in 1977. The growth of papers dealing with neuro-endocrinology after the 1970s was exponential. Modern neuroendocrinology was born.

Chapter summary

Neuroendocrinology, as a distinct subdiscipline, found its roots once physiology, chemistry and biology coalesced out of the ancestral fields of medicine, alchemy and natural philosophy. In the earliest societies, physiological knowledge came from observing natural processes such as childbirth, injury, disease and death. Pharmacological knowledge of the medicinal uses of plants sprang from the knowledge of food and nutrition. The science of ancient Greece acted as a catalyst to create a philosophical foundation of the natural and medical sciences. The basic concept of the brain as the organ of thought and molecular interactions can be traced to Democritus, although it took almost two millennia before these concepts were understood. Many competing ideas could not be properly evaluated until the experimental methods became available. Thus, endocrinology as a field did not progress, until the emergence of Islam in the 10th and 11th centuries, and their knowledge in medicine, chemistry and pharmacology was passed to the scholars of western Europe by way of the Byzantine Empire, and later via texts available in Italy and Spain. The Christian Church was instrumental in establishing centres of higher learning throughout western Europe which led eventually to academic free thought and inter-university competition. Developments in anatomical observation, medicinal chemistry and botany helped set the stage to understand circulation and the role it played in conveying nutrients and toxins to the organs of the body. An accurate interpretation of animal taxonomy and phylogeny along with the invention of the microscope fostered growth in comparative anatomy and physiology and ushered in cell theory as a means to understand organismal physiology. Bernard's studies on the pancreas and nerves were the first notable studies in endocrinology in the mid-19th century, and by the beginning of the 20th century, accurate descriptions of nerve and gland cells were available to scientists. The first hormone, secretin, was isolated in 1902. Studies on the secretion of products in invertebrates along with observations of the structure of the hypothalamus and portal system in amphibians and other vertebrates, a theory on the neuroendocrine regulation of the principal glands of the body emerged. The first demonstration of hypothalamic-releasing factors was reported in the mid-1950s, and by the late 1960s the first neurohormones were isolated and identified. Neuroendocrinology effectively became a distinct subdiscipline by the 1970s.

2

Origin of life and the first signalling molecules

Introduction

All hormones used by living species have a complex evolutionary history. So to ask the question of where did the first hormones come from is also to ask the question of where the first life came from. A living system is characterized by an ability to reduce entropy, or to increase the order of its constituents. This is performed by the actions of both metabolism and replication. However, in order to maintain this order, it must necessarily be separated from the rest of the environment it finds itself in. Thus, there needs to be a physical partition between self and non-self. Because of this barrier, some form of communication is required between living units. Multicellular life could not have evolved without a chemical signalling system. The evolution of an intercellular chemical communication system emerged from the cells' own needs for survival, then it was subsequently adapted to be used by communities of similar living units.

The first signalling molecules would have been derived from the raw materials available to the early cells on the primitive earth. Initially, these first molecular signals would have been without the specific receptor systems, signal transduction systems and the processing enzymes as we are familiar with in modern cell systems. It is likely that the first cells with a rudimentary signalling system arose perhaps a billion years before the appearance of the last universal common ancestor (LUCA) between prokaryotes and eukaryotes. Over time, as cells developed in complexity, so did the signalling molecules.

Neuroendocrinology: An Integrated Approach David A. Lovejoy
© 2005 John Wiley & Sons, Ltd

After the development of the eukaryotic cell, and later, the multicellular organisms, came a need for these chemical communication systems to coordinate the actions of the organism. Then, the first simple endocrine and nervous systems arose. The interface between these two systems, the neuroendocrine system, developed from the increasing complexity of the nervous and endocrine systems.

We may think of the nervous, neuroendocrine and endocrine systems comprising of cells that are specialized for communication, to allow a flow of information among cell types. Indeed, 'information' has been defined by some researchers as the reciprocal of entropy. The ordered systems that characterize modern cells and their ability to relay information about themselves and the environment were ultimately derived from features found in the first progenitor cell-like structures that preceded the development of the first true living cell. Theoretically, any molecule could be used as a communicator. However, a preponderance of amino acids and their derivatives, and of fatty acids and their derivatives, has been utilized as signalling molecules.

Theories of the evolution of the first cells

The evolution of the first living cells was dependent upon the raw materials of the primitive earth. There are several theories for the origin of these biogenic materials, and can be divided into terrestrial and extraterrestrial origins. Regardless of the theory, the utilization of carbon as a basic molecular unit plays a central role. Carbon has low inherent entropy, strong covalent bonding properties and low mass. It can form straight chains, branched chains, cross-links, double bonds and ring structures. Carbon appears to be unique in that no other single element can achieve all these situations. The interaction of carbon-based molecules with other types of molecules may have generated a far greater number of different molecular species, allowing the carbon-based molecules a competitive advantage over non-carbon-based molecular species.

Prebiotic synthesis of biogenic molecules

Evidence suggests that, at least, some of first molecules necessary for the evolution of life had an extraterrestrial origin. Early spectrometric investigations showed the existence of certain organic molecules, such as formaldehyde, in interstellar space (Fig. 2.1). Such molecules may have been present during the formation of the earth 4.5 billion years ago or delivered to earth by comet and meteorites. In the last few years, controversial data implicating that life may have arisen on Mars and the presence of meteorites on earth believed to be from Mars may have introduced biogenic compounds on to the planet. These meteorites possess microscopic structures that some researchers have suggested may be fossils of cell-like organisms. However, even if life or the presence of biogenic materials did develop on Mars or elsewhere, we are still faced with the problem of how they developed.

The earth was bombarded by meteors between 3.5 and 3.8 billion years ago, allowing the opportunity for at least some of these biogenic compounds to be seeded on earth (Fig. 2.2). For example, some meteorites found in Antarctica have high concentrations of α-aminoisobutyric acid and isovaline, amino acids that are rare on Earth. The age of

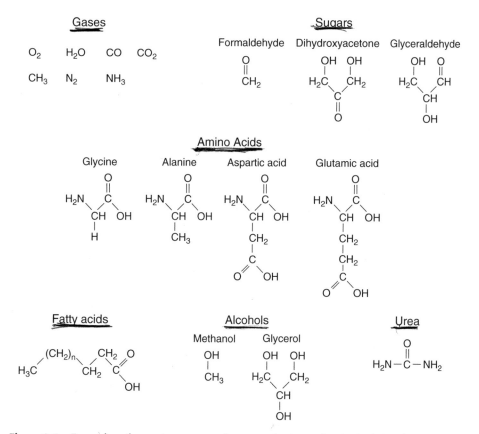

Figure 2.1   *Examples of organic compounds present in the prebiotic Earth. Such compounds were used as substrates and building blocks for more complex molecules.*

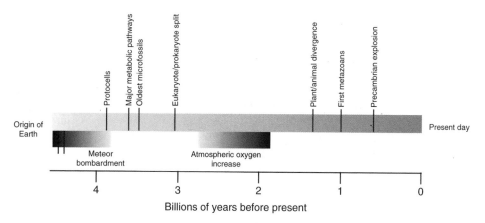

Figure 2.2   *History of the evolution of the Earth and approximate times of the major stages in the evolution of life.*

Carboniferous inclusions in Greenland and Canadian rocks are 3.5 to 3.8 billion years old, coinciding with a period of intense meteorite bombardment on earth. A number of meteors possess traces of amino acids, carboxylic and other organic acids, polyaromatic hydrocarbons, aliphatic hydrocarbons and purines. A meteorite found near Murchison, Australia in 1969 contains a wealth of organic material including polyaromatic hydrocarbons, amino acids and other organic acids, aliphatic and aromatic hydrocarbons, ureas, ketones, alcohols, aldehydes and purines and carboxylic acids up to ten carbon units long. Based on the concentration of organic material in meteorites and in comets, some researchers have estimated that several orders of magnitude greater organic carbon arrived to earth as part of meteorite and comet bombardment over a few hundred million years than is present in the entire earth biosphere at present.

A second set of theories hold that the essential biogenic materials arose on earth itself without extraterrestrial assistance. Beginning with the classic studies of Stanley Miller and Harold Urey in the 1950s, many studies indicate that methane (CH_4), ammonia (NH_3), water (H_2O) and molecular nitrogen (N_2) will readily form amino acids, sugars and purines in the presence of UV, ionizing radiation or electrical discharge. Numerous biogenic compounds could be synthesized with nothing more than a spark as an energy source, for example from lighting, and from ingredients believed to be present on earth at that time. However, over time the initial reducing character of the atmosphere changed to an oxidizing character of the atmosphere consisting of carbon dioxide and nitrogen. These gases do not support the synthetic pathways shown to occur under reducing conditions, thus life may have originated before this occurred.

Alternatively, life itself could have arisen near undersea or subterranean geological hot vents. Here, the immediate environment is primarily reducing. Some studies indicate that sulphides issuing from the vent can precipitate as membranes and absorb organic materials from solution allowing for a substrate to concentrate organic materials. Present day hot vents harbour much bacterial life, and the majority of the ancient bacterial lineages are thermophilic. Although the origin of life on earth dates to the period of intense bombardment of the early earth, some researchers have argued that each of the major impacts had the potential to completely sterilize the surface of the earth. Thus, in the million year intervals between impacts, life may have evolved on the surface several times only to be lost with each impact. Deep-sea vents or subterranean vents may have offered a protected environment where the primitive life forms could survive the impacts. A number of oxygen-hating organisms exist today and will die if exposed to oxygen levels above 0.1% of present atmospheric levels.

In some ways, the manner in which the organic materials were synthesized prebiotically is moot. The findings of organic materials in old earth rocks, in meteorites, comets or interstellar space indicate that these molecules could be synthesized. Assuming then that the first challenge of prebiotic synthesis of biogenic material has been achieved, a second hurdle of how these molecules interact to create second order complex materials becomes evident. An assortment of biogenic molecules floating about in the atmosphere or perhaps the ocean would have taken eons for the concentration of the reactants to increase to the degree where reactions could catalyse. Perhaps the approximate 800 million years that passed between the time of the origin of the earth and the first fossils present allowed sufficient time for these reactions. It is difficult to say. Alternatively, however, introduction of a matrix that could bind these biogenic molecules would increase the probability of interaction by different molecular species.

In modern cells, the extensive membranes of the endoplasmic reticulum, the plasma membrane and various organelle membranes all act as 2-dimensional matrices to anchor enzymes that aid in the synthesis and breakdown of various molecular products of the cell (Fig. 2.3). Of course in the prebiotic world, no such cells or membranes were present. Thus, the first matrices would have been composed of inorganic materials such as clays or pyrites (Fig. 2.4). For example, uracil can by synthesized under conditions believed to mimic the prebiotic earth by evaporations and mild heating of solutions of β-alanine and urea in the presence of clay-type minerals. Thymine can be synthesized in this manner by addition of acetate to the reaction. The formation of peptide and nucleotide oligomers up to 55 subunits has been synthesized on mineral surfaces. Oligomers of this length are predicted to be necessary for a viable early genetic system.

Energy is essential to allow the formation of chemical bonds and, therefore, the construction of macromolecules, such as nucleic acid polymers or proteins. Energy in the form of UV radiation, electrical discharge and atmospheric shock resulting from extra-terrestrial infall (comet and meteorite bombardment), and chemical energy were all present in the prebiotic earth. Chemical energy could be supplied in the form of condensing agents, pyrophosphate bonds, glyceraldehyde-based reactions, pyrites and activated monomers.

(a)

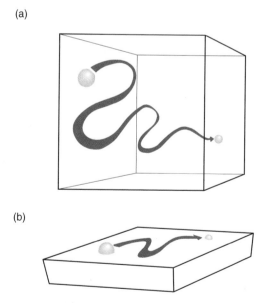

(b)

Figure 2.3 *Two-dimensional and three-dimensional diffusion. The probability of two molecules interacting with a three-dimensional matrix (a) is considerably higher than the probability of interacting on a two-dimensional matrix (b). The ability of organic ions to adsorb on inorganic substrates increases the chance of molecular interaction and therefore the synthesis of more complex organic molecules.*

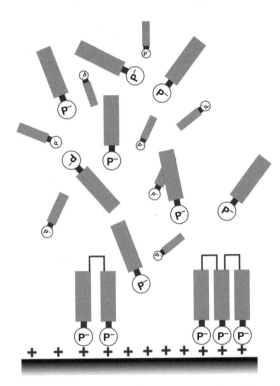

Figure 2.4   *Adsorption of organic materials onto a mineral surface. The negative charge of an organophosphate, for example, molecule can be attracted to the positive charge of a pyrite surface. The close proximity may act to induce polymerization or other reactions among adjacent molecules. The organization of the organic material on the mineral substrate acts to reduce entropy and increases the probability of molecular interaction. Modified and adapted after Deamer (1997).*

Metabolism, replication and the first signal networks

Up to this point we have imagined a prebiotic world with sufficient organic material in the form of simple molecules, energy sources and an inorganic matrix to which these molecules could adhere and combine with their molecular neighbours. These components all act to decrease entropy, a basic quality of life, but still hardly address the aspects of metabolism and replication. Indeed at this point, the formation of living cells and signalling systems are still a half billion years away!

Metabolism and replication are distinct and separable processes. Disagreement occurs with respect of which came first, metabolism or replication. One school of thought holds that life begins as a protocell with a simple metabolism. A protocell was not a living system but simply a concentration of chemicals separated from the rest of the environment by a lipid membrane of some type. Later, enzymes and proteins and finally replicating molecules (genes) were developed. Another school of thought favours the concept that replication was the more significant attribute and that replicating molecules (protogenes) came first which gave rise to enzymes and then to cells. Here, nucleic acids in the form of

RNA were the first proto-living systems. Support for this theory comes from the ubiquity of RNA as both an informational molecule in the form of genomic DNA (in retroviruses) or messenger RNA (mRNA) and as a metabolic molecule in the form of transfer RNA (tRNA) and ribosomal RNA (rRNA). Alternatively, one might imagine that both metabolic and replicating units evolved independently and in parallel but merged at sometime in the future. Here, the replicating system later entered and acted as a symbiont within the protocell where the replicants added the stability to the protocell and the protocell provided an environment conducive to increased efficiency for the replicating molecules.

Let us consider the evolution of metabolism and signalling first. Many researchers agree that self-catalysing reactions were responsible for the first cellular metabolism (Fig. 2.5). A self-catalysing reaction occurs where the formation of the final products act to stimulate or catalyse the first reactions. As a result, the relative concentration of this type of molecule increases. There are several examples of self-catalysing networks found in nature. For example, a 32-residue α-helical peptide based on the leucine zipper domain of the yeast transcription factor GCN4 acts autocatalytically to direct its own synthesis in neutral dilute aqueous solutions. Alanine can increase the formation of triose and

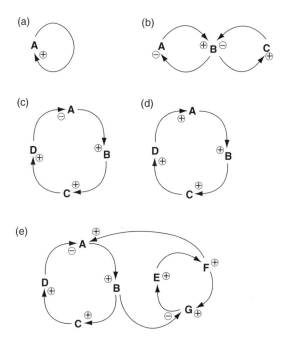

Figure 2.5 *Autocatalytic reactions. The various letters represent different chemical species. (a) Simple amplifier circuit where the formation of species **A** acts as a catalyst to increase its own synthesis. (b) An amplifier loop where **A** increases the synthesis of **B** which increases the synthesis of **C**. The species **C** then acts in a negative manner to inhibit **A**. (c) A multistep synthetic reaction where the final product **D** inhibits the synthesis of **A**. (d) A multistep amplifier circuit where the final product enhances the synthesis of the initial product. (e) Two chemosynthetic circuits that have come to interact with each other. Adapted after Loewenstein (1999).*

pyruvaldehyde from formaldehyde and glycoaldehyde 15- and 1200-fold greater respectively, than the uncatalysed reaction. Because alanine can be synthesized from formaldehyde and glyceraldehyde via a pyruvaldehyde intermediate, the reaction works autocatalytically to drive the synthesis of sugars.

Within the set of these molecular interactions, several types of competition may occur between molecular species. For example, one molecule may aid the replication of a second of which the second helps the first; one molecule may replicate first, then utilize its catalytic activity to cleave others utilizing these cleavage products for its own replication. Alternatively, some molecules may utilize other molecules as cofactors to increase the efficiency of their own synthesis although the cofactor molecule may not benefit at all. Thus, through these types of interactions, autocatalytic reactions become amalgamated into larger networks of reactions producing a simple chemical metabolism. Thus, certain species of molecules would come to dominate over others. Once the first successful amplifier loop is formed in the right environment the system may continue to grow in complexity until it is amalgamated or incorporated into another amplifier or autocatalytic circuit. A self-catalysing (or replicating) reaction would have outpaced the non-replicating or amplifying reactions. If both reactions were competing for the same subunits, then the amplifier reactions would dominate other reactions. Over time, certain reactions would be selected, whereas other reactions would eventually become extinct, so to speak. In a biological sense, one might liken the interactions of these chemicals as a 'chemical ecosystem'. This is a concept we will return in later chapters.

These autocatalytic reactions create a simple, but dynamic, local metabolism. Molecules are synthesized and broken down. Certain molecules acting to 'feed' some reactions become selected for, whereas molecules not utilized are lost. It might be argued that the autocatalytic systems represented the rudiments of the first signalling system. Here, we see the beginning of positive and negative feedback reactions and of the interaction of complex reactions with each other.

Stereoisomers

The success of some autocatalytic reactions over others likely had another significant effect on subsequent macromolecular and signalling molecule evolution. Early in molecular evolution, the selection of left-handed (levo, L) molecules over the right-handed (dextro, D) occurred (Fig. 2.6). Experiments of prebiotic organic molecule synthesis have suggested that equal amounts of both forms would have been produced. However, almost all organic molecules in modern organisms utilize L-isomers. Assuming that there were an equal number of L- and D-isomers, and that the interaction between such molecules were rare, then once the reaction did happen they tended to occur between similar isomers. Most of all biogenic molecules are inherently asymmetrical, in that they possess atoms or clusters of atoms that are unevenly spaced in three dimensions, thus unlike a crystal, which possesses a regular lattice of atoms, the interacting biogenic molecule must have a three-dimensional symmetry which is complementary to the other form. This is necessary as the attractive energy of two atoms is too weak to allow their respective molecules to be held together with the constant bombardment of surrounding atoms. A close fit to allow as many atomic interactions as possible increases the probability that the molecules will remain together long enough to allow the reaction to continue. Assuming then that the

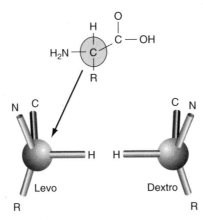

Figure 2.6 *Stereoisomers: Many organic molecules may be right-handed (dextro) or left-handed (levo). Levo and dextro forms of an amino acid, for example, are mirror images of each other. Modified after Willis and Bada (2000).*

first efficacious replicating systems were L-isomer based, then they would have outpaced D-isomer-based ones. The biological mechanism would have been subsequently L-isomer based. It had to be one or the other, hence the domination of the L-isomers.

Partitioning of the biotic world from the non-biotic world

Our prebiotic system of molecular interactions has now taken its first tentative steps towards a living system. At present, it cannot replicate, although it possesses a series of reactions that are self-perpetuating. These systems form the basis of the first metabolic systems, the first replicating or genetic systems, and the first signalling systems. But until now we are imagining a set of small molecules collected on some type of mineral substrate subject to the changes of the environment. Mechanical and temperature stresses, cycles of hydration and dehydration, not to mention the occasional comet or meteorite impact, all provide elements of instability. It is difficult to imagine how life evolved under these circumstances.

Obviously, a stable environment by which these reactions could occur might increase the probability of their evolution into more complex interactions. An essential characteristic of living cells and life in general is homeostasis. A great proportion of the neuroendocrine signalling systems are aimed at achieving this. Homeostasis may be defined as the ability to maintain a more or less steady chemical equilibrium in a changing environment. It is this physiological buffer system that maintains all chemical pathways and their feedback cycles to ensure that the appropriate molecular species are synthesized in the appropriate concentration.

In order for RNA to act as a replicating system, it first had to polymerize without enzymes. Moreover, there needed to be a plentiful source of nucleotides for the synthesis of the RNA polymers, yet there had been considerable difficulty with finding ways of synthesizing RNA subunits from prebiotic conditions. An autonomous metabolic unit required not only the presence of relatively high concentrations of organic molecules, amino acids and other organic compounds to be present but also a protected environment for these reactions to occur was needed. Both theories require a cell-like enclosure for the reactions to occur. We might envision that the reactions occurred while the molecules were diffusing through a three-dimensional aqueous environment analogous to the cytosol of a modern cell.

Most intermolecular interactions occur in membranes where the intermolecular interaction is held to two-dimensional diffusion. The Metabolic Channelling concept holds that protoenzymes and catalytic molecules bound to the surface of these substrates could accept a molecule passed along a chain of catalytic molecules (see box 'Origins of Life').

Origins of Life: 'The Molecular Embryo'
Matthew R. Edwards

Most scenarios of the origin of life, from Darwin's notion of a 'warm little pond' to the currently favoured 'RNA world', are variations of a common heterotrophic theme. This theme states simply that organic molecules (e.g. amino acids, sugars) appeared (somehow) in primitive seas and then interacted randomly to form first polymers and then protocells. Yet, in over 50 years of simulation experiments, not a single ribonucleotide or RNA molecule has come close to being produced.

In part because of these failures, some investigators have moved towards alternative scenarios, in which the primary themes are development rather than random interactions and autotrophy rather than heterotrophy. One such scenario posits that life began in ancestral metabolic complexes, in which all the catalytic entities and substrates were localized at specific sites (Edwards 1996). In these 'molecular embryos' (Edwards 1998), the individual molecular components would stand in somewhat the same relation to the developing complex as the cells and tissues to a developing organism.

The growth of ancestral metabolic complexes can perhaps best be visualized on mineral surfaces, which could have anchored nascent molecular arrays in biologically relevant configurations. Metal sulphides, in particular, would have afforded iron–sulphur clusters (e.g. [4Fe–4S]) analogous to the cores of extant ferredoxin enzymes. Such clusters might have promoted key catalyses, most notably CO/CO_2 fixation via ancestral forms of the reductive acetyl-CoA pathway (Edwards 1996; Huber and Wächtershäuser 1997). Metal sulphide surfaces might also have been involved in the basic energy transducing processes driving life, in either chemoautotrophic (Wächtershäuser 1997) or photoautotrophic (Edwards 1996) mechanisms.

The main attraction of life in molecular embryos, however, relates to the mode of catalysis. Models based on random interactions run into the following problem. A single step in a metabolic pathway is typically catalysed by a protein enzyme consisting of a specific sequence of among 20 different amino acids. The construction of this enzyme itself requires complex molecular machinery, first to transcribe a DNA strand to an mRNA and then to translate the latter on the ribosome into a peptide. Such a majestic orchestration is almost impossible to imagine arising through chance interactions alone.

In a molecular embryo, by contrast, each metabolite may have been formed already linked to a specific site in the complex. As in fatty acid synthesis, inter-mediates could then have been shuttled successively to adjacent sites for processing in pathway steps. Initially, protein enzymes for recognizing and binding intermediates would not have been needed at all, since the positions of the intermediates in the complex alone would have secured their metabolic fates. In the evolution of protein translation, it would likewise have been the relative positions of amino acids and transfer RNAs which determined the structure of the genetic code (Edwards 1996).

The origin of life in this case might be highly instructive concerning evolutionary mechanisms in general. For if the initial stages of evolution were indeed conducted in molecular embryos, then it would be reasonable to suppose, using the principle of evolutionary continuity, that analogous processes shaped all subsequent stages. Evolution might then be characterized as a continuous, dynamic interplay between the intrinsic developmental processes of organisms on one hand and their constantly changing physical, ecological and social contexts on the other. Conversely, random interactions and mutations would play, at best, a minor role.

References

Edwards, M.R. (1996) Metabolite channeling in the origin of life. J. Theor. Biol. 179, 313–322.
Edwards, M.R. (1998) From a soup or a seed? Pyritic metabolic complexes in the origin of life. Trends Ecol. Evol. 13, 179–181.
Huber, C. and Wächtershäuser, G. (1997) Activated acetic acid by carbon fixation on (Fe, Ni)S under primordial conditions. Science 276, 245–247.

In this way many molecules would have been formed without having diffused through a three-dimensional environment. Because lipids could have also been formed under these conditions, a simple hemispherical membrane could have formed around these reactions holding the metabolites locally. One might imagine these protocells breaking off from the substrate to form free-living protocells (Fig. 2.7).

The survival of these protocells would be enhanced considerably by having a membrane with the capability to be anchored both to the inorganic substrate. Protocells without this capability would drift away into regions with lower concentrations of organic materials. Their ability to grow would, therefore, be compromised. Protocells remaining within a local environment that possesses the capability to adsorb organic material would have better access to organic materials for growth. Here, one might find the beginning of a molecular system that would eventually develop into an extracellular matrix, membrane adhesion proteins and the signalling system associated with it.

The first cells

Although numerous experiments have achieved synthesis of theoretical prebiotic compounds under simulated primordial atmospheric conditions, no investigations have led to the synthesis of a self-perpetuating living system. Although many prebiotic chemical synthesis reactions have been achieved in the laboratory, the existence of a protocell, an intermediate

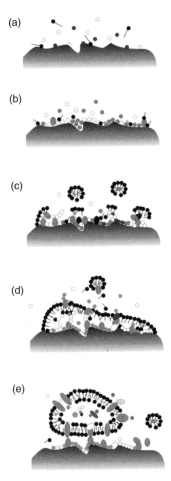

Figure 2.7   *A possible theory for the evolution of protocells on a mineral surface. Organic materials adsorb onto a mineral surface (a), then as the concentration becomes higher begin to interact with each other (b). Eventually, hydrophobic and hydrophilic molecules partition from each other (c). Hydrophobic materials, such as fatty acids, form a micelle which eventually is removed by mechanical means (d). The hydrophilic compounds trapped inside the protocell form the beginning of a simple metabolism (e).*

structure between autocatalytic chemical systems and the first living cell remains entirely theoretical. There would, of course, be no distinct stage in which a protocell would exist. The protocell was likely a long transition state between the formation of the first cluster of prebiotic and biogenic molecules and the first cells capable of independent metabolism and replication. In this early stage of cell evolution we might find the first cell signalling mechanisms.

These protocells would not be cells in the modern sense. The molecules replicating inside the protocell were completely uncoupled to any replicative ability the protocell might have had. In order to exist, the protocells had to be enclosed by a bag or membrane that could expand as the inner contents grew and which also had to be permeable to the building blocks of metabolism. Here, these chemical building blocks might be regarded as simple nutrients. However, once the level of biotic development led to the formation of biomembranes for compartmentalization, then energy could be achieved by the formation of pH or ion gradients across the membrane. The membrane must be also relatively impermeable to the larger products of metabolism. The membrane, therefore, has a dual function: to achieve environmental isolation of the autocatalytic reactions and to serve as a substrate to allow the reactions to occur. Because the membrane at this state is essential for maintaining the bioavailability of the reactions, new biosynthetic pathways leading to enhanced membrane stability would be selected for.

Signalling mechanisms in protocells

At this stage of cellular evolution there are no signalling molecules *per se*. There is, however, a growth advantage to those cells capable of being permeable to nutrients. However, the growth of these protocells is random and passive. There is no directed metabolism and there is no response to stimuli. Division of the first protocells would have been arbitrary and likely mechanical due to stresses in the ambient environment. As the lipid protein baglike protocell became larger, parts might break up and form new units. Others would dissipate, with their collection of biogenic molecules spilling out to be used as new building blocks or nutrients for those protocells still viable. The nutrients would be in the form of amino acids, sugars and fatty acids and their derivatives, and could serve as the basis for the first signalling molecules. The early membranes were likely more permeable than they are today allowing for the passage of several types of molecules that are not present today. The permeability of the membranes to H_2O, O_2 and CO_2 is 10^9 times greater than to ions. Molecules such as amino acids and phosphate are ionized and, therefore, do not readily cross lipid bilayers. However, in these early systems the permeability of the membranes to these molecules may have been essential. The early protocell membrane was likely intrinsically endowed with characteristics that would allow signalling between the inner compartment of the protocell and the external environment. Without such capability the protocell would have been a transient and unstable structure (Fig. 2.8).

   The evolution of the cell membrane is key to the evolution of signalling molecules. Initially, the chief function of the ancient cell membrane was to achieve physical isolation of its collection complement of biogenic molecules from the rest of the environment. This would increase the probability of molecular interaction by restricting the space of the reactants and for providing a two-dimensional substrate for the catalysing enzymes to adhere to. Signalling molecules, however, would have had to reach this barrier in order to function. However, the plasma membrane is only about 80 Å thick but possesses over a million lipid molecules in a square millimetre. In animal cells, the membrane is 50–70% protein by weight. The membrane is a dynamic structure in which lipid molecules are constantly changing places and rotating. Proteins are in constant motion via rotation, collision with lipids and other molecules. The structure of the membrane acts to slow down the passage of water and other solutes by 10^6–10^9 times. This characteristic of the membrane in modern cells ensures that receptor proteins interact with other proteins in the cell (Chapter 5).

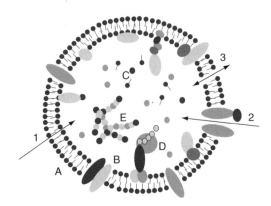

Figure 2.8   *Model of an early protocell showing some of the main characteristics: **A** – lipid bilayer; **B** – transmembrane-spanning hydrophobic amino acid chains; **C** – small organic molecules; **D** – enzyme-like polypeptides or possibly riboproteins; **E** – simple genetic material. Potential signalling abilities may have included: **1** – diffusion of gases, and small organic and inorganic molecules across the membrane; **2** – protein channels for ion diffusion; **3** – leakiness and transient openings in the membrane allowed larger organic, such as amino acids, to diffuse in or out.*

Role of amino acids and peptides

A signalling molecule, by definition, must either cross the plasma membrane or react with a membrane component in order to stimulate an intracellular response. Of the three basic classes of molecular building blocks available to the early protocells – lipids, amino acids and carbohydrates – only amino acids and lipids are sufficiently hydrophobic enough to pass through the hydrophobic core of the plasma membrane. Carbohydrates are too hydrophilic and would tend to remain in an aqueous environment. Later, after more efficient carbohydrate transporter systems were available in the cell membrane, the carbohydrate molecules were being used primarily for non-signalling functions, although sugars appear to be used, in a limited capacity, as signalling molecules in some organisms.

The first signalling molecules were likely highly present, useful for a variety of reactions, capable of crossing the primitive protocell membrane and relatively easy to synthesize. Amino acids, lipids or sugars could have all contributed to early signalling systems (Fig. 2.9). The elaboration of a signalling system would likely have proceeded through several stages. In the first stage, the putative signalling molecule is capable of passing directly through the primitive membrane of the protocell. Here, it perhaps acts more as a nutrient than a signalling molecule, and its entry into the cell confers some type of growth or stability advantage to the cell, although, as we will see in subsequent chapters, many signalling molecules are, in fact, nutrients. In the first case, the molecule acts as a simple building block for the synthesis of more complex compounds. Our signalling molecule may also be synthesized by the protocell itself in addition to being present in the environment. In any case, the concentration of this molecule would be higher in the cell

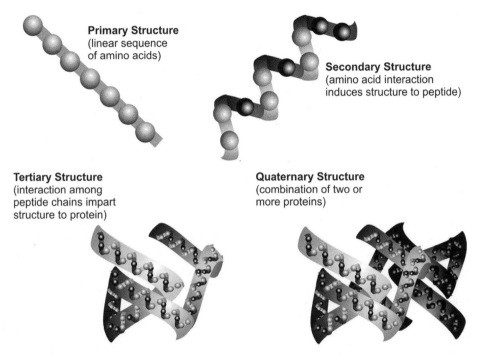

Figure 2.9   *Information content in peptides and proteins.*

than in the environment and would have a tendency to leak out across the membrane. Assuming that such a molecule could enhance the growth of a cell, then one would expect increased development and growth in areas where the concentration of this molecule is higher or, in other words, near the vicinity of other protocells. These molecules may have acted as the first autocrine and paracrine factors. There are a number of candidates for these early signalling molecules.

Sugars do not generally play a significant role as direct signalling molecules. The reasons are not completely clear. Sugars have not figured prominently in prebiotic synthesis experiments, nor have they been found in meteorites. Thus, sugars may not have been among the first generation of prebiotic compounds synthesized and utilized for the early protocells. Their synthesis may have occurred later with a combination of geochemical and early biochemical syntheses. Later synthesis of sugars and its high-energy component would have provided the early systems with a selective advantage. Perhaps it was only then when such sugar-based molecules as ATP and nucleic acids were used in protobiotic systems.

In the first part of protocell evolution, many researchers agree that RNA would have been more likely as a replicating molecule and early genome than DNA because of its ability to form three-dimensional structures and act as an enzyme. However, RNA is not a robust molecule and easily breaks down. The lack of sugars in prebiotic synthesis mixtures, or in meteorites, may indicate that a genetic material existed before RNA. This early stage genetic material may have included inorganic material peptides, or peptide-nucleic acids. Regardless of the first genetic material, the development of an efficient genetic system was necessary before any organism could evolve. Some authors have argued that these protocell would have utilized amino acids and peptides as the first autocatalytic system instead of nucleic acids because the number of amino acids is mathematically more favourable. Experiments have indicated that amino acids can be easily synthesized from components existing in the prebiotic earth. These peptides could have acted as an initial genetic system. If this did occur, it may help explain why more signalling molecules are based on amino acids and their derivatives than any other molecular system.

However, because longer chains of protein and RNA form globular structures, DNA took over the role of RNA as carrier of genetic information. DNA is a better template over RNA as it does not fold into globular structures and, therefore, is a more efficient template thermodynamically. Moreover, using DNA as a template would increase the length of the genes. The evolution of DNA may have followed these main steps: (1) synthesis of deoxyribonucleotides, (2) replacement of uracil with thymine, (3) DNA polymerase, (4) DNA repair mechanisms, (5) DNA recombination and (6) a mechanism for transcription and gene expression. The nucleotides dATP, dCTP, dGTP and dUTP are all synthesized from the corresponding ribonucleotide diphosphate. Thymine likely was added later as it is synthesized from dUMP. The first DNA synthesis may have occurred via a pre-existing RNA polymerase. Changing a single amino acid in the active site of RNA/DNA polymerase and on reverse transcriptase can relax the specificity of rNTPs and dNTPs, for example.

Histone-related proteins were also likely present in the earliest living cell. The histones are among the oldest proteins known. About 100–200 amino acids long, they are present in all prokaryotes and eukaryotes. The relationship between DNA and histones may be the earliest DNA–protein relationship. Some evidence suggests that the earliest transcription factors were derived from histones.

By the end of the protocell stage the basic rudiments of intracrine and exocrine signalling mechanisms may have been in place. Intracrine signals refer to those signals from one part of a cell to another, whereas exocrine signals refer to those signals secreted from inside the cell to outside the cell.

The first living cells

Understanding the set of events that led directly to the formation of the first living cells has been essentially a mind game as there is no experimental evidence for most of these events. If the earliest fossil-like structures, and the presence of organic material in 3.5–3.8-billion-year-old rocks is evidence of the first living cells, then there was considerable time between the formation of the first cells and the divergence of the eukaryotes and prokaryotes. Studies of the 2.7-billion-year-old shales from western Australia contain metabolic breakdown products of the 5-carbon ring hopanoid structures found in bacteria and the 4-carbon ring sterol structures unique to the eukaryotic organisms. This suggests that the lineages leading to eukaryotic and prokaryotic organisms diverged at least about 500 million years after the development of the first cells.

A comparison of shared characteristics between eukaryotic and prokaryotic systems might also provide clues as to what the earliest signalling systems look like. However, because of the longer generational times of the eukaryotes, in comparison to the prokaryotes, the eukaryotic cells may have a higher probability of containing vestiges of early molecular systems. The prokaryotes may represent a vastly derived organism bearing little resemblance to the early protocells thus the oldest common ancestor between the prokaryotic and eukaryotic lineages may have been endowed with some eukaryotic properties.

Despite this, some deductions can be made. For example, it is likely that the LUCA between prokaryotes and eukaryotes had some photoreceptive ability as evidenced by the use of the structurally similar photosensitive protein, opsin, in both lineages. The origin of the G-protein-coupled receptor, a key receptor molecule for sensory systems in the form of photoreception or chemoreception, may have dated to this period. Chemoreceptive ability in the form of amino acid and sugar receptors exist in both lineages. Signalling systems in the form of protein kinases are widespread among all organisms. The histidine protein kinases of prokaryotes and some eukaryotes appear to have a distant evolutionary history with the serine/threonine and tyrosine protein kinases found throughout the eukaryotes. Thus, before the divergence of the lineages leading to prokaryotes and eukaryotes, the early cell already needed to solve the problem of specificity between different types of signals.

Exocrine signalling between individuals or signalling between the organism and the environment, can impart a nutrient or some chemical building block that can be used by the cell, but it also conveys information. At an early stage in evolution, the cell needed discriminate between pools of information. For example, the information conveyed by sensory systems in the form of light, temperature or some chemicals is used to direct a set of responses that indicate whether the present environment is appropriate for a particular response. This might involve some locomotion, quiescence or activity. Another set of signals command a physiological change with the cell such as division. In the earliest living cells both mechanisms likely started out together, but diverged as the metabolic and sensory capability of these cells became more complicated. It was advantageous to have the receptor systems of these two information pools to be structurally different so as to avoid crosstalk between the two systems. Thus, G-protein-coupled receptor systems became utilized fundamentally as sensory systems and intercellular communication systems, whereas protein kinase-based systems became used more as growth, metabolic and transforming factors for the cell (Chapter 5).

There may have been a common origin of locomotion, cell divisions and sexual reproduction for the use of cytoskeletal elements. An internal support for the cell would have provided increased mechanical stability to the cell, and also acted as a foundation on which to allow movement, cell division and eventually multicellularity.

Whilst the first cell signalling systems were associated with nutrition and biogenic precursors, those controlling locomotion would have provided an organism with considerable selective advantage if it could move towards a food source. It is unclear how this may have evolved. Regardless of the mechanism of unicellular locomotory mechanisms, cytoskeletal elements are essential. It has been suggested earlier that cytoskeletal elements could have been among the first proteins to evolve, as this would have increased the integrity of the membrane structure. This may have acted as a foundation for the development of cilia or flagella-like structures. Then two events may have occurred. Either such formation led to the organisms having a selective advantage over all others caused great proliferation and dominance over the other organisms. Once the organism had this ability, it could then move towards a food source, initially at random, then more specific as sensory systems and integration of sensory systems were developed.

Oxygen, metabolic rate and metabolism

At some time in earth's history, the atmosphere took on an oxidizing character. It is not clear how this happened, but when it did, it set the foundation for all modern organisms to develop. One theory suggests that the rise of cyanobacteria, with their photosynthetic ability, led to the formation of oxygen in the atmosphere and effectively poisoned most of the species residing in the primitive earth at the time. More recently, however, it has been suggested that the initial oxygen concentrations arose chemically by the breakdown of water into hydrogen and oxygen by solar radiation, principally UV radiation. Hydrogen escapes into space, whereas oxygen being heavier is retained by earth's gravity. However, oxygen is toxic to all living things. Radiation contributes to the damage of biological tissues primarily by the formation of highly reactive molecular species such as peroxide (H_2O_2), superoxide radical (O_2^-) and the hydroxide radical ($OH^\bullet$). There becomes a relationship between the cellular systems to protect against radiation and those that protect against oxygen toxicity. The first organisms were probably chemoautotrophs, but as the oxygen concentrations increased in the atmosphere they developed the tolerance to oxygen. Aerobic organisms today survive the high concentrations of atmospheric oxygen because of the number of oxygen-detoxifying systems present in the cell. Extant oxygen intolerant species cannot survive because they lack these detoxifying systems. The LUCA has been thought to have trace amounts of oxygen to respire and may have had the ability to switch between aerobic and anaerobic respiration. Oxygen scavenging chemicals, such as vitamin C, vitamin E and melatonin (Chapter 8), may have had their origins around this time. In addition, oxygen-detoxifying enzymes, such as superoxide dismutase, catalase and glutathione peroxidase, may have also had their origins during this time. The regulation of these systems is among the functions of the neuroendocrine control of stress (Chapter 9). The chronic exposure to these radicals is thought to contribute to the ageing process (Chapter 7).

We can envision then three basic types of early cells characterized by their ability to respire. One type would be primarily anaerobic, whereas another would possess both anaerobic and aerobic respirations. A third type, ancestors of the cyanobacteria, evolving after LUCA, had a photosynthetic ability and exploited the comparatively high levels of carbon dioxide in the atmosphere. Eukaryotes and multicellular organism were derived from these organisms that had developed an aerobic respiratory ability. Initially, the cyanobacteria ancestors would have been at an advantage for growth and development as they would be primarily dependent upon sunlight as an energy source. Radiation and development of the primitive heterotrophs would lag as they would be dependent upon essentially the random capture of chemical nutrients for energy.

Proliferation of the early cyanobacteria led to the increased formation of atmospheric oxygen as evidenced by the change in O_2 isotopes in the rock formations of that period. This increased O_2 led to the restricted growth of those organisms that did not possess the biochemical means to detoxify O_2 and would have facilitated the growth of a likely obscure group of organisms requiring O_2 for growth. In this early ecosystem the ancestral heterotrophs and photoautotrophs now develop a co-dependency on each other. We will return to the concept of dynamic equilibrium between plants and animals in Chapters 12 and 13. This increase in the concentration of atmospheric O_2 increased the selection pressure and subsequent survival of the first symbiotic event where an anaerobic organism ingested an aerobic organism, a type of purple bacterium. This ingested aerobic cell became the ancestor of modern mitochondria (Fig. 2.10).

A second symbiotic event led to this proto-eukaryotic cell lineage ingesting a cyanobacterium-type cell. This would have endowed the host cell with photosynthetic capacity. The change in planetary ecosystem, from increased O_2 concentrations, likely had significant effects on early organisms, selecting for the vast proliferation of aerobic cells. Each rise in atmospheric oxygen has been linked with a major radiation of organisms. Some calculations, based on protein sequences, suggest that many genes have originated from this point. Increased metabolic efficiency utilizing O_2 may have led to a sudden decrease in generation time, and increased mutations and gene duplications since the early repair mechanisms were not as evolved.

The reactive oxygen species such as superoxide and hydroxyl radicals have been implicated in molecular mutation events and in higher organisms, ageing. Because of the twin effects of increased metabolic rate and higher mutation rate, evolutionary change within these organisms may have increased. Efficient utilization of O_2 would have given these organisms a selective advantage and, therefore, signalling systems involved with energy production and regulation may have evolved at this point as well as defence systems associated with oxidation.

Part of the defence system may have involved the early cysteine-rich peptides and proteins. These small proteins, with their ability to bind a number of metal ions, have some antioxidant activity. Cell systems expressing these cysteine-rich proteins were selected for. These proteins evolved into the metallothioneins, a group of cysteine-rich proteins ubiquitous in eukaryotes and multicellular organisms that play a role in oxygen toxicity, metabolic stress and metal ion homeostasis. The genes of these peptides have been shown to increase in number during oxidative and metal ion stresses and may have acted as a genetic foundation for the evolution of cysteine-containing signalling peptides.

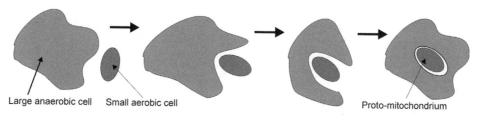

Large anaerobic cell   Small aerobic cell   Proto-mitochondrium

Figure 2.10 *Increase in cellular complexity by symbiosis. The formation of organelles occurs by the ingestion or infection of other cells. Over time, a symbiotic relationship is formed. Intracellular or intracrine signalling pathways are required to coordinate the actions of the new organelle with the actions of the rest of the cell.*

Elaboration of cellular membranes

The formation of atmospheric oxygen induced a number of adaptive changes in the eukaryotic cell lineage. Assuming that the early cells were synthesizing their own lipids and there were a combination of ester and other type lipids, then likely once there was an increased ability to synthesize these lipids, additional membrane structures may have formed in one of these early cell lineages. This would have increased the efficiency of reactions to occur, thus driving the eukaryotic lineage. The lipid structure of the nuclear envelope is similar to the endoplasmic reticulum and the plasma membrane. Changes in lipid synthesis pathways likely allowed for the growth of additional membranes. Changes in the lipid pathways may have occurred initially by an extension of the isoprenoid pathway. Elements of the isoprenoid pathway are found throughout eukaryotic and some prokaryotic organisms and contribute to a vast family of bioactive molecules (Fig. 2.11). After the appearance of free oxygen, cholesterol could be synthesized. Such changes could therefore have led to further development of the cell membranes and the appearance of endocytosis and pinocytosis.

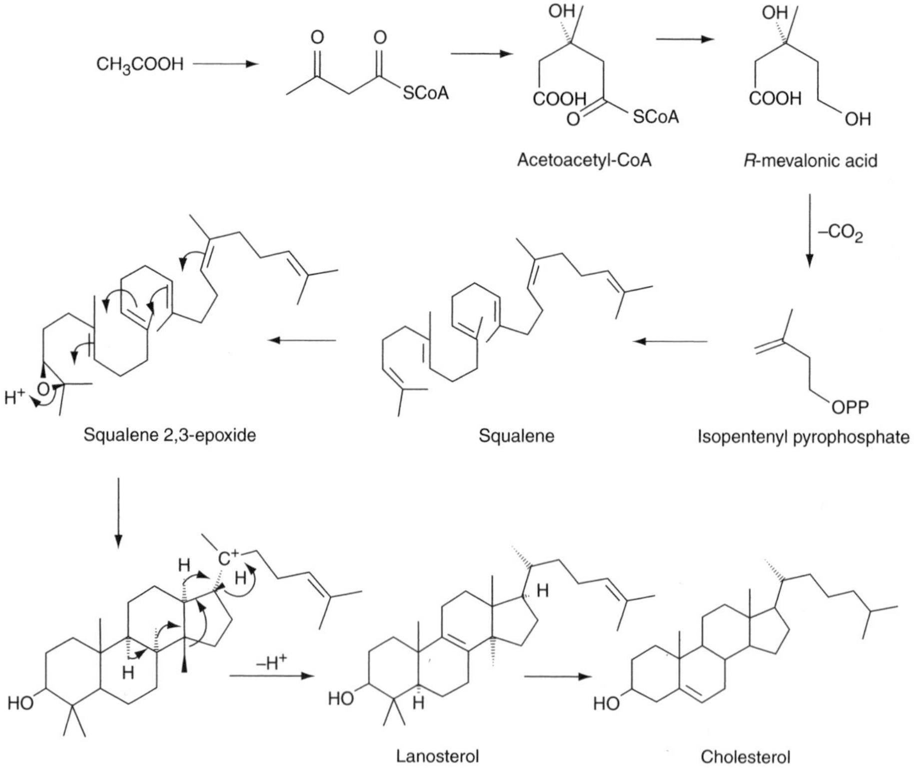

Figure 2.11   *Steroid synthesis pathway. Modified and adapted after Morgan (2004).*

The first true signalling molecules

There was of course no particular time at which signalling molecules suddenly appeared. It was a gradual shift from the random attachment of biogenic molecules to a biotic matrix to one where plasma membrane proteins and cytosolic proteins co-evolved with environmentally available ligands under selection pressure. By the appearance of the earliest true cells, the cell had the capability of synthesizing proteins, and thus the cell membrane would have become invested in those proteins that were thermo-dynamically more favourable to be oriented at the membrane–cytosol interface. Others would have been inserted across the membranes. Now, we have the beginnings of two new signalling mechanisms. In one case, polypeptides sticking out of the external face of the membrane acted as signalling molecules would could be cleaved in released into the environment. In a second scenario, the polypeptide could act as a simple receptor to bind a nutrient or early signalling molecule. The interaction of these molecules may have resulted in changing the catalytic activity of the polypeptide or perhaps introduced a pore in the cell to allow an exchange between environmental and cytosolic materials. Here, we may envision an early ion channel-type receptor or a catalytic receptor.

Our hypothetical early cell has clearly defined intracrine and exocrine signalling mechanisms largely due to the partitioning of the cytosolic and biotic components from the external and mostly abiotic environment. Intracrine signals refer to those signals utilized by the cell to coordinate actions from one part of a cell to another, whereas exocrine signals refer to those signals secreted from inside the cell to outside the cell. As we will examine in Chapters 12 and 13, exocrine signalling refers to secretion of signalling molecules outside an organism, such as pheromones. Because our ancestral cell is a distinct organism, exocrine signalling here also means outside the cell. Endocrine-type signalling has yet to evolve. Exocrine signalling capability however was essential for autocrine and paracrine signalling mechanisms to evolve. Autocrine signalling occurs when the chemical released from the cell binds to a receptor on itself or an identical cell, whereas paracrine signalling involves the chemical binding to a receptor on a *different* type of cell (Fig. 2.12).

The early cells possessed passive and facilitated transport mechanisms (Fig. 2.13). Pores in the membrane produced by proteins allowed for the passive diffusion of small charged ions such as Na^+, K^+, Cl^- and Ca^{2+} across the membrane. Proteins with a specific binding site for a particular ligand could actively transport the chemical across the membrane. Calcium is unusual in that as a free ion it is reactive and can be highly toxic. In its inorganic insoluble form it is not toxic and can play a role in structural support. It is not clear when the regulatory mechanisms for calcium evolved but it is likely that LUCA had the ability to detoxify and utilize calcium. The ocean contains potentially lethal concentrations of calcium. Molecular mechanisms required to bind calcium and create insoluble forms such as calcium carbonate needed to exist for the earliest organisms to survive. These early calcium-regulating systems were the foundation of later calcium channels, binding proteins and hormonal systems. We will return to the role of calcium in Chapters 5 and 6.

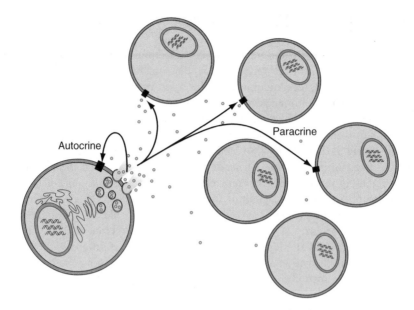

Figure 2.12   *(Autocrine and paracrine signalling systems.) Autocrine and paracrine signallings occur by diffusion. Autocrine interactions refer to the release of a signalling agent and the subsequent activation of a specific receptor on the cell that released the hormone, or one identical to it. Paracrine signalling refers to the activation of cell types that are distinct from the cell that that released the signalling agent.*

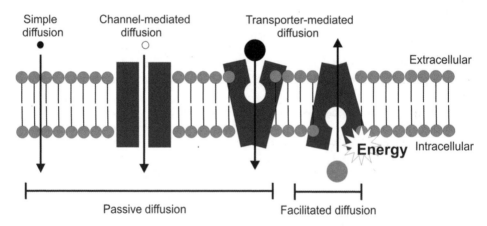

Figure 2.13   *Passive and active transport of molecules and ions.*

These early eukaryotic-like cells possessed a cytoskeleton, which was a structure attached to the membrane and its organelles, and allowed vesicular transport to take place. The cytoskeleton may have been the most important development for the evolution of the eukaryotic cell. The cytoskeleton allowed the evolution of the processes of endocytosis, the process of the uptake of liquids or solid particles into the cell by an invagination of the cell membrane, and exocytosis, the process by which the cell fuses with the plasma membrane to expel its contents. The cytoskeleton likely evolved from the beginnings of the first protocellular structures after it acquired a rudimentary ability to synthesize oligopeptides that were capable of polymerizing into longer changes. Attached to protein elements within the membranes, these polymerized protein structures offered stability from mechanical stress and provided a scaffolding upon which to attach biosynthetic enzymes. We will discuss the role of this extracellular matrix in the evolution of the metazoans in the next chapter.

The evolution of the first signalling molecules heralded a fundamental shift in the evolution and the organization of life (Fig. 2.14). Once cells could communicate with one another,

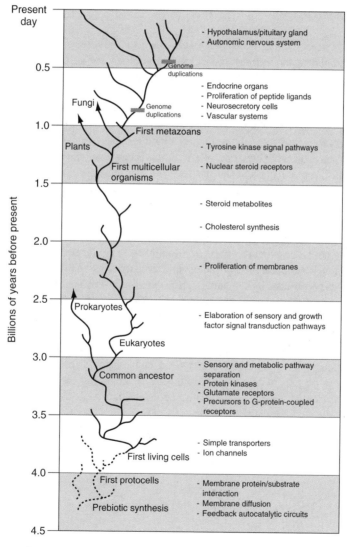

Figure 2.14 *Evolution of signalling systems in the Metazoa.*

it led to the development of sharing resources, division of labour and specialization of cells. If the first cells evolved about 3 billion years ago and the first multicellular organisms evolved about 1 billion years ago, then it took 2 billion years for cell to develop multi-cellularity but only less that 0.5 billion years later came the proliferation of organisms typified by the Ediacaran and Burgess faunae as part of the Precambrian explosion (Chapter 2). Microbial communities in the form of stromatolites may have existed 3.5 billion years ago indicating the potential for signalling events to occur at this time. Thus now the foundation of signalling was a requirement for the beginning and development of the metazoans, which set the stage for the evolution of this species, and beyond.

Chapter summary

The origin of the signalling molecules that are part of the neuroendocrine and endocrine systems are found at the earliest stages in the prebiotic evolution of life. Some of the amino acid-type signalling molecules, such as glutamic acid, may have also had an extraterrestrial origin. The combination of prebiotic synthesis from terrestrial and extraterrestrial sources may have provided the essential raw material for the development of non-living cell-like structures called protocells. Protocells may have had a number of primitive signalling systems including ion channels, passive and active transport and plasma membrane protein–substrate interactions. Energy sources for the protocells may have included ion gradients and the use of pyrophosphate from environmental sources. The formation of autocatalytic and amplifier circuits as a non-biotic mechanism for the synthesis of key compounds may have acted to increase the survivability of the cell. These autocatalytic reactions, acting as a simple metabolism, incorporated the first intracellular positive and negative feedback mechanisms. A true living cell began when the protocells developed metabolism and the ability to replicate into more or less exact copies. The genetic encoding of key biosynthetic pathways enabled the same signalling mechanisms to be utilized by the same cell populations. The success of eukaryotic cells was stimulated by the ingestion or infection of an anaerobic cell that eventually developed into mitochondria. By the formation of the earliest eukaryotes, over 3 billion years ago, all major intracellular signalling pathways were in place. The formation of multicellularity was stimulated by the ability to communicate with each other via secretory products. Cell populations may have been selected for their ability to exist in colonies during periods of harsh conditions such as changing oxygen levels, drought or temperature extremes. Metazoans began once cells could effectively communicate with each other, and functionally differentiate.

3

Rise of metazoans and the elaboration of signalling systems

Introduction

It took over 2 billion years from the formation of the first cell to the appearance to the first multicellular organism. Once this happened, it took only a half billion years for all the modern phyla of metazoans to evolve. There were several key events that were required before the primitive unicellular organisms had the potential to evolve into the complex species of today. Aggregation and adhesion of cells led to the formation of colonial groups. Cells living in such close proximity to each other were subject to the secreted chemicals of their neighbouring cells, effectively bathing in the ingredients of the secreted chemicals. This had an effect of changing the developmental pattern of some of these cells, opening up a new potential for evolutionary change. Such events may have been also responsible for the formation of haploid gametes. Then, in combination with these events, an increase in genetic material allowed for considerably greater stores of information for greater developmental complexity. With each of these steps came a need for new types of signalling molecules conveying specific information. As organisms became larger, selection for the need to coordinate the actions of all resident cells occurred. Thus, the nervous and neuroendocrine systems were born.

Neuroendocrinology: An Integrated Approach   David A. Lovejoy
© 2005 John Wiley & Sons, Ltd

Colonialism and multicellularity

There were likely several evolutionary attempts made that led to multicellularity. There were essentially two ways to create multicellularity. A single cell can divide and all subsequent cells stick together or several solitary cells can aggregate to form a colony (Fig. 3.1). The formation of colonial cell groups probably occurred shortly after the earliest cells developed the ability to regulate its own growth and survival. Assuming that these early cells could adhere to the substrate, but with little or no independent locomotor

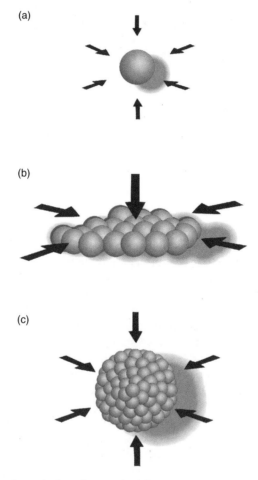

Figure 3.1   *Transition from single cell to a colonial arrangement. (a) In a single cell, interaction with the environment is three dimensional. The cell can obtain all needs via diffusion and active transport. (b) As the colony becomes larger and it exists as a monolayer, the interaction with the environment is reduced and therefore some specialization of cell types may occur. (c) Once an organism has achieved true metazoan status, then the internal layers of cells are dependent upon the outer layers of cells for nutrients.*

ability, say in the form of amoeboid or cilia-based movement, then the local concentration dividing cells increased through subsequent mitotic divisions. Initially, locomotion may have been entirely random by the shearing of cells from the substrate by mechanical forces, and subsequent drifting in an aqueous medium. Later, the development of flagella and cilia selected for a population capable of movement allowing for new niche exploitation. Now populations of cells included substrate-anchored and terrestrial-type forms on one hand, and free-living aqueous forms on the other. Colonialism evolved again in the aqueous forms. However, due to mechanical and ionic forces on the membranes, each type of organism solved the problems of colonialism in different ways. Although in modern life forms, aquatic origin organisms tend to show division and adhesion, whereas aggregation appears to be more common in terrestrial colonies. However, this likely reflects the ability for locomotion of extant forms. The earliest cells may not have had this ability.

The overall coordination of key functions within a colony is a necessary prerequisite for multicellularity. The first step in the development of a complex organism is the establishment of a pattern of cells with different states that can differentiate along alternative pathways. One mechanism of pattern formation is based on positional information. The ability of daughter cells to adhere to each other after division subjects the cells to different gradients of chemical signals. This differential gradient effects the development of the adhering cells and, therefore, changes the potential direction of the cell's development. Altering the developmental pattern of the cell then leads ultimately to the evolution of specialized cell types within a colony (Fig. 3.2). Among extant organisms, the volvox and slime moulds display aspects of colonial living. This division of labour is essential for the development of the early multicellular organisms. The increased interaction in a dense gradient of early signalling molecules led to different developmental cell types.

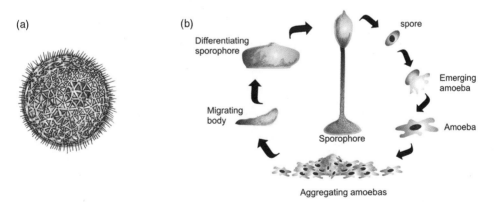

Figure 3.2   *Colonialism in organisms. (a) Volvox; (b) slime moulds. Modified and adapted after Margulis and Schwartz (1988).*

Signalling problems associated with colonial systems

Once a population of cells began to live in a matrix of aggregated cells, then the availability of environmental nutrients and signalling factors is restricted to those cells living inside the matrix, as opposed to those cells resident on the periphery of the colony. Energy flow in the form of nutrients limited the size of the earliest organisms. Thus, a certain amount of specialization was required before the aggregates could assume a three-dimensional structure. As we will see in Chapter 6, a comparatively large part of the neuroendocrine system is directed towards energy flow regulation. It is unclear how this happened in evolution, but clearly the enormous development of novel species during the Precambrian explosion is evidence that it did happen.

Some clues regarding the physiological significance of the Precambrian explosion may be found within the Ediacaran biota (Fig. 3.3). This assemblage of species, first discovered in the Ediacara Hills of Australia in the late 1940s, is now known from several sites situated in Canada, Mexico, Russia, the United Kingdom and the United States. The specimens have resisted virtually all attempts to be classified within the constraints of modern taxa. The oldest of these fossils date to about 600 million years ago. Before this period, the only fossils are of a millimetre scale and are relatively rare. The sudden appearance of the Ediacaran biota suggests a major new development of multicellularity. These species appeared to exist more or less into Cambrian times, or about 540 million years ago. The Ediacaran species appear to consist of more or less symmetrical soft-bodied objects possessing a series of repetitive subunits with no apparent locomotor structures or evidence of encephalization. They have been likened to some jellyfish and fern fronds. Thus, these species appear to represent a radiation of multicellular organisms that were primarily sedentary. One theory suggests that these species were adapted for an autotrophic lifestyle by becoming symbiotic with a photosynthetic species, such as algae, that occurs in many extant organisms. Their large size indicates that they had some type

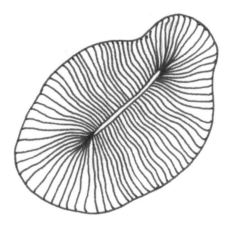

Figure 3.3   *Example of Ediacaran species. Redrawn after McMenamin (1988).*

of intra-organismal signalling ability, likely in the form of diffusible chemical signals, as there is no evidence that a vascular system existed in these species.

Debate has continued over whether the first multicellular organisms were autotrophic or heterotrophic. Let us take a moment to imagine the obstacles that the first multicellular organisms would have faced. At the single cell stage of evolution, heterotrophy was not too much of a problem as many biotic compounds released as excretions of other cells or from dying cells were likely sufficient to nourish even relatively complex protistans. However, energy requirements for a multicellular organism increase greatly with the complexity of the organism. A significant problem is the transport of nourishment to all cells. This would not have been a major problem with a hypothetical colonial organism consisting of a monolayer of attached cells. However, once the colony or organism develops a bilayer of cells, but is still restricted to the substrate, there remains a cell surface that is not exposed to the environment. Thus, a polarity in the cell structure is required such that food sources are only absorbed along one surface (Fig. 3.4).

As the organism becomes more complex, resembling a ball structure, the cells in the interior must derive all of their nutrients from the surrounding cells. Thus, here is a beginning of the division of labour where the surface cells become more specialized for taking in nutrients and the internal cells develop specializations to synthesize more nutrients than is required in order to feed their cellular neighbours (Fig. 3.5). One might imagine that here the importation of nucleosides and other building blocks for ATP, for example, would be preferential. The surface cells would then export more of these molecules than required. If this hurdle is met then the organism can grow larger as long as cells are receiving sufficient nutrients.

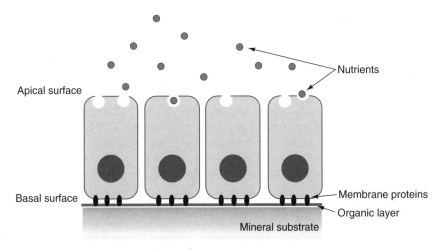

Figure 3.4 *Development of polarity in early cells. A colony of cells adhering on a mineral substrate has only on surface from where to obtain nutrients. Cells become selected for are more efficient at obtaining nutrients on their apical surface.*

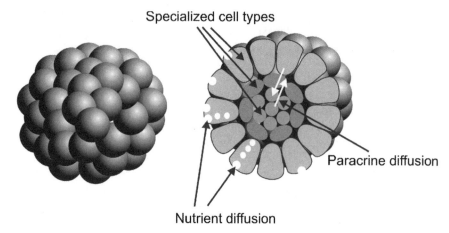

Figure 3.5   *A cross section of a hypothetical primitive metazoan showing the differentiation of cell types as a result of the spatial location of the cells.*

This ability to feed, however, suddenly becomes limited when the food requirements of our proto-multicellular organisms is greater than what can be supplied in the immediate local environment. Here, then, it becomes advantageous for the organism to move to new environments. This can be partially obtained by having passive movement, for example, drifting with the currents if the organism is free living, but eventually the complexity of the organism will be constrained unless it can acquire a higher energy food source. Eventually, the organism requires locomotion. Therefore, several modifications of the organism are required before it can evolve into a relatively macroscopic creature.

Alternatively, we might imagine then that our proto-multicellular heterotrophic organism is coexisting along with autotrophic organisms. Then, through a symbiotic arrangement, photosynthesizing organisms become incorporated with our little ball of heterotrophic cells. This then solves the problem of a food source. The organism is free to remain sedentary or drift by passive movement. The Ediacaran biota then may have represented a great radiation of such passive sedentary autotrophic/heterotrophic symbionts. The Ediacaran species did not appear to have any type of vascular system, and so we might surmise that the primary mode of signalling occurred through paracrine type diffusion. At this point there were no predators, but a lot of space with sufficient but limited nutrients. These species were, therefore, not under any selective pressure to become mobile to obtain nutrients or to compete with other members of the community.

Fortunately, for the first multicellular organisms that remained as strict heterotrophs the great radiation of heterotroph/autotroph symbionts acted to enrich the local environment with organic matter resulting from excretions, secretions, death and decay. Such an environment set the stage for the radiation of the true Metazoa. The first heterotrophs were likely filter or deposit feeders, sessile at first, and later mobile. When the first mobile heterotrophs did evolve, they could exploit the relatively large number of sessile and complex organisms associated with the Ediacaran species. It was a huge biological smorgasbord with only a few feeders.

The elaboration of hormone pathways

The primitive heterotrophs at the beginning of the Ediacaran evolution were simple relatively shapeless organisms that moved with the help of flagella or cilia-like structures, perhaps much in the way that the modern placozoans move. *Trichoplax adherens*, the only known member of the phylum Placozoa, is a tiny metazoan about 1–2 mm in diameter (Fig. 3.6). It has no defined shape and moves using cilia, and by amoeboid-like movement along the substrate. It has no mouth or gut cavity and appears to obtain its nutrients by absorption from the environment. It possesses only three known tissues: a dorsal surface, a ventral surface and an interior containing mesenchyme cells. Although assignment of the Placozoa as the most basal metazoan known has been debated, because it may be a degenerate and derived organism, it may resemble the early metazoans and be used as a model as such. If they did exist, such organisms were not likely predators of the Ediacaran-like species. However, it is likely that they could capitalize on the richer concentrations of nutrients found in the Ediacaran communities, allowing the photoheterotrophic metazoans to flourish.

Signalling systems in extant species

The phylogenetic relationship of the placozoans to the Porifera (sponges) and Radiata (Ctenophora or comb jellies, and Cnidaria, which include sea anemones, corals and hydra) is not well understood but considerably greater genetic and tissue complexity was required before the primitive heterotrophs could develop into an active predator of

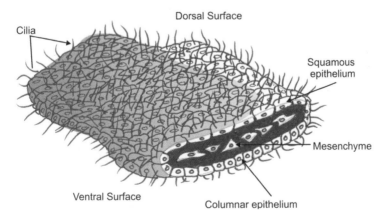

Figure 3.6   Trichoplax adherens. Adapted after Margulis and Schwartz (1988).

macrofauna (Fig. 3.7). Unfortunately, nothing is known about any signalling systems the placozoans utilize, although a number of guesses can be made. There is a considerable difference in the complexity of signalling differences between sponges and the phylogenetically younger cnidarians.

Unlike the Placozoa, sponges possess a number of features suggesting a primitive system that acts to coordinate sensory stimuli. Evolutionary developments of the Metazoa such as extracellular matrix molecules, cell surface receptors, the nervous signal transduction molecules and immune molecules are all found in Porifera. Cell adhesion recognition proteins are found in Porifera but are missing in the fungi and viriplanatae. Sponges do not possess a nervous system or cells that behave in a neuronal fashion.

Multicellularity, as we have discussed, can be achieved by direct cell-to-cell contact, or by an indirect interaction via the large extracellular matrix molecules (Fig. 3.8). The formation of an efficient signalling system is also dependent upon cell-to-cell contact.

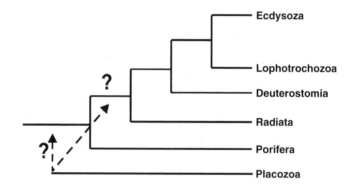

Figure 3.7   *Phylogeny of the phylogenetically oldest lineages of metazoans.*

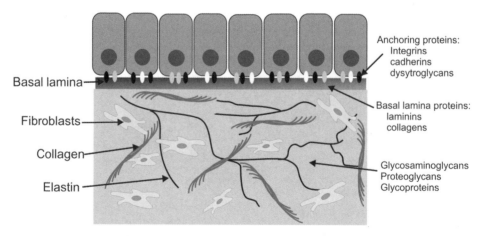

Figure 3.8   *Some of the major structural components of the extracellular matrix.*

Sponges have complex extracellular matrices. They also possess collagen and their receptors are similar to phylogenetically younger metazoans. In sponges, collagen is regulated by myotrophin and an endothelial monocyte activating peptide-like hormone that occurs in other metazoans. Sponges show rudimentary electrical signalling abilities. For example, the species *Rhabdocalptus dawsoni* can reduce its exhalant water current in response to electrical stimuli. This response is coordinated through the sponge by an unpolarized cell-to-cell conduction. Larvae of the demosponge *Reneira* have the ability to sense light intensity via a posterior ring of monociliated epithelial cells containing photoreceptors (Fig. 3.9).

We might predict that ion channels are among the oldest types of intracellular proteins that play a role with cell signalling. Ligand-gated channels may, therefore, represent one of the earliest types of hormone receptors. At present, four such receptors are known. These include the γ-aminobutyric acid (GABA) receptors, responsive to the transmitter, GABA, and the glutamate receptors, NMDA, AMPA and kainate that bind glutamate and glycine (Chapters 5 and 11). Coincidentally, channel receptors, being predicted to be one of the oldest classes of receptors, can be activated by glutamate, GABA and glycine (Fig. 3.10). As we saw in an earlier section, glutamate and glycine are amino acids that are not only easily synthesized by prebiotic conditions but have also been found in meteorites, suggesting that these amino acids were present at the beginning of the early development of life. Glutamate receptors, glutamate and GABA are an intrinsic part of neurotransmission between nerve cells in higher metazoans. Despite this, ionotrophic receptors have yet to be found in Porifera. The sponge, *Geodia cydonium*, does, however, possess a protein that has structural similarity to the metabotropic glutamate receptor and shows some specificity for binding ligands similar to glutamate and GABA.

Thus, despite not having a coordinating nervous system, sponges have the ability to coordinate organismal responses via cell-to-cell transmission of signals. Computer modelling studies have suggested that once an organism possesses a cell that is capable of conducting an electrical stimulus, it can increase the adaptivity of behaviour without the

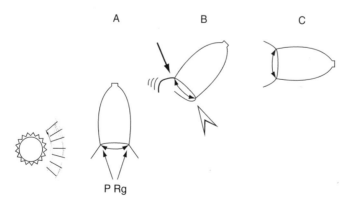

Figure 3.9 *Photoreception in a sponge larva. Cilia, associated with a ring of photoreceptive cells at the base of the larvae, act to propel the organism away from sunlight (A, B and C show the various positions of the organism). Reprinted with permission from Leys and Degnan (2001).*

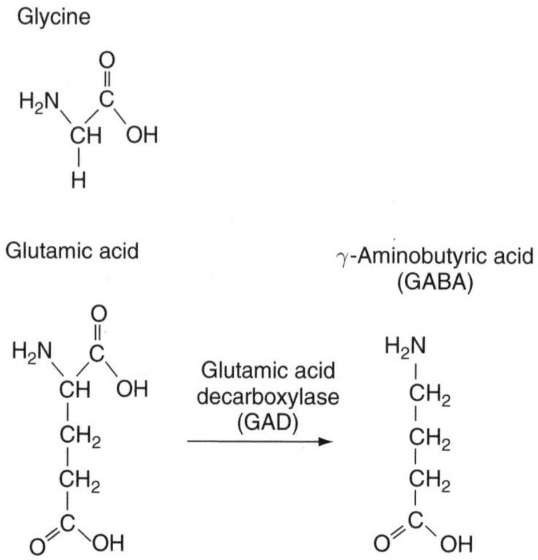

Glycine

Glutamic acid γ-Aminobutyric acid
                                                        (GABA)

Glutamic acid
decarboxylase
(GAD)

Figure 3.10   *Glycine, Glutamate and GABA.*

need of specific genetic or developmental information on how to organize the construction of the system. Ultimately, this can lead to a new niche adaptation of the organism.

Phylogenetic studies support the divergence of the Cnidaria, Ctenophora and Porifera before the bilaterians. In the Cnidaria, hydra is the most-studied animal at the molecular level (Fig. 3.11). Hydra is diploblastic having only endoderm- and ectoderm-derived

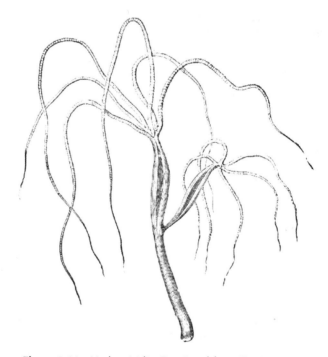

Figure 3.11   *Hydra viridis. Reprinted from Figuier (1888).*

tissues. However, hydra is highly derived in that it lives in freshwater whereas most cnidarians are marine forms. Hydra lacks a free-living larva that is present in virtually all members of the Hydrozoa. Thus, hydra may not be representative of the cnidarians in general. The interstitial cell compartments in hydra functions much like bone marrow in a vertebrate. It consists of multipotent stem cells that give rise to four classes of differentiated products such as nerve cells, gametes, secretory cells and nematocytes. Homeostasis within the interstitial cell compartment requires communication between cells of this compartment and epithelial cells via signalling pathways.

The nervous system of hydra consists of a variety of nerve types that express particular genes encoding neuropeptides. Currently, over 800 different peptides have been found in the adult hydra and 40 have been sequenced. Although it is likely that a number of these do not have a direct biological action, and instead represent transient proteolytic cleavage products during the degradation process, many do have a distinct signalling role. One of the peptides that is of particular interest is Hym-355, a peptide that stimulates neuronal differentiation in hydra. This peptide has structural similarity to the vasotocin family of peptides found in chordates although the precursor is organized much differently than that of the vasotocin family of peptides (Chapters 5 and 6). Hym-355 is expressed throughout the nervous system, but it is not known if it possesses similar functions to vasotocin (Fig. 3.12). It may be an example of convergent evolution in peptide structure, although instances of actual peptide structure convergence are rare. One of the hallmarks of neuroendocrine cells is the presence of a family of enzymes called the prohormone convertases (PC) (Chapter 5). These enzymes act in a post-translational manner to cleave the peptide precursor into smaller bioactive fragments. A protein with over 50% sequence identity to the human PC-3 and furin (a PC homologue) has been identified in *Hydra vulgaris*. PC-like proteins have also been found in yeast suggesting that a PC-like ancestor was present at the onset of metazoan evolution.

A number of researchers have questioned that why so many apparent peptides are present in hydra. One reason suggested for the preponderance of peptide signalling molecules in hydra, and perhaps other phylogenetically older metazoans, is the lack of relatively complex biosynthetic pathways that occur in species with a much richer genome. Peptides can be encoded directly by genes whereas small signalling molecules such as steroids, monoamines or thyroid hormones, for example, require a number of specific enzymes to direct the synthesis. However, given the similarity in a number of complex biosynthetic pathways found in animal, plant and fungal kingdoms, there is no reason to assume that hydra and other basal metazoans should not have this ability. The apparent reliance on peptide signalling systems may instead reflect the chemical nature of the signalling system. Without a vascular system, the use of steroids and other small lipophilic molecules may be limited by their diffusion ability across cells. Small hydrophilic molecules on the one hand may be readily lost to the exterior. Peptides on the other hand are relatively amphiphilic (Chapter 5), and can be degraded by only a few enzymes. Hydra also appears to lack the larger polypeptides of the growth factor family found in triploblastic organisms and in particular vertebrates. In hydra, such polypeptides may not be adequately encoded, transcribed or translated by the simpler systems resident in basal metazoans. The peptides of hydra control diverse mechanisms such as muscle contraction, neuron differentiation and the positional value gradient. Early in metazoan evolution, cell-to-cell communication may have been based on these small molecules rather than on the growth factor-like polypeptides that control differentiation and development in higher animals.

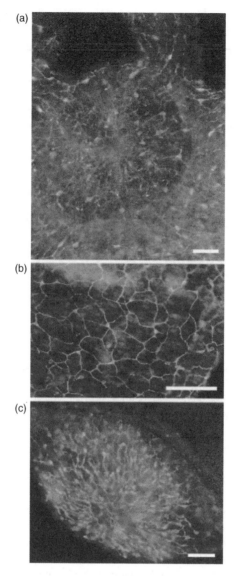

Figure 3.12   *Nerve net in hydra. A network of nerve cells is seen in (a) hypostome, (b) peduncle and (c) basal disc after visualization with an anti-vasopressin antiserum (see text for additional details). The scale bars represent 100 μm. Reprinted with permission from Morishita et al. (2003), Elsevier Ltd.*

Unlike the situation found in triploblastic organisms (possessing endoderm, exoderm and mesoderm) the peptides of hydra bind few G-protein-coupled receptors and instead interact primarily with receptor kinases and other types of receptors. In vertebrates, such small peptides are usually associated with G-protein receptor activation, but in Cnidaria only a couple of these receptors have been identified. The evolution of more advanced diploblastic animals and eventually triploblastic bilaterians, resulting from genomic and

subgenomic duplications, led to a greater number of endocrine G-protein-coupled
systems being utilized. After the Radiata, G-protein-coupled receptors appear to have vastly
developed. In humans, for example, as much as 2% of the genome appears to be associated
with the encoding of G-protein-coupled receptors.

There is evidence for some non-peptide signalling systems in hydra. In vertebrates, the
endocannabinoids are a family of neuromodulatory arachidonic acid-derived signalling
molecules that bind to G-protein-coupled receptors (Chapter 5). Hydra possesses anandamide, the same structure that is found in phylogenetically younger metazoans such as
vertebrates, and a set of specific binding sites for this ligand. The receptor has not been
identified and, therefore, is not known whether it is a G-protein-coupled receptor.
However, the presence of the anandamide precursor and enzyme activity consistent with
the biosynthetic pathway is also present in hydra. Thus, the endocannabinoid signalling
system appears to have developed early in metazoan evolution. Exogenously administered
serotonin (5-HT) and dopamine (Chapter 5) are bioactive in hydra, although the endogenous
molecules have not been isolated, and therefore it remains unclear as to whether these
molecules actually comprise a signalling pathway in the species. Moreover, the receptors
mediating the serotonin and dopamine response in hydra are not known.

However, a number of signalling systems have been characterized in hydra. Receptor
tyrosine kinase (RTK) signalling systems are found in hydra (Fig. 3.13). This includes
members of the HTK-7 insulin receptor family where the highest levels are found in the
non-dividing ectodermal epithelia cells in the bases of the tentacles. Currently, the ligand
is not known; however, exogenously added bovine insulin will stimulate cell division,
but not differentiation. Other RTK genes are *shinguard* and *lemon* of which the latter is
a homologue to the human *cck4*, chicken *klg* and drosophila *Dtrk* genes. *Shinguard* has
no known homologues in other animals. A homologue of endothelein-converting enzyme
has also been found in hydra. Moreover, hydra appears to have some endothelein signalling

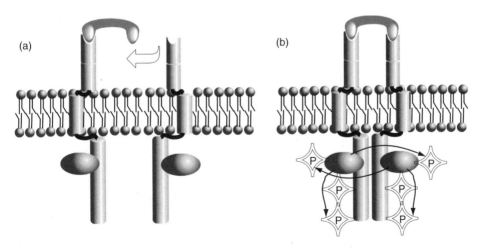

Figure 3.13   *Receptor tyrosine kinase. (a) The ligand binds to one of the two receptor subunits
which leads to homodimerization of the two subunits. (b) Accessory proteins phosphorylate
each other, then phosphorylate additional tyrosine sites along the intracellular domain.
These sites in turn initiate the signal transduction cascade.*

capacity (Fig. 3.14). In the presence of human endothelin 1 or 3, but not 2, hydra will contract to about half of its length. Transforming growth factor β (TGFβ) superfamily members play prominent development signalling roles in all phylogenetically younger metazoans (Fig. 3.15). Homologues to the TGFβ Type I receptor and to the SMAD transcription factors are found in corals. Bone morphogenic protein (BMP) is a peptide

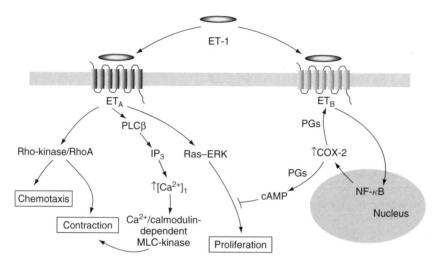

Figure 3.14   *Endothelein signalling mechanism. Modified after Hui and Friedman (2003), Cambridge University Press.*

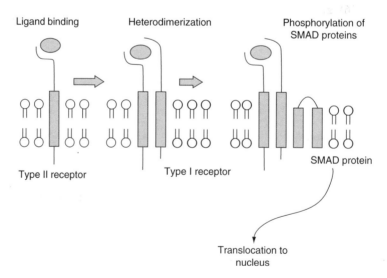

Figure 3.15   *Basic mechanism of some receptor serine/threonine kinases. The binding of the ligand to the receptor initiates heterodimerization of the two receptor subunits. This causes phosphorylation of the SMAD proteins and the subsequent translocation to the nucleus. There the SMAD proteins will interact with one of a number of different factors to initiate or inhibit transcription.*

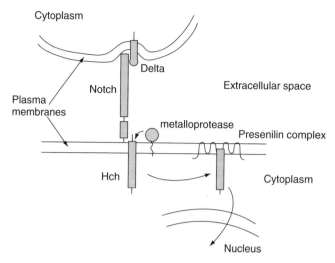

Figure 3.16 *Basic mechanisms of notch signalling. Upon binding of notch to the delta ligand, a metalloprotease cleaves an itch subunit, and frees the cytosolic domain of the protein. It then interacts with the presenilin complex then is subsequently translocated to the nucleus.*

structurally related to TGFβ and is expressed in the vertebrate brain. A homologue of BMP is found in a sea anemone and at least two BMP members are present in hydra. Their roles are not clear, however. Components of the downstream signalling pathway for notch (Fig. 3.16) are present although neither the receptor nor the ligand for the pathway has been found yet. Nuclear receptors belonging to the steroid superfamily of receptors appear to be functional in hydra. A receptor most closely related to the nuclear orphan receptor, COUP (chicken ovalbumin upstream promoter) is found, and treatment of hydra with retinoids results in patterning alterations. The receptors for retinoic acid (vitamin A) are related to the steroid receptor superfamily. Thus, elements of all or most of the key molecular pathways appear to be present in hydra.

Distinct signal transduction pathways

Greater complexity within the Metazoa is dependent on the increased division of labour and hence the formation of more specialized tissues. But, increased specificity of the ligand for its receptor and the subsequent downstream signal transduction events were a perquisite for this. Until there could be a clear set of specific responses for each type of signalling molecule, the size a multicellular organism could reach was limited. Unrestrained molecular cross talk between different signalling pathways would have led to chaos in development. Thus, once these molecular problems were solved then the organism could evolve into more complex forms. The cell-to-cell interactions that were so crucial in the evolution of the Metazoa are also, therefore, essential in the coordination of embryonic development. It was important, however, to keep signalling systems associated with sensory systems from those that mediated growth and differentiation. Only a few signalling pathways are involved in and are responsible for most of metazoan development.

Hedgehog, wingless-related (wnt), two signalling systems originally discovered in *Drosophila*, and named after the phenotype, TGFβ, RTK, notch, janus kinase (JAK) and nuclear hormone (steroids, retinoic acid) pathways play key roles in numerous developmental processes. Hedgehog, wnt, TGFβ, notch and nuclear receptor signal pathways are found in diploblastic organisms such as those of the Radiata, but have not been found in unicellular eukaryotes or in plants. A RTK is found in *Monosiga brevicollis*, a choanoflagellate. The choanoflagellates are thought to be a sister lineage to the Metazoa. Thus, the RTK appear to have their origins before the rise of multicellularity.

The G-protein-coupled receptors are not typically used in signalling pathways associated with growth and differentiation. Instead, they play a significant role with regard to sensory pathways, such as chemoreception and photoreception, and pathways associated with the flow of sensory information. For this reason, the elaboration of G-protein-coupled receptors may have been associated with the elaboration of sensory systems in triploblastic and bilateral animals. Although G-protein-couple receptors predate the appearance of the first metazoans they appear to be poorly represented in the genomes of the early metazoan taxa. Only one type of G-protein-coupled receptor homologue has been found in a sea anemone and only another in *Hydractinia*. Complex sensory systems with efficient coordination of locomotion and prey capture were not required until there was competition for the autotrophic species by the heterotrophs. This subsequently led to the heterotrophs exploiting each other as food sources and the beginning of predator–prey interactions.

The wnt pathway plays a role in the dorsal–ventral axis during embryonic development (Fig. 3.17). Only a single gene encoding its receptor, frizzled, is present in hydra. The wnt ligand and its receptor appear to be a primary component of the axis forming circuitry in the hydra polyp. The 'frizzled' protein has a structural similarity to the G-protein-coupled receptors in that it possesses a heptahelical membrane-spanning region, but it does not complex with G-proteins. The development of a functional wnt pathway in Radiates, but a lack of G-protein-coupled receptors may indicate that although the heptahelical transmembrane receptor evolved early in cell evolution, there was a long evolutionary lag phase before it became associated with G-protein signal transduction systems. Wnt ligands, and their receptor, frizzled, may therefore represent an evolutionarily older signalling system.

The formation of different developmental types in cells and increased complexity of genetic material causes a subsequent increase in complexity on the cells proteome (the total of all expressed proteins within a cell), and hence increases the number of intracellular molecules available for interaction during different states. One might imagine that with the proliferation of potential signalling molecules and the increase in intracellular pools of protein, there would be considerable cross talk between the various receptor systems. In the early evolution this was probably the case. But later certain pathways could be selected for in different cells or cells in different developmental states.

With the advantage of hindsight, it might make physiological sense to keep receptor systems processing sensory and information-based signalling systems separate from those systems involved in tissue development morphology. Cross talk between sensory systems and systems associated with growth and differentiation could lead to the instability of the evolving organism. Having receptor systems utilizing a completely different molecular system minimizes the chance for cross-communication. In Chapter 2 we discussed how this separation occurred early in cell evolution, but after the rise of multicellularity

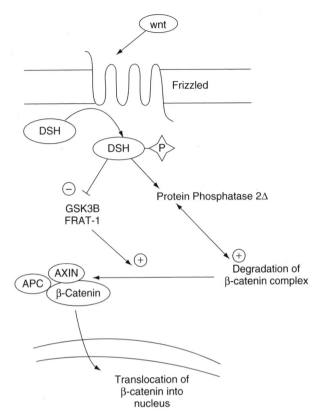

Figure 3.17 *Wnt signalling pathway. Although the wnt receptor, 'frizzled' is a heptahelical plasma membrane protein it does not couple with G-proteins.*

physiological separation of information pools becomes even more essential. Another means of avoiding receptor transduction cross talk is by the compartmentalization of signal transduction systems into protein complexes. A number of proteins utilized in a particular signal transduction pathway are bound together as an aggregate referred to as a proteosome. This may inhibit cross talk between unrelated signalling systems as many of these proteins would be unavailable for interaction with other systems. The formation of the proteosome, however, occurred long before the development of the first metazoans.

Signalling systems are not linear. They can branch at many different levels during the cascade leading to many interacting pathways in the same manner exemplified by the autocatalytic circuits described in Chapter 2. There are many ways of achieving specificity of signalling systems within a cell. This specificity can be regulated at the level of the receptor system, the signal transduction system or the complement of transcription factors present in the nucleus at the time of the receptor–ligand interaction.

At the receptor level, the affinity, and the kinetics of interaction that ligands and receptors have for each other, can generate different signal transduction pathways. This might include the activated receptor–ligand complex associating with another identical receptor–ligand complex (homodimer), or with a dissimilar receptor complex (heterodimer) (Fig. 3.18).

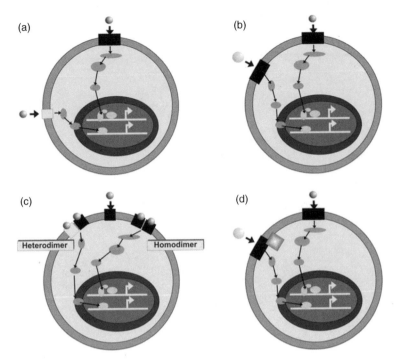

Figure 3.18 *Mechanisms of receptor specificity. (a) The same ligand can bind two different receptors to activate separate signal transduction pathways. (b) The same receptor may be activated by different ligands to activate different signal transduction pathways. (c) A ligand may induce a receptor to heterodimerize or homodimerize. Depending upon its dimerizing partner it may activate different pathways. (d) The same receptor may change its affinity for different ligands in the presence of a receptor activity modulating protein (RAMP).*

Alternatively, the receptor may interact with other proteins that act to change the affinity of the receptor for the ligand or perhaps a regulatory protein that acts to initiate the signal transduction system.

The same receptor can potentially activate a number of different signal transduction pathways in various cells and tissues. The combinatorial activation by different signalling pathways results in the regulation of specific genes. Various complements of transcription factors are expressed in different cells, thus even with the same signal and same signal transduction pathway a different response can be achieved.

Nervous systems and rudimentary neuroendocrine systems

The evolutionary origin of the neuron is unknown but appears have been born during the emergence of the diploblastic metazoans. The phylogenetically oldest members of the Metazoa, Placozoa and Porifera, do not possess nerve cells but the epithelial cells of these phyla do appear to conduct electrical stimuli. Both groups of animals are asymmetrical with considerable morphological variation among individuals of a given species. A developmentally unpredicted morphology places a severe constraint on the development of the nervous system.

Symmetry as a prerequisite for the evolution of the nervous system

The formation of symmetry was likely a prerequisite for the nervous system as the spatial organization of the nervous system relative to non-nervous tissue was essential for the coordination of organismal responses to a stimulus. Cells differentiating into neurons had to do so in the same temporal and spatial position in order for the neuronal axons to make contact with the appropriate target consistently among individuals. Evidence suggests that such symmetry in body form evolved before a nervous system. Cnidarians do possess a defined nervous system, but it is possible to produce nerve-free hydra by selectively destroying stem cells from the interstitial cell compartment. This is called the epithelial hydra. Because these animals are unable to capture and ingest prey themselves, they will die if left unattended. This animal can be maintained indefinitely by hand-feeding. However, these animals can maintain their normal axial patterning, budding and regenerate. This suggests that pattern formation and body morphology could exist before the nervous system. If an organism was simple enough to derive nutrients by diffusion, then the nervous system was not necessary. Only paracrine and autocrine signalling was needed. We might imagine this basal organism to be symmetrical and sessile and feeding opportunistically.

Symmetry in development is controlled by a series of patterning genes. These include the homeobox-containing genes, a family of genes originally grouped together by the presence of a conserved region of the gene (homeobox). The appearance of the first homeobox-related genes that encoded positional information and, therefore, the ultimate morphology of the organism evolved before the appearance of a nervous system. Once the first neurons and nervous system did evolve, then the hox-related genes encoded their development. The Pax genes are members of the homeobox gene family that is involved in organismal development and pattern selection. One of the fundamental roles of the Pax genes is the development of the nervous and sensory systems. These genes appear to have evolved relatively early in metazoan history as evidenced by their presence in cnidarian species. The Pax B gene in hydra, for example, is related to Pax 2, 4, 5, 6 and 8 of vertebrates. In chordates and several invertebrate phyla, Pax 6 has been associated with the formation of the eye, despite its structural dissimilarity among these phyla. The hydra is the phylogenetically oldest species that possesses an eye or photoreceptive organ. Transgenic rats possessing a null mutation for Pax 6 from both parents fail to develop not only eyes but also noses, suggesting a role of Pax 6 with olfaction as well. A Hox-like gene, *cnox-2Am*, cloned from the staghorn coral *Acropora millepora* and its orthologues in other cnidarians and placozoa resemble Gsx and to a lesser extent Hox 3/4 proteins. The expression pattern of this gene resembles that of the Gsx orthologues in *Drosophila* and vertebrates where it is expressed in a spatially restricted portion of the nervous system.

Selective pressures on the emerging nervous system

The next phylogenetically younger group of species include those of the superphylum Coelenterata, which consists of the Ctenophora (comb jellyfish) and Cnidaria (hydra, corals, jellyfish, anemones). Neurons more or less in their modern form are already present in this group. Evidence suggests that these phyla evolved during the time of the Ediacaran assemblage of species and represented the first heterotrophic metazoans. The first symmetrical metazoans, however, were likely far less complex than hydra or other cnidarians, and may have resembled some ctenophoran species. Observations of the epithelial hydra (p. 79) and the initial symmetrical organization of the Metazoa suggest that a mouth structure leading to the extracellular digestion of food material occurred first before an elaborate nervous system developed. The topology of the earliest symmetrical metazoans could have followed two main forms. They may have developed a bell shape as shown by the Cnidaria or a tube shape as is found in most other metazoans. In the bell form, only a single opening is required but a physiological method is required to ingest the food material and expel undigested material through the same opening. Alternatively, in tube forms, a method to ingest the food material and allow passage through the interior was required. Thus, both morphologies required additional mechanism for feeding. In our hypothetical bell-shaped creature, however, it would have the benefit of having a larger surface area and, therefore, able to remain in the water column, thus benefiting from planktonic food sources. In addition, the mechanisms of opening and closing the mouth component in order to ingest food would have had the secondary effect of taking in water and expelling water. Thus, the same mechanism used for feeding could be used for locomotion in these species. The symmetrical regulation of the oral aperture likely necessitated the symmetrical arrangements of nerve cells around the aperture, leading eventually to a nerve ring that is found in radiate species.

However, it is not clear which topological arrangement evolved first. Although the radiate animals, with the exception of the Echinodermata (starfish, urchins, sea cucumbers) that are secondarily radial, are the phylogenetically oldest species, they may have only exploited a pelagic niche once a feeding and locomotory mechanism evolved. The initial evolution of our hypothetical tubelike creature may have lagged a bit, relative to the sessile Ediacaran assemblage of species, for example, until a sensory system and locomotor system became associated with the mouth (Fig. 3.19). This creature likely exploited the habitats on the substrates in the limnoral regions of seas and lakes.

These first animals had sensory systems in the form of chemosensory and photosensory systems as evidenced from the existence of such sensory systems in sponges. But the sensory system would not have been coordinated with ingestion or digestion. It was likely coordinated with locomotion to a limited degree so that the organism could move towards a potential food source in the case of the bottom-dwelling tube organism. It was really a more complex form of positive chemotaxis. In order for coordination between sensory locomotion and digestion to occur, a new class of cells, neurons, needed to evolve.

The first neurosecretory cells

One of the great mysteries is how the first nerve cells evolved. The Porifera and Placozoa do not have nervous systems. The next phylogenetically oldest phyla are the Ctenophora and Cnidaria both of which have well-differentiated neurons and elaborate nerve nets. Metazoans displaying a transitional state between these two arrangements have not been found. Thus, our understanding of the first of the first steps in neuronal evolution is largely conjecture.

Direction of movement

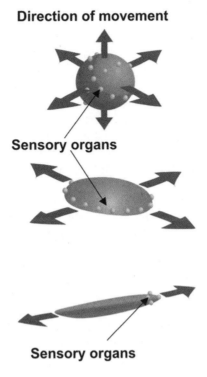

Sensory organs

Sensory organs

Figure 3.19 *Relationship between sensory systems, symmetry and locomotion.*

Some clues as to this initial evolution may be found by examining the nervous system of the phylogenetically oldest metazoans that do possess a nervous system. Sometime after the development of the Placozoa and Porifera but before the Coelenterata, there may have been a diversification of sodium channel protein genes and their functional attributes allowing for the eventual formation of an action potential. In jellyfish, swimming motor neurons possess different classes of sodium channels as determined by their kinetics. One might imagine then that the first such cells started as simple sensory cells such as a chemosensory, photoreceptive or mechanoreceptive cell that released its chemical signals in response to a robust depolarizing current. Hydra possesses sensory cells in the tentacles. The sensory cell has cilia on the apical surface that act as the receptive component of these cells. Each cell has one or two thin unmyelinated axons that extend into the nerve net region. The axons possess regions of clusters of dense-cored vesicles and synapses on to other neurons, nematocytes and epitheliomuscular cells. It has been suggested that this multifunctional neuron may be a modern representative of a primitive stem cell that gave rise evolutionarily to the sensory cells, motor neurons, interneurons and neurosecretory cells of higher animals. Once the basic electrical properties of the cells evolved, then they could differentiate into various types. Thus, the neuroendocrine secretory cell likely evolved at the same time as the nervous system.

Increase in genetic complexity and the rise of triploblastic organisms

Evidence supports the occurrence of sudden increase in the amount of genetic material after the rise of the diploblastic phyla that evolved during Ediacaran times. This increase appears to be the result of genome duplications, where the entire complement of all genetic material is duplicated, or a series of large subgenomic duplication events, where a considerable portion of the genetic material has duplicated. These duplications added considerably to the genetic raw material that was available to increase the physiological and morphological complexity of later evolving species. Five key developments in metazoan evolution appeared to have their origin in this set of genome duplications. This includes the development of the triploblastic organism possessing mesoderm along with ectodermal and endodermal tissue, a nervous system incorporating synaptic transmission, a vascular system, the formation of a bilateral organism, and cephalic integration of sensory systems leading to the development of a brain.

The endocrine system in its modern form was born with the development of a vascular system. Until a viable vascular system had evolved, the size and metabolic potential of an organism was constrained by the limited ability of oxygen and nutrients to diffuse into the tissues. Internally, physiological coordination and differentiation of tissues were limited by the diffusion of secreted chemical signals into the surrounding tissues. Paracrine and autocrine diffusion was the primary mode of intercellular signalling.

Precambrian explosion and the emergence of modern life forms

Almost all extant species have their origins from the Precambrian explosion, a 6–10 million year period over which occurred the rapid evolution of numerous metazoans. The evolutionary origins of virtually all extant triploblastic taxa can trace their origins to this period in prehistory. The sudden radiation of the Metazoa from this point seems to have been associated with several biological and environmental factors such as triploblastic development, genetic complexity and patterning genes, sensory systems and bilateral symmetry along with sufficient concentrations of free oxygen in the oceans.

The increase in genetic material through genomic or subgenomic duplications discussed earlier appears to have occurred well before the great radiation of species of the Precambrian explosion. One theory suggests that the Precambrian explosion may have been due, in part, by the sudden development of body plans upon which all modern organisms are based. There was a sudden allowance to make the genetic programming of body plans possible. Here, as system by which an embryo sets aside a package of cells that are destined to grow into an adult such that the body plan of the adult has no connection with the body plan of the embryo. There is a separation of the germinal and somatic cells. It has also been suggested that the amount of time spanned by the Precambrian explosion was insufficient to develop new genetic material in the form of duplication events by the emerging species. Thus all species, despite the great variability in morphology, possessed similar genomes. However, with an enhanced nervous and neuroendocrine system these organisms could adapt behaviourally to the environment and in comparison to evolutionarily older organisms exploit new habitats and niches much quicker. This ultimately impacted on morphological patterns encoded by the patterning genes. With the presence of mobile predatory organisms the nervous, vascular and hence endocrine and neuroendocrine systems took their modern forms.

Chapter summary

The rise of elaborate signalling systems played a major role in the evolution of multi-cellular organisms. Environmental conditions led to the selection of primitive cells that could survive in a colony. The increased interaction among these cells in the form of secreted products led to a quasi-dependence of these cells on their neighbours. Various forms of colonialism probably evolved several times at different stages of cellular evolution. Eventually, however, the single-celled organisms reached a level of sophistication that allowed the formation of metazoans. The increase in metazoan complexity in the earliest stages was dependent on both the accurate and specific interpretation of chemical signals secreted by a neighbouring cell and also the evolution and development of functionally distinct cells and tissues. The evolution of symmetrical body morphology was a prerequisite for functional nervous systems and the accurate control of somatic processes by the nervous system. The first symmetrical organism was likely radial, sessile and fed primarily opportunistically. Electrical coupling among cell types was the chief manner in which cell function could be coordinated. Increased diversity of sodium channels from one or more genome expansion events led to the first primitive nerve cells. These cells were a combination of sensory neurons, motor neurons and neurosecretory cells. This early nervous system, encoded by elements of homeobox genes formed a neural network interspersed among the somatic cells. The gene expansion events that led to the formation of symmetry and the nervous system also appears to be responsible for an increase in the complexity of intercellular signalling mechanisms. The oral aperture being useful for primarily feeding then later for locomotion was the evolutionary impetus for the formation of a nerve ring. This oral nerve ring became the forerunner of the central nervous system. By the evolution of the radiate species, the fundamentals of modern neuroendocrinology had been developed.

Adenosine: The signal of life
Imogen R. Coe

The evolution of early signalling systems are likely to taken simple compounds, already in use for other purposes, such as metabolic byproducts or cellular building blocks, and co-opted them for additional roles such as intercellular communication. Examples of these compounds that are still in use as signalling compounds in both simple and complex organisms are cAMP in *Dictyostelium* and the purine nucleoside, adenosine, in virtually all eukaryotes. Adenosine is a truly remarkable and almost unique compound that is a catabolic by product, an anabolic building block, an intracellular modulator of signalling pathways, an autocrine and paracrine hormone. It is produced both intracellularly and extracellularly and has diverse functions in both situations. Extracellular adenosine can interact

(Continued)

with G-protein-coupled purinergic receptors to activate a variety of complex signalling pathways which can regulate a multitude of physiological responses particularly in the central nervous and cardiovascular systems. Intracellular adenosine is involved in complex metabolic pathways where it can be phosphorylated to form AMP, a key regulatory molecule (e.g. AMP kinase, or cAMP, a chemoattractant in simple organisms) and ATP, the major energy currency of cells. In addition, ATP is used in the synthesis of nucleic acids, DNA and RNA, and cells that are undergoing rapid division or are energetically demanding (muscle, brain) require a lot of adenosine to meet their metabolic and synthetic demands. Adenosine can also be catabolized to various breakdown products which are recycled or released. Since adenosine is a hydrophilic molecule, it cannot traverse the lipid bilayer and therefore crosses cellular membranes via integral membrane proteins known as transporters. Purinergic G-protein-coupled receptors appear to not have arisen until after the deuterostome and protostome lineages diverged suggesting adenosine's role as a classic G-protein-coupled signalling agent was acquired later in evolutionary history. However, nucleoside transporters are found in both prokaryotes and all eukaryotic organisms studied to date and in their capacity as modulators or regulators of adenosine concentrations both inside and outside the cell, they are important components of pathways responsible for regulating and responding to changes in cellular physiology.

The nucleoside transporters cloned to date comprise a novel family of integral membrane proteins which show no sequence or structural similarity to any other known family of transport proteins (such as the glucose or neurotransmitter transporters). There are two major superfamilies of nucleoside transporter, the equilibrative (ENTs) and the concentrative (CNTs), which have no structural or sequence similarity to each other. The origin of two completely different families of proteins that catalyse movement of the same substrate is unclear but not unprecedented (e.g. glucose transporters). The ENTs allow for facilitated diffusion of nucleosides down their endogenous concentration gradient while the CNTs utilize the inherent energy in a cation concentration gradient to drive transport of nucleosides. In mammals, the cation of choice is sodium although in some invertebrates and prokaryotes, proton gradients are used. A number of isoforms for each transporter subtype exist which appear to have arisen due to gene duplication events which have occurred at various times during evolutionary history. Evolutionary divergence has lead to different transporter isoforms that are differentially expressed and have different substrate specificities. For the ENTs, in addition to a number of isoforms which are derived from different genes, splice variants of individuals genes also exist. The physiological significance of splice variants is currently not clear. Nucleoside transporters are responsible for the uptake of nucleoside and also nucleoside analogues that are routinely used in anti-cancer and anti-viral therapies (e.g. ara-C used in the treatment of leukaemia, AZT used in the treatment of AIDS). For this reason there is considerable interest in the expression and regulation of nucleoside transporters in human cells. We believe that an increased understanding of the structure, function and regulation of nucleoside transporters in a variety of organisms will provide insight into the physiological role of these important proteins in basic homeostatic cellular mechanisms and in improving drug uptake in a clinical setting.

4

Elaboration of
neuroendocrine systems

Introduction

The metazoan central nervous system is required to organize incoming sensory information, the coordination and stimulation of motor mechanisms and the coordination of physiological processes. The nervous system acts to transduce environmental information into a chemical signal readily understandable by the non-nervous cells of the organism. The information flow is, therefore, primarily outgoing. Although communication within the brain is achieved by nervous signalling in the form of synaptic couplings, feedback mechanisms from non-neural tissues must necessarily be non-nervous and endocrine in nature, as non-nervous cells do not possess the ability for synaptic communication. A functional and efficient nervous system requires feedback input from the cells, tissues and organs of the animals in order to coordinate sensory information from the environment with the metabolic requirements of the organism. Thus a neuroendocrine interface between the nervous system and non-nervous cells must have developed at the earliest stages of the central nervous system evolution. As we saw in Chapter 3, the first neuron was derived initially from a non-neural secretory cell, and subsequently acquired a combined neuronal, neurosecretory and motor neuron function well before each of these functions became differentiated into distinct neuronal lineages.

An organism with an enhanced locomotory system capable of moving faster and capturing more complex prey requires a nervous system that can coordinate more complex

Neuroendocrinology: An Integrated Approach   David A. Lovejoy
© 2005 John Wiley & Sons, Ltd

movements in a shorter time frame. Decisions, therefore, need to be made quicker. This requires a more efficient nervous system. It also requires a greater energy input to the cells and a more efficient utilization of energy by the organism.

Early evolving bilateral metazoans utilized a nervous system with an increasingly more efficient synaptic transmission, enhanced by paracrine neurosecretory mechanisms. Triploblastic tissue organization, bilateral symmetry and segmentation all evolved around the same time, and collectively appear responsible for developing the nervous/neurosecretory nerve net present in the radiates into a system with a cephalic brain and ventrally oriented nerve cords and ganglia found in most bilateral metazoans. This allowed for the formation of specialized neurosecretory structures, and together with the development of a vascular system came the first true neuroendocrine system. A dorsal–ventral inversion occurred in an ancestral deuterostome lineage that led to the development of the dorsal nerve cord found in Chordates.

Elaboration of nervous system and development of organismal complexity

The elaboration of central nervous system complexity results from the increase in the absolute number of neurons, the number of differentiated neuron types, the complexity of individual neurons and the arbourization of their processes. Generally, within invertebrates, the elaboration of the nervous system was accomplished by increasing the degree of complexity of individual neurons. In the earliest Chordates, however, the elaboration was characterized by an increase in the number of neurons leading to clusters of functionally related cells.

Three main clades of bilateral organisms emerged around the time of the Precambrian explosion (Fig. 4.1). These were the Deuterostomia (echinoderms, hemichordates and chordates), the Ecdysozoa (arthropods) and the Lophotrochozoa (molluscs, annelids and platyhelminthes). It is not clear which lineage emerged first. The acoel organisms previously belonged to an order within the phylum Platyhelminthes, which include the flatworms; however, recent investigations of the 18S ribosomal subunit DNA sequences support a reclassification of this group as a separate phylum and the most basal of the triploblastic and bilateral organisms. The acoels appeared to have evolved well before the Precambrian explosion, suggesting that after the initial formation of the triploblastic and bilateral organisms, there was a long lag phase before the more complex predatory species came to be. An analysis of the neurosecretory and nervous system elements of this group of species provides some clues as to the evolution of the bilaterian nervous system from the radiate nervous system.

Nervous and neurosecretory systems in the first bilateral organisms

The nervous system in the earliest metazoans was a simple neural network in the form of a nerve net as exemplified by that found in cnidarians and particularly hydra. This arrangement is an intermingling of nerve cells throughout non-nervous tissues. H.G. Wells and associates in their book, *The Science of Life*, published in 1931 described the

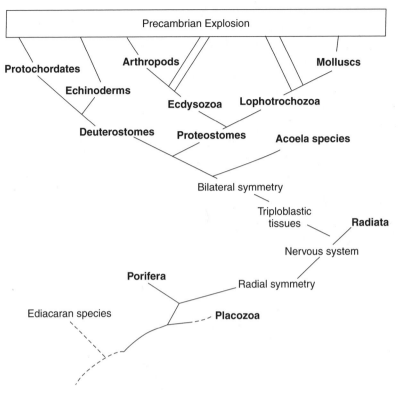

Figure 4.1   *Phylogeny of the Metazoa.*

cnidarian nervous system as 'a nightmare telephone system in which there is no proper exchange but only a tangle of wires; where the raising of one receiver would call up hundreds of subscribers, or indeed, if you spoke loud enough into it, every subscriber in the system'. Because there is no vascular system of these animals, the nervous system acts as both a nerve network employing synaptic-like transmission (though less efficient) and a neuroendocrine system utilizing paracrine secretion of endocrine modulators. Hence, there is the need for the nervous system to be arranged throughout the tissues in a netlike manner. A nerve ring around the oral aperture coordinates tentacular activity primarily for feeding, as in the case with anemones, but is used for locomotion as seen in hydra and jellyfish. In our hypothetical ancestral radiate metazoan, the mechanisms under the control of the nervous/neurosecretory system were primarily food capture and locomotion. Reproduction, growth and development could proceed without the need of a nervous system. Osmotic regulation and respiration could be achieved entirely at a cellular level.

One of these basal radiate lineages underwent a major increase in the amount of genetic material in the genome. This led to the first triploblastic organisms. Most, if not all, of these transitional organisms appear to have disappeared because all triploblastic organisms are bilateral (with the exception of the Echinodermata) although ontologically all begin as more or less radial forms. We might imagine then that the first triploblastic organisms resembled the general body form of the Cnidaria initially. They would have possessed a nerve net like the Radiata and employed similar neurosecretory cells. However, the phylogenetically oldest lineages of bilateral organisms have a segmented nervous system connected by a nerve cord running between the segmentations. Segmentation or metamerism might be defined as the repetition of a structural unit along an anterior–posterior axis, which is physiologically integrated with the rest of the body. Although the origins of segmentation are obscure, it remains unclear whether the segmentation present in chordates, annelids and arthropods began from a common ancestor or if it evolved separately in each of these lineages. In any case, segmentation had the effect of extending our hypothetical basal triploblastic organisms from a spherical structure to a simple wormlike creature (Fig. 4.2). The nerve net of the proto-triploblastic organisms then became extended as the set of nerves and neurosecretory cells were reproduced in each segment, where each neural unit was connected by a nerve cord. Thus, within each segment a cluster of neuroendocrine cells, a forerunner of a segmental ganglion evolved and

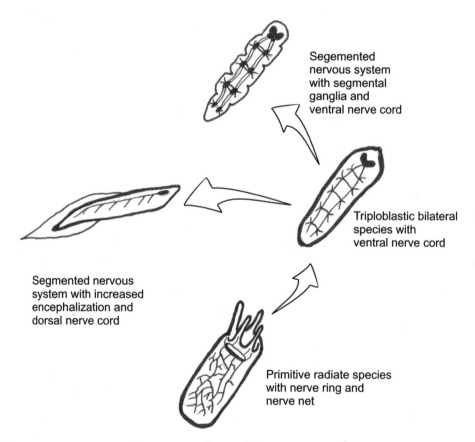

Segemented nervous system with segmental ganglia and ventral nerve cord

Triploblastic bilateral species with ventral nerve cord

Segmented nervous system with increased encephalization and dorsal nerve cord

Primitive radiate species with nerve ring and nerve net

Figure 4.2   *Evolution of the nervous system.*

eventually came to specifically modulate the actions of the epithelial secretory cells within each unit, in a manner analogous to how the autonomic nervous system regulates tissues in chordates.

Acoelomorpha and Platyhelminthes as model systems

A model for this type of this hypothetical organism might be similar to the flatworms of the Acoelomorpha and Platyhelminthes lineages (Fig. 4.3). The Acoelomorpha includes the acoelan and nemertodermatidan species that were formally grouped with the phylum Platyhelminthes but now appear to be a separate and phylogenetically older phylum. The nervous system of the acoels includes a simple brain formed by clusters of nerve cells that lack a neuropile. They also possess a variable number of longitudinal nerve cords (Fig. 4.4) and do not possess a stomatogastral nervous system. The planarians are a group of flatworms within the order Tricladida of the Platyhelminthes. This phylum appears to have evolved early in metazoan evolution some time after the separation of the first lophotrochozoan species. The platyhelminths consist of well over 12 000 species of which about one-quarter are free-living and the rest have a parasitic life history. The platyhelminthan nervous system has a distinct segmental pattern, defined by the 'orthogon', a ladder-like organization of longitudinal nerve cords connected by transverse commissures at periodic intervals. It is comprised of a brain and paired longitudinal nerve cords and a peripheral nervous system consisting of a number of smaller nerve cords and plexuses (Fig. 4.5).

The platyhelminths are characterized by a greater degree of encephalization of their brains. In general, a brain differs from a ganglion in that a brain subserves the entire body whereas a ganglion is only associated with the functions within a particular segment.

(a)   (b)

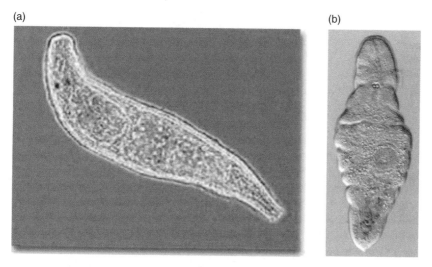

Figure 4.3 *Representative Platyhelminthes and Acoelomorpha species (a) Dalyellia, a platy-helminth; (b) Flagellophora, an acoelomorphan species. Images courtesy of Nikon Corp. (a) and Dr. Matthew Hooge University of Maine (b).*

(a) (b)

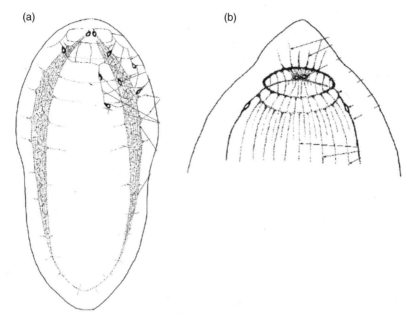

Figure 4.4 *Nervous system of acoelomorphan species. (a) 5-HT immunoreactive fibres and cells in the nervous system of* Meara stichopi; *(b) 5-HT immunoreactive fibres and cells in the central nervous system of* Nemertoderma westbladi. *Both species belong to the Nemertodermatida, which is thought to be a sister taxa to the acoela in the Acoelomorpha. There is no obvious neural lobe in these species. Modified with permission from Raikova et al. (2000). Reprinted by the permission of Harcourt Publishers Ltd.*

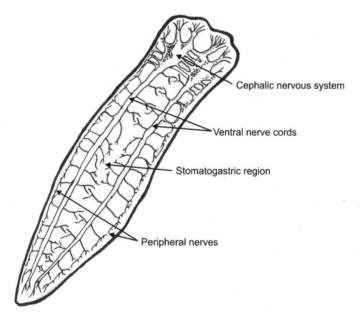

Figure 4.5 *Planarian nervous system. Adapted and modified after Kershaw (1988).*

A brain is bilobular and has functionally specialized components in comparison to the more homogenous arrangement of a ganglion. A 'cephalic ganglion', as a forerunner of the brain, appears not to exist in any metazoan species nor is it likely to have existed in extinct species. It is likely that the brain was derived from the integration of a number of sensory systems and the systematic coordination of feeding and locomotory mechanisms, and, therefore, may have always possessed a functional heterogeneity within its parts. The fibroblast growth factor (FGF) pathway may be important for the development of the brain in vertebrates. The planarian, *Dugesia japonica*, possesses an FGF receptor-related gene, *nou-darake* (*Djndk*). Loss of function of this gene results in the ectopic expression of the brain in the trunk region, suggesting that this gene plays a role in the restriction of the brain development to the head region. Thus, the diffuse nervous system of the radiates may have developed into the brain, ganglia and nerve cord type of higher metazoans by the formation of genes controlling the proliferation of neurons in particular regions of the body and the subsequent migration of the cells and processes.

The neurons of the planarian brain resemble those of vertebrates much more than those of phylogenetically younger and more complex ecdysozoan species such as insects. The planarian neurons possess multipolar morphologies, dendritic spines, a single axon and synaptic boutons. Some authors have argued that the planarian brain may, therefore, resemble the ancestor of the vertebrate brain. A recent gene microarray study of this same species revealed the presence of 205 head-specific genes. Of these, 33 represented homologues of genes expressed in both vertebrate and invertebrate nervous systems. Thus, the nervous system for the three main groups – Deuterostomia, Ecdysozoa and Lophotrochozoa – appears to have had a common origin.

Both the Platyhelminthes and the Acoelomorpha lack a coelom and circulatory system. Thus, any long distance control of growth and development is controlled by the nervous system using neurosecretory paracrine secretions. Planaria utilize cholinergic, serotonergic and dopaminergic signalling systems in their brain. In addition, flatworms appear to contain a large number of bioactive peptides. Peptidergic material is highly expressed in the brain and in the longitudinal and transverse fibre tracts. Peptides are particularly highly expressed in innervating fibres to the musculature of attachment organs, feeding and copulatory structures. Immunoreactive evidence for over 30 different peptides has been obtained, although only 6 have been sequenced. The characterized peptides can be classified into FMRFamide-related peptides and neuropeptide F-related peptides. Neuropeptide F appears to be a homologue of Neuropeptide Y, a peptide found in vertebrates that regulates anxiety and feeding. If so, it suggests that the NPY/NPF ancestor evolved before the Precambrian explosion and during the genome duplications that ultimately lead to bilateral triploblastic morphologies.

Nervous and neuroendocrine systems in phylogenetically younger invertebrates

Nematodes may represent a lineage that evolved early in metazoan prehistory, but well after the initial genomic duplications. The phylogenetic placement of the nematodes is controversial. Although analysis of the 18S subunit places the phylum within the Ecdysozoa, more comprehensive studies support their placement as a basal bilateral metazoan. However, the use of *Caenorhabditus elegans* as a model species has added much to our knowledge to the evolution of the nervous system and hormonal signalling systems. A complete sequence analysis of the *C. elegans* genome has revealed the existence of at least 130 putative peptide receptors in the form of G-protein-coupled receptors. In one study 92 putative peptide genes were identified. Although some of these peptides appear to be homologues of known gene families such as FMRFamide and allatostatin, most cannot to be readily identifiable in other metazoan lineages. Peptidergic opioid signalling systems appear not to be used in *C. elegans* as the genes are not present in the genome. An opioid signalling system is functional in planaria, although it is not known if the endogenous ligand is peptide or non-peptide based. In any case, however, despite the simple morphology of *C. elegans* and other nematodes, they appear to utilize a rich peptide and receptor signalling system.

The general organization of the nervous system of ecdysozoan species is similar to that seen in acoelomorphs and other lophotrochozoan species (Fig. 4.6). The nervous system consists of a bilobed brain and two ventral nerve cords that run the length of the organism connecting the paired ganglia within each segment reflecting the common evolutionary origin of the ecdysozoan and lophotrochozoan lineages. Transverse nervous elements connect each ganglion within the pair at each segment. In insects, the brain is derived from the fusion of the ganglia found in the first three segments of the head. Fusion of ganglia also occurs in the thoracic and abdominal segments. Neurosecretory cells are

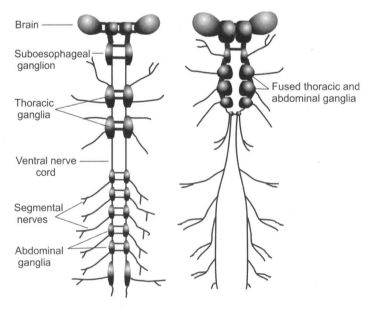

Figure 4.6   *Examples of insect central nervous systems. Modified after Gullan and Cranston (1994).*

present in the brain and at each ganglion. Neurons are differentiated into sensory neurons, interneuron, motor neurons and neuroendocrine cells. The visceral or sympathetic nervous system consists of stomatogastric, ventral visceral and caudal visceral subdivisions. The systems innervate the anterior and posterior gut, a number of the endocrine organs including the corpora allata and corpora cardiaca, reproductive organs and the tracheal system.

The neuroendocrine cells of an insect are found throughout the nervous system and are part of a peripheral hormonal feedback system analogous to the hypothalamus–pituitary–peripheral gland system of chordates (p. 106). The neuroendocrine cells of insects produce most of the known insect hormones with the exceptions of juvenile hormone (JH) and ecdysteroids that are produced by non-neural tissues. The corpora cardiaca are paired neuroendocrine glands located behind the brain on either side of the aorta. They store and release a number of neuroendocrine agents including prothoracicotropic hormone (PTTH). The prothoracic glands consist of diffuse neurosecretory tissues located in the head or rostral thorax. The corpora allata are small glands derived from epithelium and are located on either side of the foregut (Fig. 4.7).

Similar to organisms that have evolved before the ecdysozoan species, and apparently ubiquitous among the Metazoa, neuropeptides are the largest class of signalling molecules. These neuropeptides are discussed in detail in upcoming chapters. Insects have apparently lost much of the pathway following the conversion of arachidonic acid to other biosynthetic compounds. Depending upon the species, they produce little or no arachidonic acid (Fig. 4.8). This has presumably led to the loss of the cannabinoid receptors as well (Chapter 5). All ecdysteroids found in insects are derived from steroids such as cholesterol. Insects cannot synthesize steroids *de novo* and, therefore, all steroid precursors must be obtained in their diet. Once obtained, they are converted into a number of different steroidal structures including the ecdysteroids. Insects do, however, have a well-developed isoprenoid pathway leading to numerous bioactive compounds. Many of these products are used as internal and external signalling agents (Chapters 12 and 13).

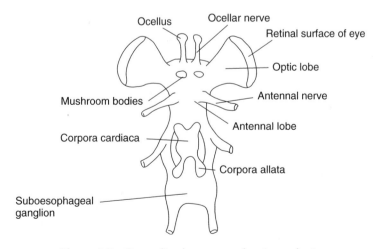

Figure 4.7   *Generalized structure of an insect brain.*

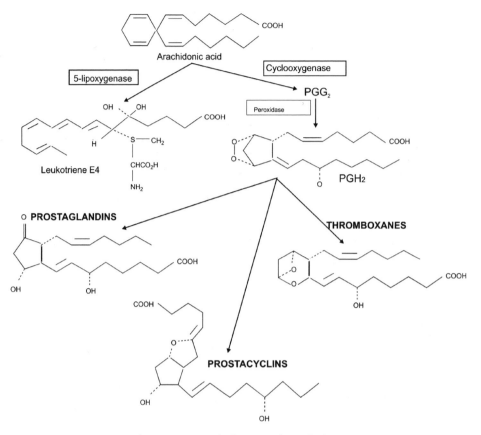

Figure 4.8   *Arachidonic acid metabolites.*

Insects possess true endocrine and neuroendocrine systems having a well-developed circulatory system consisting of haemolymph that traverses through the insect via a set of muscular pumps. Thus, many of the neurosecretory products of the various neuroendocrine glands can gain access to all main regions of the organism's body. The vascular system in two major lophotrochozoan phyla – the annelids and molluscs – are similar in the basic arrangement and may reflect a common origin. There is, therefore, the development of major organs that utilize a neural and vascular interface. For example, the major neurohaemal organs of the American cockroach are the retrocerebrocomplex and thoracic and abdominal perisympathetic organs. These organs are the major storage and release sites of neurosecretions produced in the central nervous system. In molluscs, the cephalopods (octopus and squid) possess the most complex nervous system (Fig. 4.9). In octopus (*Octopus vulgaris*), a peptide with a strong structural identity to the vertebrate GnRH was recently reported. Immunoreactive fibres were found in the subpedunculate lobe that controls the optic gland activity terminate on cells of the optic gland. The optic gland in

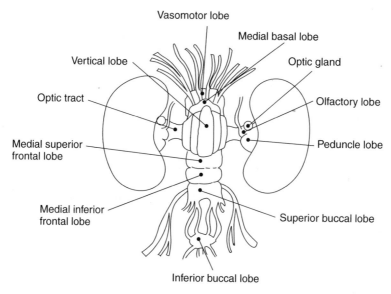

Vasomotor lobe

Medial basal lobe

Vertical lobe

Optic gland

Optic tract

Olfactory lobe

Medial superior frontal lobe

Peduncle lobe

Medial inferior frontal lobe

Superior buccal lobe

Inferior buccal lobe

Figure 4.9 *Generalized central nervous system of* Octopus vulgaris.

octopus is an endocrine gland that plays a role in the maturation of the gonads (Chapter 10). It remains to be determined, however, if the subpedunculate lobe and optic gland complex is homologous with that of the vertebrate hypothalamo–hypophysial complex.

Nervous and neuroendocrine systems in the deuterostomes

The first deuterostomes also evolved early in metazoan ancestry, likely well before the Precambrian explosion. A chordate-like fossil has been found among the assemblage of Burgess shale fossils suggesting that by the time of the Precambrian explosion, the deuterostome lineage was already well developed. *Xenoturbella bocki* is a marine deuterostome with a ciliated vermiform morphology that has been recently established to have a phylogenetic relationship to both the Echinodermata and Chordata. It possesses a nerve net structure that resembles aspects of the nerve net found in echinoderms and hemichordates, but it does not have a brain. It also lacks a through gut, defined gonadal organs, excretory structures or a coelomic cavity. It may, therefore, be similar to the most basal deuterostomes. In echinoderms, one of the closest deuterostome relatives, there is no central component such as a brain or a collection of central ganglia. Here, the nervous system is centrally organized and reflects the condition found in the Radiata. Although the radial morphology of the echinoderms is thought to be a derived condition from a bilateral ancestor, the echinoderm lineage has its origins shortly after the appearance of triploblastic organisms, and therefore may still reflect, in part, radiate patterning mechanisms.

Ancestral chordate nervous system

Current theories favour the idea that the basic body plan of chordates and non-chordates are similar in that the dorsal nerve cord of chordates is homologous to the ventral nerve cords of most invertebrates (Fig. 4.10). An ancestor of the chordates underwent a dorsal–ventral inversion in the body plans to change the ventral nerve cord to a dorsal orientation. In hemichordates (e.g. acorn worms), no notochord or dorsal hollow nerve cord has been identified. A nerve net is present in the epidermis that contains sensory neurons, interneurons and some motor neurons. A nerve net is thickened to form a dorsal solid nerve cord in the proboscis and both dorsal and ventral nerve cords in the trunk. A neurocord that does have a central lumen is formed by invaginated nervous tissue in the intermediately located collar region and connects the dorsal nerve cord of the proboscis and trunk. The neurocord contains motor neurons and interneurons and it may be homologous with the dorsal hollow nerve cord of other chordates.

Among the urochordates, tunicate larvae have a comparatively well-developed nervous system. A cerebral vesicle present in the rostral part of the organism has a gravity-sensitive

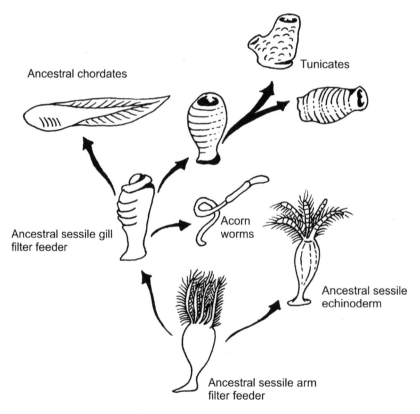

Figure 4.10 *Protochordates.*

organ called a statocyst and possesses a simple photoreceptive organ called an ocellus. The cerebral vesicle is continuous with a neural tube that extends through to the tail of the larvae and lies dorsal to the notochord. These organ systems act together to guide the larvae towards gravity and away from light in order to find a place to attach and begin metamorphosis to the adult form.

In adults of the cephalochordate, Branchiostoma (*Amphioxus*), a dorsal hollow nerve cord is present dorsal to the notochord and is divided into a dorsolateral sensory zone and a ventral motor zone. Ocelli formed by a ganglion cell and one pigmented cell are distributed along the dorsal nerve cord. At the rostral end of the nerve cord is a cerebral ventricle. A cluster of photosensitive cells lies at the rostral end of the cerebral vesicle.

Evolution of the chordate brain

The ancestral vertebrates were soft-bodied deuterostomes that left virtually no fossil record. The most primitive vertebrates would have had a notochord that was derived from the roof of the primitive gut. The nerve cord running dorsal to the notochord was expanded at the rostral end. Sensory receptive structures for senses including terminal and/or olfactory, visual pineal parapineal photoreceptive, taste octaval and lateral line were present in some of the early vertebrates but likely evolved at separate and distinct times. The earliest chordate ancestor likely would have had the four basic division of the central nervous system: forebrain, midbrain, hindbrain and spinal cord (Fig. 4.11). The telencephalic component of the forebrain was likely rudimentary and may not have been present at all. The forebrain function was likely more homologous to that of the basic function of the diencephalon. The diencephalon may have had a retinal apparatus, infundibulum and a simple photoreceptive pineal–parapineal complex. The rostral extent of the ventral motor neurons would have marked the rostral border of the midbrain.

There are two basic features that characterize the organization of the nervous system of chordates. The first includes the regional control of cell proliferation in the radial dimension. For example, in some non-chordate invertebrates the nervous system is diffusely distributed over the body as a series of ganglia or an interconnected nerve net. However, in most chordates, on the other hand, there is a differential regional expansion of a particular radial sector of the nervous system. After induction by the root of the primitive gut, the dorsal part of the nerve net in invertebrate chordates thickens to form the dorsal nerve cord as it does the neural plate in vertebrate chordates. A second feature of the chordate nervous system involves the regional control of cell proliferation in the rostro-caudal dimension. Rostral expansion of the dorsal nervous system leads to the development of the brain. Founder cell populations of neurons are established in the neural plate lying dorsal to the archenterons roof that will each give rise to a specific part of the nervous system. Further regional development and differentiation is controlled by homeobox genes in chordates and non-chordate invertebrates. The neuromeric organization of the brain is a manifestation of the homeobox gene specificity of regional development.

(a)

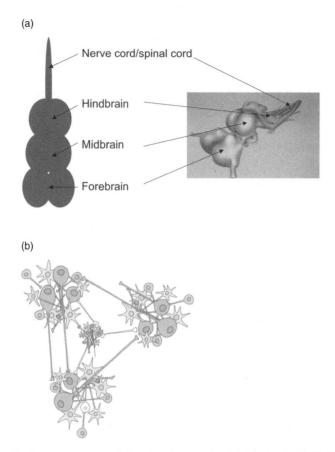

(b)

Figure 4.11 *Basic arrangement of the chordate brain. (a) The brain is divided into three main regions that can be found in all chordates. The brain is bilateral consisting of both left and right halves. One side is basically a mirror image of the other. This means also that the neuroendocrine cells are similarly divided. (b) Cell groups are generally organized in clusters or nuclei. There are extensive connections among the cells within the nucleus. In addition there are a number of projections to other nuclei.*

The greatest majority of synapses are made between nearby neurons 1–2 mm away. In fact, as much as 90% of the synaptic connections are likely local. If connections were made without regard to how close they are, the extra wiring would crowd the skull leaving no room for the neurons. As a result, the brain is left as a series of functional nuclei or neuronal centres. There are a number of levels of organization to the brain. Cortical structures are homogenous, highly repetitive throughout the cortex and exist in a layered pattern. Nuclear structures consist of a few hundred to several million cells. Nuclei of cells are a clusters of cells and the nuclei itself can occur in clusters. The hypothalamus is one such cluster of nuclei and exists both in layers and as a series of nuclei.

Peripheral and autonomic nervous systems

From the appearance of the nerve nets in the early metazoans, neurosecretory cells were interspersed among the non-nervous cells of the periphery. By the time the triploblastic and segmented animals evolved, this peripheral nervous system along with neurosecretory nodes became associated with ganglia in each segment as exemplified by the general lophotrochozoan and ecdyzoan nervous systems. Thus, this peripheral neurosecretory component developed into a significant component of the neuroendocrine system. As previously discussed, members of the Acoelomorpha, one of the most primitive triploblastic metazoans, do not possess a stomatogastric nervous system, although this system is present among other lophotrochozoan and ecdyzoan species. This may suggest that digestion in the earliest metazoans came under nervous control at a later point in evolution. The autonomic nervous system of vertebrates has been the best studied, although investigations suggest that the stomatogastric nervous system of invertebrates may be analogous to the vertebrate system.

In vertebrates, the autonomic nervous system is divided into two branches, the sympathetic nervous system and the parasympathetic nervous system (Fig. 4.12). The sympathetic

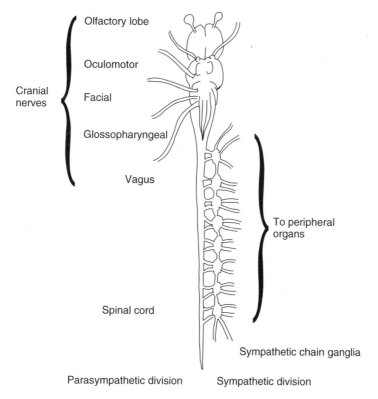

Figure 4.12   *Divisions of the autonomic nervous system in vertebrates.*

nervous system is involved in the expenditure of energy and responses to threat and homeostatic challenges whereas the parasympathetic nervous system conserves and stores energy and is associated with digestion and growth. Preganglionic sympathetic neurons synapse onto post-ganglionic neurons that innervate the target organs. Preganglionic neurons use acetylcholine as their neurotransmitter, which subsequently act upon nicotinic receptors on the post-ganglionic neurons. The post-ganglionic neurons use norepinephrine as their neurotransmitter that activate α- or β-adrenergic receptors on the target organs. Activation of the sympathetic nervous system activates papillary constriction, inhibits saliva, dilates lung bronchii in terrestrial vertebrates, accelerates heart rate, constricts cutaneous blood vessels, inhibits digestion and stimulates the conversion of glycogen to glucose. Most parasympathetic neurons are located in the brainstem and travel along the vagus nerve. Some are located in the sacral spinal cord and are associated with the control of eliminative and sexual functions. The parasympathetic ganglia are distal from the spinal cord and are located close to their target organs. The parasympathetic pre-ganglionic fibres utilize acetylcholine and act on nicotinic receptors at the post-ganglionic junctions similar to the sympathetic nervous system. However, the post-ganglionic parasympathetic neurons also use acetylcholine but bind to muscarinic receptors on their target organs.

Blood–brain barriers

Although endocrine, and peripheral paracrine feedback to elements of the simple nervous system in primitive metazoans provide the necessary regulation of the nervous system, a brain with vastly developed integrative regions must be protected from non-specific endocrine signals. This is particularly true in organisms possessing a high metabolic rate and efficient circulatory system. In animals with complex nervous systems, a number of additional neuroendocrine interfaces have developed, and more importantly much of the brain has become protected by non-specific, blood-borne chemical signals and hormones.

The brain is protected in part from noxious elements in the blood stream by a barrier that restricts the diffusion of many types of molecules from the blood into the brain (Fig. 4.13). A blood–brain barrier is found throughout the deuterostome and protostome species. The blood–brain barrier ensures the integrity of the neuronal cells by protecting and partitioning neuronal function from non-neuronal function. Without the blood–brain barrier, paralysis and death occurs. This barrier is not a single structure but a multiple structure located at several sites within the brain. The blood–brain barrier is formed by the capillary endothelium. The brain capillaries are comprised of flattened endothelial cells surrounded by a basement membrane and a thin adventitial layer. The endothelial cells of the capillary have tight junctions between the cells eliminating most spaces between cells. The basement membrane surrounding the endothelial cells has most of its surface covered with glial cells. Cerebral blood vessels are lacking significant fenestrations or pores or a vesicular transport system.

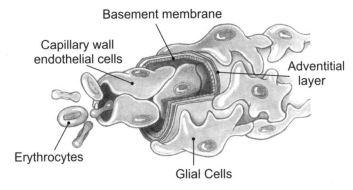

Figure 4.13 *Basic components of the vertebrate blood–brain barrier.*

Transport of hormones across the blood–brain barrier

The limited movement of molecules across the blood–brain barrier may involve passive diffusion or active transport. Water, for example, moves readily across the blood–brain barrier by diffusion. Many lipophilic molecules such as steroids, eicosanoids and some fatty acids, as well as some drugs such as barbiturates and alcohol move across the barrier in relation to their lipophilicity. D-Glucose is readily transported across the barrier by a specific transporter protein that does not recognize L-glucose. The endothelial cells of the blood-brain barrier are metabolically active and can metabolize a number of molecules including biogenic amines present in the blood. For example, dopamine does not readily cross the blood–brain barrier; however, its precursor, L-DOPA, if present in the blood stream, enters the endothelial cells where it is converted to dopamine and subsequently passed into the brain. A number of large neutral amino acids required for the synthesis of neurotransmitters and proteins are transported into the brain by specific carrier proteins. Active transport systems exist in the brain to transport extracellular K^+, salts and weak organic acids from the brain into the plasma. A number of recent studies have suggested that there exist several types of molecular scavenging systems in the blood–brain barrier that act to protect the brain against xenobiotics and other noxious or bioactive compounds. These mechanisms appear to be present in cartilaginous and ray-finned fishes suggesting a highly conserved mechanism.

Although the blood–brain barrier functions, in part, to protect the brain from noxious xenobiotic compounds, it also restricts the entry of many of the endogenous hormones and molecules from entering the brain. Many of the signalling molecules used outside the brain are the same as those used as neuromodulators or neurotransmitters inside the brain. Therefore, it is necessary for the brain to partition these two pools of messengers. However, it is also necessary for the neural circuits of the brain to be receptive to those signalling molecules that are acting as feedback systems to neurologically or neuroendocrinologically controlled physiological circuits, for example. Most of these signalling molecules are peptides of which many appear to gain entry to the brain. Although it has been argued that these peptides could gain entry via the circumventricular organs (p. 104), the majority appear to cross the blood–brain barrier directly. The surface area of the circumventricular organs in mammals is less than 0.02% of that of the blood–brain barrier surface area. Some studies indicate that less than 5% of the total neural uptake of some peptides occurs through the circumventricular organs. Thus, many regions of the blood–brain area appear to allow both the passive diffusion and active uptake of peptides into the brain. Peptides such as met-enkephalin, interleukin-1a, neuropeptide-Y and melanocyte-concentrating hormone (MCH) appear to gain entry into the brain via a saturable transporter mechanism. Corticotrophin-releasing factor (CRF), on the other hand, appears not to have a carrier protein into the brain but has a saturable transporter to allow passage out of the brain. Peptides of the calcitonin family, amylin, adrenomedullin, calcitonin-gene-related peptide and calcitonin may gain entry via specific receptors in circumventricular organs.

Recent evidence suggests that other factors may be involved in the movement of molecules across the blood–brain barrier. The organic anion transporting polypeptides (OATPs) are a large gene family that mediate the transport of a wide variety of amphipathic organic solutes. They can have substrate preferences for bile salts, steroid conjugates, thyroid hormones, anionic oligopeptides, drugs, toxins and other xenobiotics. Some of these OATPs are preferentially or selectively expressed in a particular tissue such as the liver, but others may be expressed throughout the blood–brain barrier, choroid plexus and other organs.

Invertebrate blood–brain barriers

Blood–brain barriers are found in representative species of both the Ecdysozoa and the Lophotrochozoa. There is no evidence of blood–brain barriers in the most basal metazoans and so the blood–brain barriers of each of the three main lineages of bilateral organism may have evolved independently as the need arose. The blood–brain barrier of arthropods is derived from an accessible polarized glial layer. The glial perineurium forms the blood–brain interface in crayfish whereas the perineurium of the peripheral nervous system is relatively permeable. In insects, the blood–brain barrier is made up of occlusive (pleated sheet) septate and tight junctions between perineurial cells, glia and perineurial cells and possibly also between glia. In immature dipterans, septate junctions are present, but without the tight junctions, whereas both junctional types are found in the imago stage. A blood–eye barrier also arises early in pupal life. Neurexin IV has been identified as a molecular component of the *Drosophila* septate junctions and is also essential for the axonal insulation in the peripheral nervous system in embryos and larvae. The vertebrate gene homologue of neurexin IV is *caspr* or *paranodin* and is also localized in septate-like junctional structures. They are located in the paranodal region of the nodes of Ranvier, between axons and Schwann cells. In the cuttlefish, *Sepia*, the blood–brain barrier is achieved by a number of mechanisms. About 90% of the brain microvessel wall of *Sepia* is covered by a glial sheath without intercellular clefts thus limiting the number of potential leakages. *Sepia* possesses a novel junctional type different from other vertebrate and invertebrates occluding junctions. This junction may act as a fine mesh molecular filter. This unusual structure appears not to be a classical tight junction, but may involve the condensation of extracellular materials that creates a molecular sieve. Despite the unique morphology, the *Sepia* blood–brain barrier appears to be as tight as the endothelial barrier of mammals.

Cerebrospinal fluid and the choroid plexus

In vertebrates, cerebrospinal fluid (CSF) is a clear, colourless, acellular fluid that surrounds the brain and fills the ventricles. It contains a small amount of protein, glucose and K^+, but a large amount of NaCl. There are no substances in the CSF that are not found in the blood plasma. The CSF resembles an ultrafiltrate of the plasma, although the amounts of dissolved substances in the CSF are not always proportional to each other relative to that found in plasma. CSF is present in *Amphioxus*, a cephalochordate, but it is not known if it is present in the urochordates. A homologue of CSF in ecdysozoans or lophotrochozoans appears not to exist. Once CSF did evolve in chordates, its composition has changed little throughout the various classes. The CSF plays a significant role in the neuroendocrine interface between the brain and blood. Neurohormones may be secreted directly into the CSF where they can be taken up by specialized cells (tanycytes) in the ventricles and transported to other regions of the brain. There is no diffusion barrier between the brain and CSF, thus material in the CSF can gain entry into neural tissues by both passive and active uptake mechanisms. There is, however, a barrier between the blood and the CSF, composed of tight junctions of the cells. The movement of substances from the blood into the CSF resembles that from the blood to the brain. However, the surface of the blood–CSF barrier is a tiny fraction of the surface area of the blood–brain barrier. Despite this small interface, there is evidence that some peptide hormones can gain entry into the brain by passing across the blood–CSF barrier. The CSF also removes the waste products of metabolism, xenobiotics and secreted hormones and neurotransmitters from the brain via an interface with venous blood. The CSF appears to have evolved as a means to maintain the chemical and hormonal environment of the brain however in terrestrial vertebrates, the CSF has a secondary function as a protective cushion against cranial injury.

The CSF is produced primarily by the choroid plexus, a convoluted layer of epithelial cells with villi on their apical surfaces. The choroid plexus is found along the CSF-contacting surfaces of the ventricles. *Amphioxus* and hagfish do not appear to possess a choroid plexus, although they do have specialized regions of the brain that produce the CSF. Material in the CSF can be taken up by pinocytotic mechanisms, active transporters and internalization of ligand-bound receptors. The cells of the choroid plexus, which do not have a blood–brain barrier, play a particularly important role in the uptake of insulin-like and growth-factor–like hormones. This will be discussed in later chapters. The size of the choroid plexus does not corroborate with brain size, and is particularly large in both basal actinopterygians and basal sarcopterygians.

Neurohaemal and circumventricular organs: Neurovascular interfaces

There are a number of regions of the brain where the blood–brain barrier is incomplete or non-existent. In these regions, the capillaries may be fenestrated allowing relatively unrestricted movement of larger and more hydrophilic molecules out of the capillaries. Regions of the brain without a blood–brain barrier include the median eminence, neuro-hypophysis, organum vasculosum of the lateral terminalis, pineal body and subfornical organ (Fig. 4.14). These structures are situated around the third ventricle and hypothalamus and are referred to as circumventricular organs. The area postrema, present in the brainstem also lacks a blood–brain barrier. These regions play a role both in the active uptake of larger proteins and hormones from the blood, and also the release of brain proteins, peptides and other molecules into the blood. The median eminence, neurohypophysis, and the organum vasculosum of the lateral terminalis appear to play a role mostly in the release of neural signalling molecules into the periphery. Thus the circumventricular organs play a critical role as informational interfaces between the blood, neurons and the CSF.

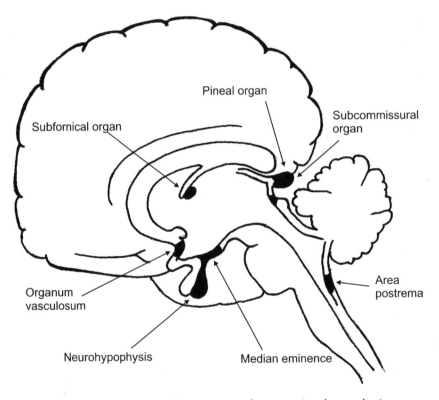

Figure 4.14 *Position of circumventricular organs in a human brain.*

The number of circumventricular organs varies considerably among vertebrates. Anamniotes typically have four or five, reptiles and mammals have six, and birds have nine. All vertebrates possess a pineal complex and subcommissural organ. Both are implicated in biological rhythms (Chapter 8). A pineal complex appears to be present throughout the vertebrates with the possible exception of the crocodilian, caiman. A pineal complex does not occur in hagfish, suggesting that it may have arisen after the bifurcation of the Myxini from the vertebrates, but before that of the origin of the lampreys. The subcommissural organ may be the brain's phylogenetically oldest gland and perhaps the earliest gland to differentiate in ontogeny. The subcommissural organ secretes a glycoprotein that aggregates to form Reissner's Fibre. This structure grows and extends along the cerebral aqueduct, IV ventricle and central canal. The glycoproteins move caudally along the fibre binding epinephrine, norepinephrine and possibly dopamine eventually transporting them to the central canal of the spinal cord where they enter the systemic blood. Thus the subcommissural organ/Reissner's Fibre complex appears to play a role in the clearance of monoamines from the CSF as a bound protein–ligand complex.

The subfornical organ and the area postrema appear to be the phylogenetically youngest organs. The subfornical organ is found in the lungfish (*Lepidosiren*). The subfornical organ in mammals, which is called the subseptal organ in birds and turtles, is associated with water balance and blood pressure. However, the development of the subfornical organ is highly variable among amphibians. The area postrema is also widespread among the vertebrates and has been implicated in food aversion and blood pressure. This organ is found in both cartilaginous fish (Chondrichthyes) and also in the phylogenetically older ray-finned fishes, the brachiopterygians (*Polypterus* and *Erpetoichthyes*).

A number of additional circumventricular organs are present in the vertebrates. The paraventricular organ is present in all vertebrate classes except mammals and appears to play a role in blood pressure and volume. The paraventricular organ is not differentiated in the lungfish and the caecilian (*Typhlonectes*). Birds uniquely possess a lateral septal organ that secretes vasoactive intestinal peptide (VIP) and also the subtrochlear organ of which the function is not understood. A saccus vasculosus is found throughout the Chondrichthyes and in the freshwater ray (*Potamotrygon*) but not in the primitive freshwater teleost, *Osteoglossum*. The OVLT of the dogfish (*Etmopterus*) contains neurosecretory fibre terminals and is considered the neurohaemal organ in this group. The paraphysis is found in the dogfish (*Mustelus*) and the Osteoglossiformes (*Osteoglossum* and *Gnathonemus*).

Caudal neurosecretory system (CNSS)

In fishes, a caudal neurohaemal organ, the urophysis, is also present outside the blood–brain barrier (Fig. 4.15). This structure, present in the terminal segments of the spinal cord, is responsible for the release of the peptide hormones, urotensin-I and urotensin-II, into the blood stream. The structure appears to be lost in the tetrapod lineage sometime after the divergence of the lungfishes (dipnoi) but before the amphibia.

A caudal secretory system analogous to the neurohypophysis appears to have evolved early in vertebrate evolution. It is unclear whether this system existed in taxa phylogenetically older than the petramyzontiformes (lamprey) as two of the principal hormones secreted from the CNSS, urotensin-I and urotensin-II, has not been found in the hagfish, *Eptatretus*

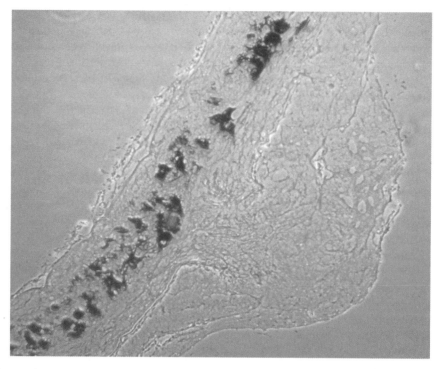

Figure 4.15 *Immunoreactive urotensin-I neurons in the urophysis of a rainbow trout. Photomicrograph courtesy of Dr. Nicholas Bernier, University of Guelph.*

stouti. Clusters of neurosecretory cells immunoreactive for urotensin-I or urotensin-II have been found in the caudal segment of the lamprey, *Petramyzon marinus*, the holocephalan, *Hydrolagus colliei*, the elasmobranchs, *Squalus acanthias* and *Dasyatis sabina*, the skate *Raja binoculata*, *Heterodontus japonicus* and *Cephaloscyllium umbratile*. Coincidental with the bifurcation of the sarcopterygians and actinopterygians, CNSS development follows two distinct anatomical arrangements. In the actinopterygian lineage leading to higher bony fish, the CNSS has been extensively elaborated and plays a significant role in the regulation of interrenal cortisol release, ion and fluid homeostasis. Among the sarcopterygians, the CNSS is eventually lost, although in the lungfish, *Protopturus annectens*, immunoreactive urotensin-I/CRF in the terminal segments of the spinal cord has been reported. A fundamental change in the urotensin-I system apparently occurred afterwards as a CNSS has not been found in amniotes. The phylogenetic loss of the CNSS coincides with the evolution of the terrestrial vertebrates.

Hypothalamus–pituitary gland complex

As discussed in Chapter 1, the discipline of neuroendocrinology began with the understanding of the neural regulation of the pituitary gland and has provided the model upon which to understand general neuroendocrine principles. Among the vertebrates, niche adaption appears to have played a role in the relationship of pituitary morphology and its hypothalamic regulation. Thus, a comparison of the structure and function of the pituitary gland is essential to the understanding of the neuroendocrine responses to physiological stimuli by the different classes of vertebrates. The pituitary gland contains a number of physio-trophic hormones (Table 4.1) that act to regulate, virtually, all physiological responses in the body. These will be discussed in detail in the upcoming chapters. For much of the discussion in this book the hypothalamus will receive the most attention. The hypothalamus has receptors for temperature, glucose, salt and virtually all hormones. It has been said that virtually any signalling molecule found in the brain can also be found in the hypotha-lamus. This neural crossroads is necessary to perceive everything that is happening in the body. The hypothalamus receives input in the form of synaptic input from the rest of the nervous system, hormonal and neural hormone input and a number of physiological con-ditions indicated by ions metabolites and temperature.

The functional cell clusters of the hypothalamus that we recognize as being essential for the regulation of pituitary hormones vary as a function of topological changes in the chordate brain. However, for virtually all chordates, all the essential releasing factors appear to have been conserved, although data is lacking for the hagfish. Homology between hypothalamic nuclei from one species to another is often not known until the presence of a particular releasing factor is found.

Ontologically, the cells expressing the releasing factors tend to develop just before the pituitary hormones do. This has been particularly well studied in mammals. The parvocellular neuroendocrine cells of the hypothalamus are all generated simultaneously from the proliferative neuroepithelium surrounding the third ventricle. Both neuroendocrine and non-neuroendocrine cells are formed about the same time. In rats, at e11 all neuroendocrine cells are located centrally. By e12 neurons in the rostral and dorsal parts of the periven-tricular zone appear, then by e14, the caudal cells begin to appear. The CRF cells of the paraventricular nucleus (PVN) appear between e11 and e16, whereas the neurosecretory CRF cells appear around e12–e14. The growth hormone releasing hormone (GHRH) cells of the arcuate nucleus appear around e11–e15 and the neurosecretory cells follow about a day later. Somatostatin cells develop around the same time. TSH-releasing hormone (TRH) cells appear around e11 and may continue until e15 whereas the formation of the neurosecretory TRH cells are in place between these times. The dopaminergic cells

Table 4.1 *Hormones secreted by the adenohypophysis*

Cell type	Hormone secreted
Gonadotrophs	Luteinizing hormone (LH)
	Follicle-stimulating hormone (FSH)
Lactotrophs	Prolactin
Mammolactotrophs	Prolactin, growth hormone
Somatotrophs	Growth hormone
Somatolactotrophs	Somatolactin
Thyrotrophs	Thyrotrophin (thyroid hormone-stimulating hormone, TSH)
Corticotrophs	Adrenocorticotropic hormone (ACTH), β-endorphin

develop between e11 and e17 although the neurosecretory component is usually in place by e15.

Pituitary gland development

Establishing a satisfactory ontological and phylogenetic pattern for pituitary gland development and evolution has been problematic. The ontogeny of the pituitary gland has generally been described as a fusion of neural and epithelial tissue. In this model, the neural component of the pituitary derives from a ventral extension of the diencephalon that differentiates into the tissues comprising the median eminence, infundibular stalk, and pars nervosa. This neural component fuses with epithelial tissue arising from an invagination of pharyngeal tissue in the roof the mouth. This pocket, termed 'Rathke's pouch', was observed originally by Rathke in the early 19th century. The epithelial component of the pituitary leads to the formation of the adenohypophysis, which typically includes the pars distalis, pars intermedia and pars tuberalis. The differentiation of these tissues follows distinct patterns in the different vertebrate lineages. In tetrapods, the pars nervosa differentiates into a distinct infundibular stem forming the neurohypophysial lobe, and expanded median eminence. Along the actinopterygian line, the median eminence becomes less pronounced concurrent with a simplification and eventual disappearance of the portal system.

However, it has been difficult to reconcile this model of development with the phylogenetic pattern of pituitary-like structures present in species evolving before the vertebrates. In the cephalochordate, *Amphioxus*, a structure termed 'Hatschek's pit' appears to have some similarities to Rathke's pouch. It is an evagination of the pharynx, however does not fuse with tissues of the central nervous system. Attempts to show the presence of pituitary-like hormones in this structure have been inconclusive with some researchers showing immunocytochemical evidence, whereas others have not. In the tunicate, *Ciona intestinalis*, a neural gland lying ventral to the brain and connected to the buccal cavity by a canal has thought to represent a homologue of the vertebrate pituitary gland. The neural gland is part of a complex that includes the neural gland, brain and dorsal strand (Fig. 4.16). A relationship with the pituitary gland has been strengthened by immunocytochemical evidence of prolactin-like and adrenocorticotropic hormone (ACTH)-like molecules in the dorsal strand. Within the cerebral gland both proopiomelanocortin (POMC) mRNA, and gonadotropin-releasing factor (GnRH) peptides have been isolated.

Recent studies incorporating molecular and developmental approaches have led to the postulation of a new model of pituitary development where the pituitary gland is neuro-ectodermal in origin. In *Xenopus*, cells transplanted from the anterior neural ridge differentiated into ACTH-expressing cells in the anterior pituitary. Additional studies in toads (*Bufo*) have indicated that only the anterior neural ridge appears to be solely responsible for the formation of the adenohypophysis. The pituitary cells appear to arise from the sensory layer of the anterior neural ridge. Tissue derived from the posterior regions, the anterior end of the neural plate appear to develop into the hypothalamus and infundibulum. During development, the anterior aspect of the neural ridge migrates ventrally under the forebrain and fuses with the infundibulum. Rathke's pouch may not be pharyngeal in origin but rather deriving from the neuroectoderm. In the developing chick, the ventral aspect of the neural ridge appears to be homologous with that of the amphibian anterior neural ridge.

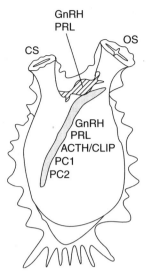

Figure 4.16 *Neural complex in a tunicate. A number of hypothalamic and pituitary hormones and processing enzymes have been found in the neural complex suggesting a relationship with the chordate hypothalamus–pituitary system. See text for further details. CS – cloacal siphon; OS – oral siphon. Reprinted from Kawamura et al. (2002) by the permission of Elsevier Science (USA).*

In mammals, cells of the rostro-medial end of the neural plate give rise to the hypothalamic tissue whereas cell groups anterior to this structure later form Rathke's pouch and cells of the adenohypophysis (Fig. 4.17).

As far as we know, the same basic cell types are present in the adenohypophysis (pars distalis) of all vertebrate species. However, studies of cartilaginous fish and the agnathan pituitary are relatively rare, and therefore some speculation exists. Assuming that the basic cell types are present some observations can be made. In the ancestral condition, the

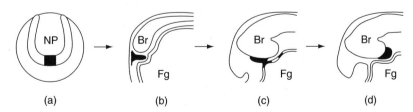

Figure 4.17 *Pituitary ontogeny. Migration of the adenohypophyseal primordium in a toad. The primordium begins at the anterior ridge of the neural plate (a), separates (b), then forms a transient structure (Rathke's pouch) with the foregut (buccal cavity) (c), before coming to its final position, juxtaposed with the neurohypophysis (d) NP – neural plate; Br – brain; Fg – foregut. Reprinted from Kawamura et al. (2002) by the permission of Elsevier Science (USA).*

various cell types of the pars distalis were mixed together. In vertebrates that have developed a portal system, the cell types tend to remain mixed. In species where direct neural connections have been made, the cell types become segregated.

In mammals, the expression of various pituitary hormones follow a particular spatio-temporal pattern and show their appearance after the formation of the neurons synthesizing the releasing factors in the hypothalamus. In rats, the mRNA for the α- glycoprotein subunit appears by embryonic day (e) 11 and is confined to the ventral part of the anterior wall of Rathke's pouch. The POMC and β-thyroxine-stimulating hormone (TSH) subunit messages appear by e14 followed by the β-luteinizing hormone (LH) and β-follicle-stimulating hormone (FSH) subunits in the ventral part of the anterior lobe around e16–e17. By e18, cells expressing growth hormone (GH) and prolactin (PRL) appear in the dorsocaudal aspect of the anterior lobe.

Evolution of the pituitary gland

For both the hagfishes and the lampreys there appears to be a complete separation of the pars distalis from the rest of the hypothalamus. Diffusion of the hypothalamic-releasing factors appears to be the main route of communication between the hypothalamus and pars distalis. However, a simple portal system may be present although this is unclear. In hagfishes, the pars nervosa is a relatively undifferentiated part of the hypothalamus where the axonal termini of neurosecretory cells impinge on a vascularized region at the hypothalamus wall. In lampreys, the pars nervosa becomes more differentiated into a discrete lobular structure. Hagfishes and lampreys may also utilize the systemic blood as a route for releasing factors to regulate the pars distalis. Ectopic transplantation of the hagfish pars distalis in other regions of the body, for example, does not appear to compromise the normal physiology of the these animals. The various cell types in the pars distalis are relatively intermingled.

The class Chondrichthyes or cartilaginous fish are the phylogenetically oldest group of gnathostomes or jawed vertebrates. The cartilaginous fish include the subclasses Elasmobranchii (sharks, skates and rays) and Holocephali (chimaeras). The cartilaginous fish evolved 50–100 million years after the lineage leading to the lampreys and about 400 million years before present. The elasmobranchs and holocephalans diverged early in chondrichthyan evolution, but still possess a number of related features. The elasmobranch pituitary consists of a fused pars nervosa and pars intermedia (Fig. 4.18). In this situation where there is considerable intermingling of pars nervosa and pars intermedia, it is referred to as a pars neurointermedia or neurointermediate lobe. There is a well-developed portal system that connects most of the pars distalis with the hypothalamus. The elasmobranch pars distalis consists of a second lobe ventral to the main body. This structure is called the ventral lobe and is connected to the rest of the pituitary by a thin stalk of tissue. The ventral lobe does not appear to have either a vascular or nervous connection to the rest of the brain. Releasing factors are secreted into the systemic blood to communicate with the ventral lobe. The structure of the pituitary in holocephalans is similar to that of the elasmobranchs (Fig. 4.19). The main difference lies in the structure of the ventral lobe. In holocephalans, the ventral lobe is called a buccal lobe and is found in the roof of the mouth. It is separated from the brain by a layer of cartilage. Like elasmobranchs, the hypothalamus appears to communicate with the buccal lobe by secreting releasing factors into the systemic blood.

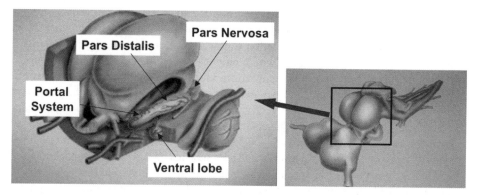

Figure 4.18 *Elasmobranch pituitary gland. Cutaway showing the elongated pars distalis and portal system. The ventral lobe containing the gonadotropins is separate from the rest of the pars distalis.*

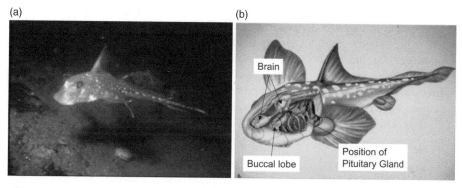

Figure 4.19 *Holocephalan pituitary. (a) Pacific ratfish,* Hydrolagus colliei; *(b) cutaway showing the position of the buccal lobe. Photograph (a) courtesy of Dr. Debra Murie, University of Florida.*

Although there are few studies to draw upon, the location of cells in the pituitary gland in the cartilaginous fish appears to have some organization. For example, the gonado-tropes are located primarily in the ventral lobe of elasmobranchs (or the buccal lobe of holocephalans). Although there is some interdigitation of the pars nervosa with aspects of the pars distalis, there is currently no evidence that there is any direct neural link between the hypothalamus and pars distalis. However, given the organization of the neurosecretory cells of the hypothalamus and the presence of interdigitation in cartilaginous fish, there is the distinct potential that some form of rudimentary neural connection may exist. If so, one might also expect that some of the basic pituitary cell types are organized to a limited degree in clusters of related cells.

Around 350 million years ago, vertebrate evolution followed two main pathways. One group of fishes exploited a niche associated with the substrates on the ocean bottoms whereas another group exploited a pelagic niche. The bottom-dwelling group were selected for robust and limb-like fins and developed into the lobe-finned fishes (Sarcopterygii) and ultimately to land animals. The pelagic adapted lineage developed into the ray-finned fishes (Actinopterygii). Pituitary evolution followed separate morphological patterns in each group. Jawed vertebrates began with a pituitary structure similar to chondrichthyan fishes where there was a portal system and a more or less distinct pars distalis and pars nervosa. In the lobe-finned fishes and tetrapods, the portal system became more developed, whereas in the ray-finned fishes the portal system was lost and a direct neural connection developed (Fig. 4.20). The coelacanths appear to be the only extant members of this phylogenetically old group of lobe-finned fishes. The pituitary structure is most similar to the elasmobranchs; however, the ventral lobe resembles the holocephalan buccal lobe in many respects. These species have a functional portal system that connects the hypothalamus with the pars distalis. The pars nervosa and pars intermedia are probably structured in a similar manner as that in the elasmobranchs.

Recent evidence suggests that the Dipnoi (lungfish) and amphibians shared a direct common ancestor. The pituitary gland has a combined pars neurointermedia and pars distalis arrangement, a functional portal system but no ventral lobe of the pars distalis. The overall structure of the lungfish pituitary is more similar to tetrapods than other fishes.

The evolutionary pressure that led to the evolution of the amphibians and eventually the tetrapods is not well understood, although there are some theories. Based on fossil evidence, the earliest amphibians appear to have evolved around before the Devonian period, over 400 million years ago. At this time the continental land masses were coming together creating vast areas of shallow seas. This was also a time of immense radiation of the fishes and therefore, the number of predators. Thus, some theories suggest that some of the slower-moving bottom-dwelling fishes tended to exploit niches along calmer

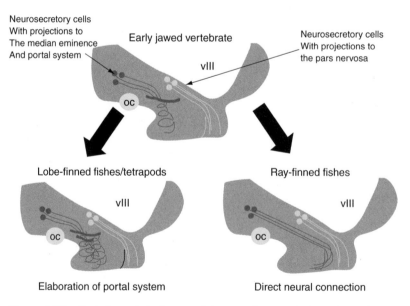

Figure 4.20 *Evolution of pituitary and the portal system in jawed vertebrates.*

waters along the shoreline to escape the pelagic predators and to utilize other food sources where there was less competition. Eventually, they evolved the ability to leave the water and eventually hunt on land to exploit those food sources. Today, teleost fishes such as mudskippers, climbing perch and walking catfish have all developed the ability to leave the water and spend time on land. Endocrine changes in these organisms would have been associated with osmoregulation and metabolism. This may explain, in part, changes that occurred in the morphology of the pars nervosa in tetrapods.

The amphibia consist of three distinct subclasses: Urodela (salamanders and newts), Anura (frogs and toads) and Gymnophiona (caecilians). Both the Anura and Gymnophiona appear to be derived from a urodele-like ancestor but all three lineages have been separate for at least 250 million years. A much greater elaboration of the portal system occurs in the amphibian groups. A distinct lobular pars nervosa becomes apparent in the amphibia with less intrusion into the pars intermedia. Amphibians may possess an additional pituitary-related structure with a similar origin as the pars tuberalis. This structure possesses TSH-positive cells and is found in the caudal region of the pars distalis.

The earliest amniote tetrapods evolved about 30 million years after the evolution of the first amphibians. This group includes the mammals, reptiles and birds, and refers to the amniotic egg present in all groups. The early amniotes began to radiate extensively in the Carboniferous and early Permian times, displacing the non-amniotes (early amphibians) from those habitats and niches. Evidence suggested that virtually all of the early amniotes were carnivorous. The extensive radiation of insects at this time is thought to have been a food source that was exploited by the early amniotes thus acting to stimulate this radiation of species. Moreover, higher levels of atmospheric oxygen, postulated to exist at that time by some geophysiologists, may have facilitated the adaption of vertebrates onto land. Physiological changes that accompanied this adaption included changes in respiratory mechanisms, diuresis and excretion, reproduction and integration of sensory systems.

There are four subclasses of reptiles: Chelonia (tortoises, turtles and terrapins), Rhynchocephalia (tuataras), Crocodilia (alligators, crocodiles, caimans and gharials) and Squamata (lizards and snakes). The general arrangement of the reptilian pituitary is more or less similar in most of the groups. Differences are most apparent within the pars nervosa morphology. The phylogenetically older reptile groups such as the chelonians (turtles) and rhynchocephalians (tuataras) tend to have a pars nervosa with some interdigitation of the pars intermedia. In all reptiles there is an expanded portal system and generally a mix of pituitary cell types instead of clusters of similar cells.

The reptiles, dinosaurs and birds form a clade of related species, and thus all groups share a set of common pituitary morphologies. Birds underwent a great radiation in relatively recent times once the ability of flight was established. The evolution of the birds is not as well understood as some phylogenetically older groups and consequently there is no consensus on their phylogeny. To date, the pituitary glands of well over 100 species of birds have been examined. A pars intermedia has not been found in birds although the hormone melanocyte-stimulating hormone (MSH) is present in the domestic chicken. It is not clear if the lack of pars intermedia is a derived characteristic for birds as only a relatively few species have been examined. However, the lack of a pars intermedia is not unique as some mammals such as whales and elephants also do not possess a pars intermedia. In birds and some reptiles like the caiman, the median eminence is divided into anterior and posterior parts. Within mammals, there is extensive development of the pars nervosa but a considerable regression of the pars intermedia. In addition there is considerable elaboration of the portal system (Fig. 4.21).

The net effect of the evolution of the pituitary gland in the sarcopterygians and tetrapods was the development of an elaborate portal system; by contrast, the portal system was lost completely in the actinopterygians. The Chondrostei, the group that includes sturgeons and paddlefish, is the phylogenetically oldest group of ray-finned fishes and bears a number of structural similarities to the elasmobranchs. The pituitary gland structure is also similar in that they possess a portal system and a neurointermediate lobe but do not possess a ventral or buccal lobe however. The brachiopterygians (bichirs and redfish) have a pituitary structure that is largely similar to that of the sturgeons. The bowfin and gar are the remaining extant species of a once large assemblage of fishes, collectively referred to as holosteans. These species represent the phylogenetically youngest group of non-teleost fish. There is greater interdigitation of the pars nervosa with the pars intermedia and pars distalis. There is also a reduced portal system, and some direct neural connection between the hypothalamic neurosecretory cells and the pars distalis. The Teleostei are a vast assemblage of fish that include about 25 000 species. The pituitary gland is unusual in that cells of the pars distalis are clustered in nuclei of similar cells. There is extensive interdigitation of the neural lobe with the rest of the pituitary, and direct neural connection between the hypothalamus and pars distalis (Fig. 4.22). The teleost pituitary gland morphology represents the most-advanced structural features among the fishes. Two major changes have occurred: neurosecretory cells of the hypothalamus send their axons through the extensive interdigitations of the pars nervosa with the pars intermedia and

(a)   (b)

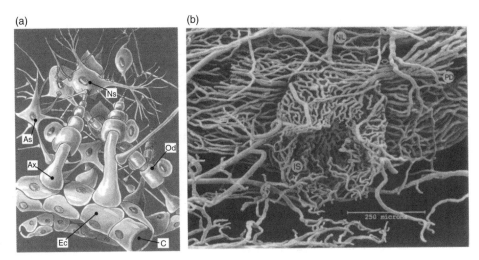

Figure 4.21 *Median eminence and vascular portal system. (a) Representation of the cell types associated with the release of neurosecretory factors into the pituitary portal system. Ns – neurosecretory cell; As – astrocyte; Ax – axon; Od – oligodendrocyte; Ec – endothelial cell; C – capillary; (b) a cast of the blood vessels from the little brown bat showing the plexus of vessels. IS – infundibular stem; NL – neural lobe; PD – pars distalis, reprinted from Anthony et al. (1998) by the permission of Elsevier Inc.*

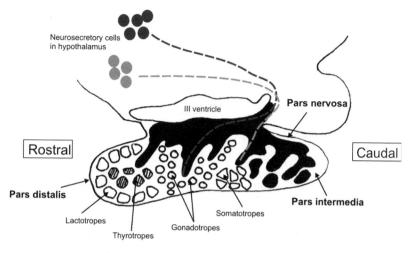

Figure 4.22 *Generalized teleost pituitary.*

pars distalis. Within the pars distalis cells have become grouped into discrete clusters. Thus, in this manner the releasing factor can stimulate the appropriate pituitary cell. However, it is important to note that the pituitary structure of phylogenetically oldest lineages of teleosts may resemble non-teleosts. For example, osteoglossomorphous fishes (*Osteoglossum* and *Gnathonemus*) possess a distinct median eminence.

Chapter summary

The nervous system acts to transduce environmental information into a chemical signal readily understandable by the non-nervous cells of an organism. A functional nervous system requires feedback input from the cells, tissues and organs of the animal in order to coordinate sensory information from the environment with the metabolic requirements of the organism. Thus a neuroendocrine interface between the nervous system and non-nervous cells must have developed at the earliest stages of the central nervous system evolution. The Precambrian explosion was characterized by the appearance of numerous grazing and predatory organisms with well-developed nervous and vascular systems, and elaborate feeding and locomotory structures. Genomic expansion events created the necessary genetic complexity for organisms to massively expand and invade new niches around this time. Coincident with this expansion, and the appearance of predators of grazers, and predators of predators, was the selection pressure for more elaborate nervous and neuroendocrine systems. The development of segmentation allowed for division of labour and specialization of the peripheral nervous system from the central nervous system and the specialization of the nervous system in each functional segment. Ventral nerve chords, that characterize the nervous systems of the Ecdysozoa and Lophotrochozoa, became a dorsal nerve cord in the chordates due to a dorsal ventral inversion. Another set of genome expansion events in a protochordate lineage led to further development of sensory systems and the brain. The most-developed species from a nervous and neuro-endocrine point of view in the Ecdysozoa, Lophotrochozoa and Deuterostomia have a major brain-neuroendocrine gland interface, and a blood–brain barrier that protects most of the nervous system from circulating chemicals.

Neuroendocrinology of Dopamine
Wendi Neckameyer

As with many other signalling molecules, dopamine has been adapted to serve in diverse physiological pathways. Dopamine is derived by the hydroxylation of the amino acid tyrosine via the actions of the rate-limiting enzyme, tyrosine hydroxylase (TH). Dopamine biosynthesis is highly conserved across species: the *Drosophila* homologue of TH, DTH, shares over 50% identity with its mammalian counter-parts; like mammalian TH, DTH requires O_2 and a biopterin cofactor, BH_4, for full enzymatic activity. Biochemical regulation of DTH is strikingly similar to that observed in mammals. The pathway for biopterin synthesis is conserved, as is the second enzyme in DA biosynthesis, dopa decarboxylase (TH hydroxylates tyrosine to form L-DOPA, which is rapidly converted by Ddc to form DA).

Perturbations in dopaminergic systems are partly responsible for Parkinson's disease and have been implicated in the etiology of schizophrenia, Alzheimer's disease, Huntington's disease, and some depressive disorders. Numerous pharmacological studies have implicated dopamine in synaptic modulation and behavioural plasticity. Dopamine also acts as a neurotransmitter in evolutionarily diverse organisms: in *Drosophila*, as well as in mammals, dopamine plays a role in learning acquisition and female sexual receptivity. It also modulates the effects of cocaine, nicotine and ethanol treatments in *Drosophila*, demonstrating the extent of the conservation for the role of DA in addiction and reward behaviour. Dopamine may act as a toxin, by forming radical oxygen and other radical species; it has been suggested that the actions of these highly reactive catechols may contribute to neurodegeneration. It is therefore not surprising that dopamine has been shown to be a marker for neuronal senescence in *Drosophila*, since dopamine levels decrease with increasing age, and deficits in dopaminergic-modulated behaviours are observed in ageing flies. Mutational analyses in *Drosophila melanogaster* have implicated the biogenic amines in determining longevity.

In addition to its fundamental role as a transmitter in nervous tissue, dopamine is vitally required during development. In mice, disruption of the rate-limiting biosynthetic enzyme, tyrosine hydroxylase, results in lethality; animals die during late gestation or immediately after birth. Dopamine and related catecholamines are involved in planula metamorphosis suggesting a role in growth regulatory signalling. *Drosophila* larvae that have been systemically depleted of DA become lethargic and aphagic, the same phenotype observed in transgenic mice able to synthesize adrenaline and noradrenaline but not DA. Dopamine is also required in *Drosophila* for normal ovarian maturation and juvenile development, as well as for the development of the normal physiology of adult sensory tissues.

Dopamine is important in the modulation of certain neuroendocrine functions; it can activate sex steroid receptors in a ligand-independent manner. Presynaptic actions of DA within the female rodent brain stimulate lordosis, the position indicative of female sexual receptivity. This role appears highly conserved, since depletion of dopamine levels via inhibition of tyrosine hydroxylase activity in *D. melanogaster* adult females renders them significantly less receptive to courting males. In the parasitic nematode *Romanomermis culicivorax*, catecholamines have been implicated in regulating copulatory behaviour; dopamine is also involved in reproductive control in bivalves. In addition to its roles in longevity and reproduction, dopamine is a key factor in the stress response; as with its other physiological functions, this role for dopamine has been conserved between *Drosophila* and mammals.

Thus, dopamine plays an evolutionarily conserved role in diverse organisms in development, behaviour, and cellular degeneration. It is likely it has been used as a signalling molecule previous to the development of the nervous system, and continues to perform this role in both neural and non-neural tissues.

5

Neurohormones and receptors: Structure, function and co-evolution

Introduction

A firm grasp of physiological processes of neuroendocrinology is dependent on understanding the underlying molecular mechanisms. Knowing the basic sequence of peptides or the chemistry of steroids, for example, is key to predicting their actions on receptors and ultimately some predictions of their physiological role can be made. Now, having said that, understanding the molecular mechanisms of a set of hormones can no more give you a complete understanding of the process than can injecting the hormone into an animal or measuring how the tissue levels change in a wild species. All approaches are required in order to understand a particular process as completely as possible. This is the 'integrated' approach to neuroendocrinology.

A comparative approach is also essential to understand a given physiological mechanism. I hope I have managed to convey this in the first chapters of this book. A comparative approach allows researchers to examine the process in one species and compare the mechanism in another species. This approach helps understand how a physiological system has changed over time, how it has been utilized by different species to exploit new niches or it may be useful to determine new functions of a hormone or physiological system. For example, amino acid sequences of functional regions of the peptide or protein vary between species or the gene copy and therefore an understanding of the primary structure allows researchers to predict within limits whether a given peptide will be active

Neuroendocrinology: An Integrated Approach   David A. Lovejoy
© 2005 John Wiley & Sons, Ltd

on a given receptor. One of the greatest recent achievements in zoology and medicine has been the sequencing of the human genome. This feat will be followed by the complete sequencing of the genomes of several other species. Knowing the structure of proteins then allows one to identify the function of unknown genes.

This chapter introduces the reader to all of the main molecular players in neuroendocrine signalling. A number of well-established signalling pathways such as wnt, hedgehog and notch, as introduced in Chapters 3 and 4, as well as integrin- and cadherin-based signalling pathways will not be discussed here. Although these pathways are significant in growth, development and differentiation clearly play a role with the overall function of neurosecretory and endocrine tissues, their role in the dynamics of neuroendocrine signalling is less well understood.

Orthology and paralogy

As we have discussed in the previous chapters, the complexity of organisms and their signalling systems is based on the amount of genetic material they possess. Obviously, organisms with more genes will tend to have a wider range of signalling molecules than those organisms with fewer genes. Because genes can duplicate for a variety of reasons, the proteins or peptides they encode for will also be present as duplicates. Over time, the functions of the new proteins will change and the proteins will have new functions. Different species have different complements of genes and proteins, and depending upon the selective pressures on that species some genes will be lost. As we try to understand and compare the neuroendocrine systems among species we are faced with trying to compare the functions of hormones, their receptors and all associated proteins as well. It becomes essential, therefore, to discriminate between proteins and peptides, which have evolved due to speciation, from those that have evolved from gene duplication, when trying to establish the functions of hormones across species.

If a number of individuals of a species are separated from the rest of the population, then over time this new group will evolve into a new species. A number of morphological, physiological and behavioural changes will result as the genes accrue mutations and their functions are modified. If we were to compare the structure of the same gene and its protein in each of the two species, we would expect to see some changes in the base sequence of that gene, and the amino acid sequence of that translated protein. But likely the gene and protein will be carrying out the same function in each species. In this case, these two genes are considered to be orthologues of each other (Fig. 5.1). For example, growth hormone in a rat is an orthologue of growth hormone in a chicken.

On the other hand, two genes may arise by a gene duplication such that all progeny of the individual with the gene duplication will now possess two copies of that same gene relative to individuals that existed before the gene duplication. Over time, the new gene and protein will take on new functions, but it may still possess some structural and functional similarity. Thus, two proteins or peptides arising from genes that were once the result of a gene duplication are referred to as paralogues (Fig. 5.2).

For phylogenetic and evolutionary purposes, the structure of a peptide can be used to predict the structure of an orthologous peptide in another species. By comparing the

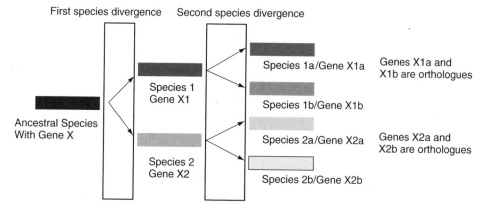

Figure 5.1 *Formation of orthologous genes and proteins.*

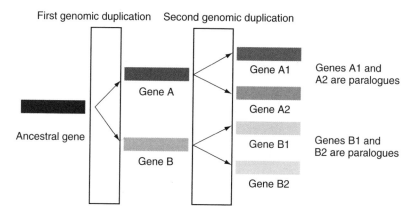

Figure 5.2 *Formation of paralogous genes and proteins.*

structures of peptides of species that diverged before and after our species of interest, we can make predictions of what the peptide sequence might be in species diverging between the species we used to compare sequences. Say, for example, you want to know what the structure of gonadotropin-releasing hormone (GnRH), the key neuropeptide regulating reproduction, is in *Tyrannosaurus rex*. Despite the optimism of some recent Hollywood films, the hormone gene cannot be cloned. Moreover, it is unlikely you will be able to obtain a *T. rex* brain in the near future to purify the hormone. However, we do know a little about the evolution of this monster – that it evolved sometime after the appearance of reptiles – and its closest surviving species are crocodilians and birds. By examining the structure of GnRH in all species diverging before and after the time of this group of dinosaurs we can predict the structures of this hormone (Fig. 5.3). We may not be able to clone the beast yet, but should we chance across a pair, we can assist the breeding efforts.

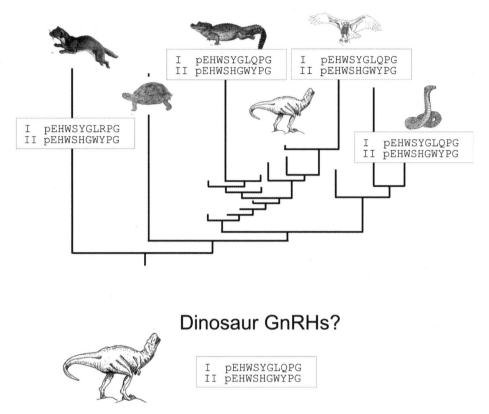

Dinosaur GnRHs?

```
I   pEHWSYGLQPG
II  pEHWSHGWYPG
```

Figure 5.3 Inferring peptide sequences in extinct species. By examining the peptide sequences in extant species, certain predictions can be made about those sequences in extinct species. Here, we could expect Tyrannosaurus rex *to have the same gonadotropin-releasing hormone sequences as those found in birds, snakes and crocodilians.*

Structural description of non-peptide ligands

Organisms synthesize an inordinate number of small bioactive compounds through either *de novo* synthesis or modifications of chemical compounds obtained through their diet. Consequently, the list of bioactive ligands and their receptors is constantly growing. Ligands such as these, by virtue of their small size, may find a number of binding sites in the vast array of receptors, enzymes and other proteins that are found. Many of these may be produced as apparently metabolic byproducts in one species, but have potent bioactive effects in another species (Chapter 13).

Small inorganic ions and gases

Calcium may well be the oldest signalling molecules used by life today (Fig. 5.4). Calcium and magnesium probably evolved as a signalling molecule with the earliest cells 4 billion

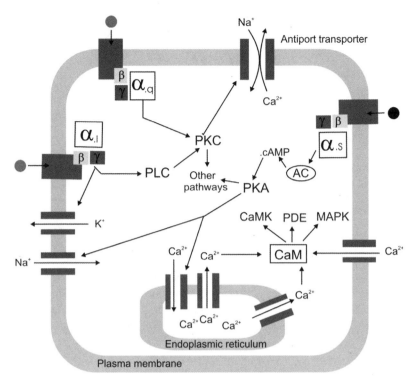

Figure 5.4   *Calcium signalling in a cell.*

years ago. Calcium can bind to plasma membrane receptors or intracellular receptors. Calcium is unusual in that as a free ion it is highly soluble but as an inorganic compound it is highly insoluble and can act as a structural support material (bones, for example). Both ions do not pass readily through membranes and, therefore, require a channel to enter the cell. Calcium's small size predicts that it will likely bind to a number of different receptors to modulate their action. One receptor that does appear to have a fairly specific binding site for Ca^{2+} is the calcium sensing receptor, a G-protein-coupled receptor that is structurally related to the metabotropic glutamate receptor family (pp. 129–130).

In the last decade or so, it was discovered that the gases nitric oxide (NO) and carbon monoxide (CO) are produced naturally by organisms and subsequently act as signalling molecules (Fig. 5.5). Nitric oxide is synthesized from L-arginine via nitric oxide synthase and requires NADPH as a coenzyme and tetrahydropterin as a cofactor. Because NO is a small and highly soluble molecule, it cannot be stored in vesicles and instead is synthesized when it is required and freely diffuses through the membranes. It is relatively unstable and readily degrades. It is, therefore, limited to local paracrine and autocrine actions. One of NO's actions is to increase the production of cGMP by guanylyl cyclase and may play a role in synaptic plasticity and also acts as a vasodilator. Carbon monoxide is produced in the conversion of heme to biliverdin by heme oxygenase in the brain, spleen and liver.

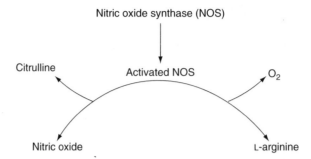

Figure 5.5   *Nitric oxide production.*

Purines

Purines, such as adenosine and adenosine triphosphate, act as neurotransmitters in addition to their role in energy metabolism (Fig. 5.6). They are stored in synaptic vesicles and released in response to action potentials throughout the nervous system. Membrane receptors for purine neurotransmitters are divided into P_1 receptors that bind adenosine,

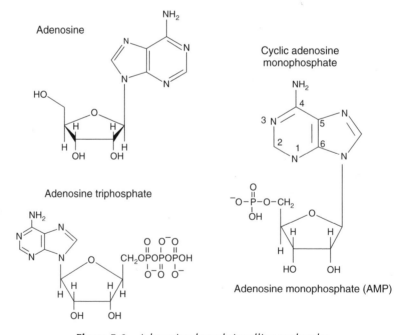

Figure 5.6   *Adenosine-based signalling molecules.*

and P_2 receptors that bind ATP. The P_1 receptors are subdivided into A_1, A_{2A}, A_{2B} and A_3 receptors. The P_2 receptors are divided into the ionotropic receptors (P_{2x1}–P_{2x7}) and metabotropic receptors (P_{2y1}, P_{2y2}, P_{2y4} and P_{2y6}). However, the P_{2x7}, P_{2y2}, P_{2y4} and P_{2y6} receptors do not appear to be present in the nervous system.

Lipid hormones: Steroids and eicosanoids

Lipid hormones are released as soon as they are synthesized. Because they are highly lipophilic, they easily pass through membranes and, therefore, cannot be stored. They are synthesized in the smooth endoplasmic reticulum and in the inner membrane of mitochondria.

All steroid hormones are derived from cholesterol via either uptake in the diet, *de novo* synthesis or both. A number of animal species cannot synthesize steroids and must take in the precursors from the diet (e.g. insects). There can be some storage of cholesterol in the form of cholesterol esters in lipid droplets that are generally abundant in steroid-synthesizing cells. In vertebrates, the rate-limiting step in cholesterol synthesis is the cleavage of cholesterol to form pregnenolone via the actions of cytochrome P450 cholesterol side cleavage enzyme (P450scc) located on the inner mitochondrial membrane. Once pregnenolone is formed, steroids may be synthesized via a Δ^4 pathway that leads to cortisol, corticosterone, aldosterone and progesterone, or a Δ^5 pathway that leads to the androgens, oestrogens or also cortisol (Fig. 5.7). Alternatively, in mammals, cholesterol can be converted to 7-dehydrocholesterol in the skin then into the active form of vitamin D via a multi-step pathway utilizing skin, kidney and liver enzymes. In plasma, steroids may be transported by carrier proteins such as specific steroid-binding proteins or via the albumins that possess a low-affinity high-capacity transport ability.

The eicosanoids are a class of highly fat-soluble ligands that are derived from polyunsaturated fatty acids with C_{18}, C_{20} or C_{22} carbon backbones. Arachidonic acid is the principal precursor and rate-limiting step for many of the eicosanoids. Phospholipase A_2 or phospholipase C and diglyceride lipase stimulate the cleavage of arachidonic acid from glycerophospholipids in the plasma membrane. Once formed, arachidonic acid can be converted to a number of different eicosanoids including prostaglandins, prostacyclins, leukotrienes, thromboxanes and cannabinoids (Chapter 4). Although the eicosanoids are highly lipophilic, they appear to utilize G-protein-coupled receptors to transduce most of their actions. There has been considerable interest in the endogenous cannabinoids (endocannabinoids) due to their psychotropic and neurological effects (Chapter 13). The cannabinoid, anandamide, and its receptor, cannabinoid receptor 1 (CB1), are ubiquitous in the vertebrates and many invertebrates. Cannabinoids act on two different receptors CB1 and CB2, the former being present predominately in the brain.

Amino acids and modified amino acids

A number of structurally unrelated hormones and neurotransmitters are classified here together as they are all derived initially from an amino acid.

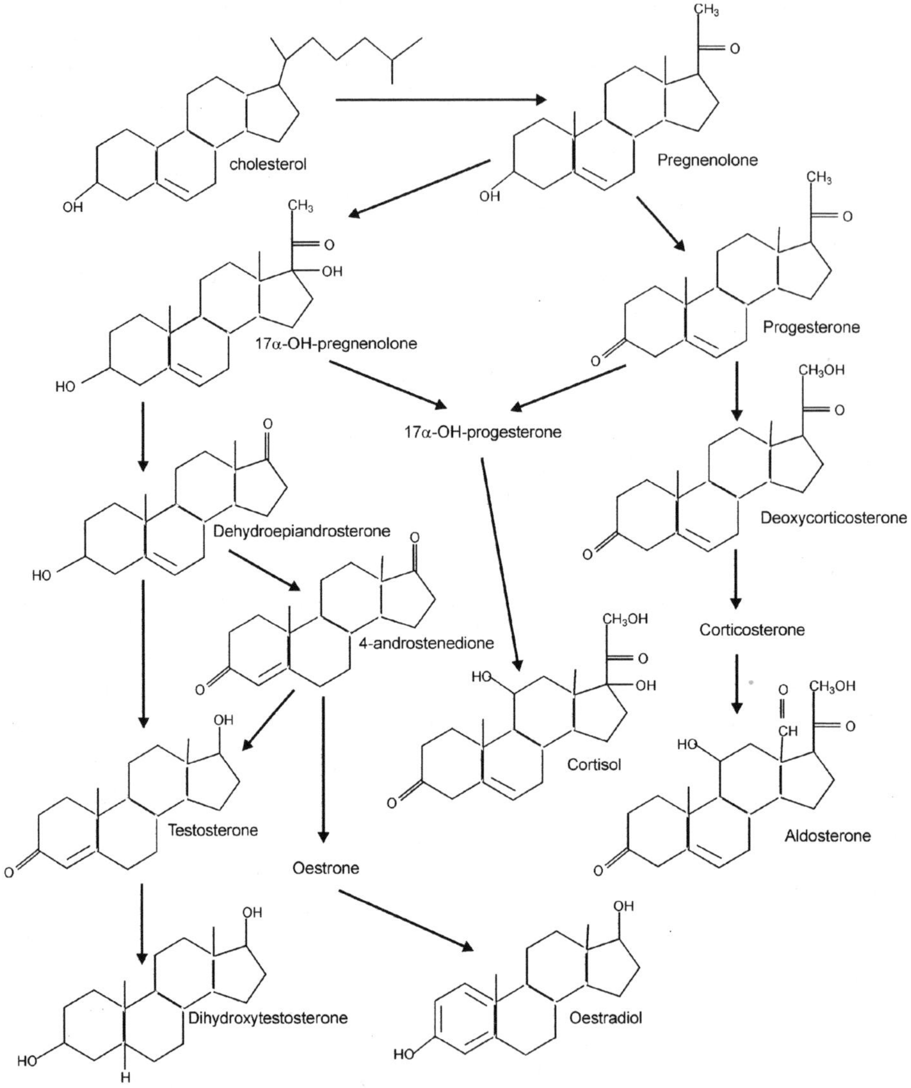

Figure 5.7   *Steroid synthesis pathways in mammals.*

Catecholamine hormones are derived initially from the amino acid tyrosine and are synthesized in the nervous system. The adrenal medulla, which is derived from nervous tissue, is the major source of epinephrine, whereas most circulating norepinephrine originates from the sympathetic nerve terminals. Catecholamines are stored in the cell after synthesis, in storage granules that are similar to those used for the storage of peptide hormones. Tyrosine is converted to dihydroxyphenylalanine (DOPA) by tyrosine hydroxylase.

Tyrosine hydroxylase appears to have its origins in the early metazoans as the enzyme is found in arthropods. DOPA is converted to dopamine by L-amino acid decarboxylase in the cytosol. Dopamine is subsequently transported into a storage granule where it is converted into norepinephrine by dopamine β-hydroxylase. In the adrenal medulla, the enzyme phenylethanolamine-*O*-methyltransferase (PNMT) is present in the cytoplasm and converts norepinephrine to epinephrine where it is returned to the storage granule (Fig. 5.8).

Dopamine, norepinephrine and epinephrine all bind to G-protein-coupled receptors. Dopamine exerts its action via at least five different types of dopamine receptors. The D1 receptor is stimulatory whereas the D2 receptor is inhibitory. The classification of the adrenergic receptors was originally based on their relative affinities to different ligands. The α-adrenergic receptors were shown to have the highest affinity for epinephrine, lower affinity for norepinephrine, then the lowest affinity for the synthetic ligand, isoproterenol. The β-adrenergic receptors had the highest affinity for isoproterenol, followed by epinephrine, then norepinephrine. However, each receptor possesses several subtypes encoded by different genes. The affinity of the receptor–ligand interaction differs considerably among the receptor subtypes and also among homologous receptors in different species.

The indoleamine hormones or monoamines, as they are frequently called, include serotonin (5-hydroxytryptamine or 5-HT) and melatonin. Melatonin and 5-HT both bind G-protein-coupled receptors. The biosynthetic pathway begins with the amino acid tryptophan (Fig. 5.9). Depending on the species, tryptophan can be either synthesized *de novo* or obtained through the diet. The indoleamine pathway appears to be phylogenetically ancient, indeed, as these hormones have been found in virtually all kingdoms of life forms (Chapter 8). Tryptophan is converted to 5-hydroxytryptophan by tryptophan

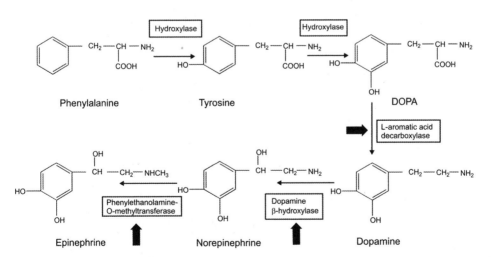

Figure 5.8 *Catecholamine Synthesis. Arrows indicate key enzymes associated with each of the hormones.*

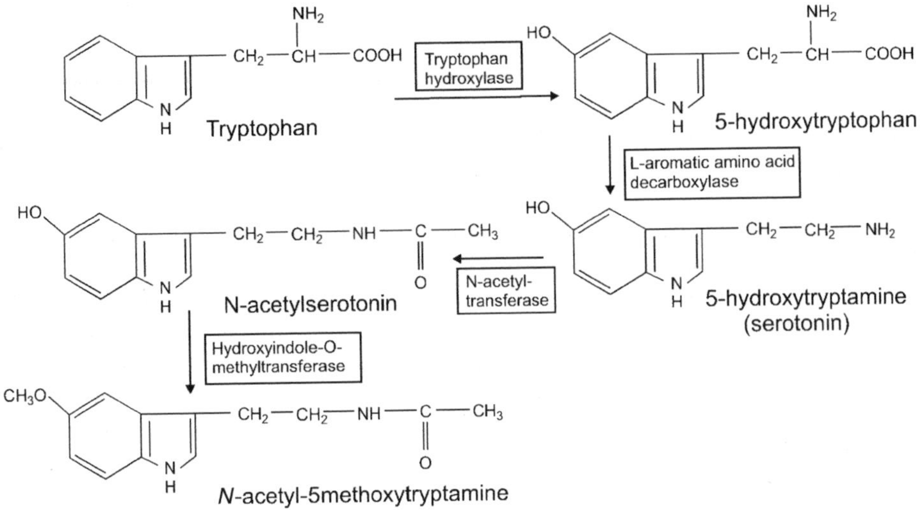

Figure 5.9   *5-HT and melatonin synthesis.*

hydroxylase, then to 5-hydroxytryptamine (5-HT) by L-aromatic amino acid decarboxylase, the same enzyme that is utilized in the biosynthetic pathway for catecholamines (p. 127). Serotonin is then converted to melatonin via a two-step synthesis involving N-acetyltransferase and hydroxyindole-O-methyltransferase. About 90% of 5-HT in the body is found in the enterochromaffin cells of the gastrointestinal tract. The remainder is found in the nervous system and in platelets. Seven basic types of 5-HT receptors have been identified and are classified as 5-HT_1 to 5-HT_7. There are 5 subtypes of the 5-HT_1 receptor, 3 subtypes of the 5-HT_2 receptors and 2 5-HT_5 subtypes. Most of the receptors belong to the G-protein-coupled receptor class and signal through adenylate cyclase or phospholipase C (p. 137). The 5-HT_3 class of receptors, however, are ion channels. The 5-HT_6 and 5-HT_7 receptors are highly expressed in the limbic system and mediate a number of the effects associated with emotionality, learning and memory. The unusually high number of 5-HT receptors likely reflects its ancient origin as a signalling molecule. Melatonin on the other hand has been utilized relatively recently as a signalling molecule (Chapter 8). In mammals, melatonin receptors may be present in the pituitary gland, regions of the hypothalamus and hippocampus, striatum and midbrain regions. The melatonin receptor is a GPCR and appears to have at least three different subtypes, although this appears to vary among vertebrate species.

Thyroid hormones are unusual in a number of respects. They are highly lipophilic, and easily pass through membranes and bind to a class of receptors similar to steroid receptors (p. 142). They are synthesized initially from tyrosine, but utilize the attachment of an inorganic ion, iodine, for full activity. Moreover, despite their hydrophobicity, they are stored in the cell via interaction of a large transport protein. The thyroid hormones are synthesized solely in the thyroid gland (Chapter 6). The thyroid gland produces high concentrations of the glycoprotein, thyroglobulin. Oxidized iodine is coupled to the phenyl rings of the tyrosine residues on the thyroglobulin. The tyrosine residues are coupled together by thyroid peroxidase to yield thyronines. The thyroglobulins along with its attached thyronines are released into the follicles of the gland for storage. Although several variants of thyronines occur, the biologically most active metabolites are T3 and T4, possessing three and four atoms of iodine respectively. The thyroid hormone receptor is a nuclear receptor of which at least two different subtypes, TR-α and TR-β, have been identified (Fig. 5.10).

The amino acid, glutamate, is widespread throughout the Metazoa and acts as a transmitter without subsequent modification. Recall from Chapter 2 that glutamate was likely a constituent of the organic material found in the prebiotic earth. Although glutamate binds to a class of G-protein-coupled receptors, there are three known types of glutamate channel receptors and are named after the ligand that was initially used to identify them. The receptors all have an excitatory action on the membrane acting to depolarize the membrane. The NMDA receptor, binding *N*-methyl D-aspartate, plays a role in learning and long-term potentiation (Chapter 11). The channel opening for this receptor has a comparatively large diameter and allows Na$^+$, K$^+$, Cl$^-$ and Ca^{2+} ions to pass readily through. The NMDA receptor also has a high-affinity binding site for glycine; however, given the level of affinity and the high concentration of glycine in tissues and fluids in the body, the binding site appears to be maximally occupied. Thus, glycine does not appear to play a modulatory role on the NMDA receptors. Phencyclidines, a class of psychotropic drugs, also known as angel dust, bind in a non-competitive manner in the ion channel effectively blocking the channel (Chapter 13). The other two glutamate receptors, AMPA (named after α-amino-3-hydroxy-5-methyl-4-isoxazoleproprionate) and kainate possess smaller ion channels allowing Na$^+$, K$^+$ and Cl$^-$ but not Ca^{2+}. The AMPA and kainate receptors have been implicated in the mediation of spinal cord reflexes and cortical-evoked potentials.

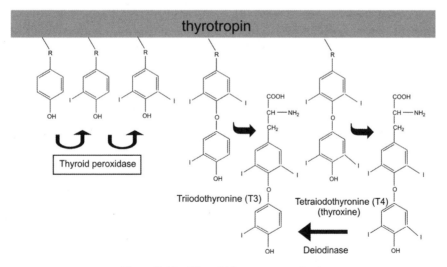

Figure 5.10   *Thyroid hormone synthesis.*

γ-Aminobutyric acid (GABA) is an inhibitor of presynaptic transmission in the nervous system and in the retina. It is synthesized from glutamate by glutamate decarboxylase (GAD). GABA signals through both ionotropic receptors ($GABA_A$ and $GABA_C$) which induce fast synaptic inhibitory responses, and metabotropic receptors ($GABA_B$) which play a role in the reduction of presynaptic transmitter release and post-synaptic inhibitory potentials. The GABA ionotropic receptors are Cl⁻ ion channels and have an inhibitory action on the plasma membrane by contributing to its level of hyperpolarization. The receptor in mammals also has binding sites for barbiturates and benzodiazepines. Neither class of drug has a direct effect on the conductance of Cl⁻ directly, but instead increase the affinity for GABA by the receptor due to allosteric effects. GABA binding to the receptor will also have a cooperative effect on benzodiazepine binding. The metabotropic GABA receptors ($GABA_B$), though highly expressed in vertebrates, have been cloned in *Drosophila*. $GABA_B$-R1 and $GABA_B$-R2 show high sequence similarity to the mammalian counterparts; however, $GABA_B$-R3 appears to be an insect-specific isoform, as a chordate receptor with sufficient sequence similarity has not been identified.

Other signalling molecules

Acetylcholine is synthesized from choline and acetate derived from acetyl co-enzyme A via the enzyme choline acetyltransferase (Fig. 5.11). Acetylcholine in cholinergic nerve fibres is taken up into the synaptic vesicles by a high-affinity transporter system. Acetylcholine binds to two classes of receptors. The nicotinic receptors are ligand-gated ion channels and are typically found at the neuromuscular junction, autonomic nervous system ganglia and in other parts of the central nervous system. Muscarinic receptors are G-protein-coupled receptors of which at least five different subtypes have been identified. The M1 receptor subtype is the major muscarinic receptor of the nervous system.

The retinoids include retinoic acid and 9-*cis* retinoic acid (Fig. 5.12). Both are derived from retinol via two-stage biosynthesis. The retinoids in mammals cannot be synthesized *de novo* and must be taken up in the diet as vitamin A. Vitamin A is cleaved to produce retinal. The retinoids bind to two classes of receptors, RAR and RXR. At least three subtypes of the RAR receptor and two subtypes of the RXR have been found in vertebrates.

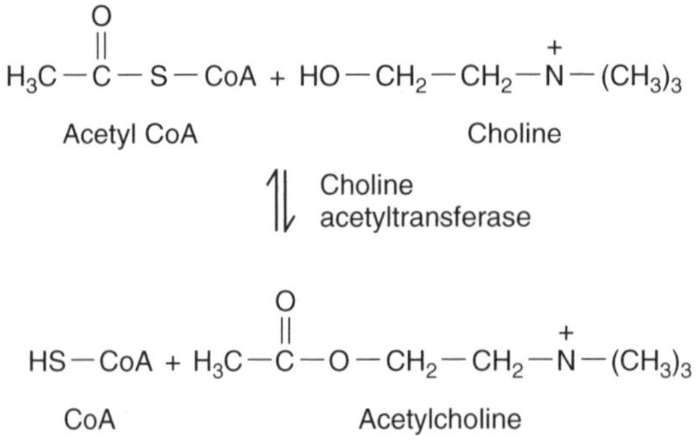

Figure 5.11   *Acetylcholine synthesis.*

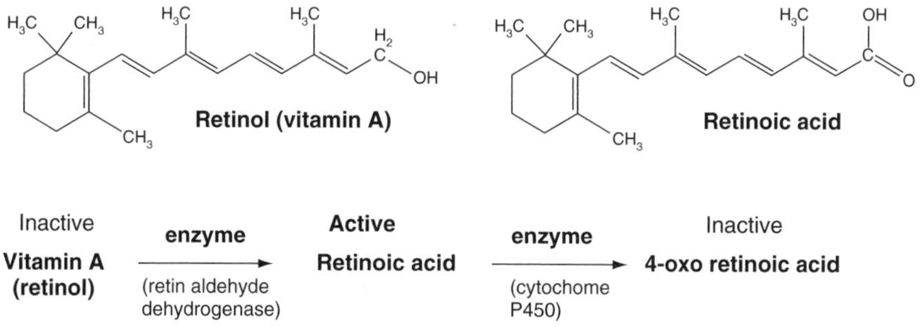

Figure 5.12 *Retinoic acid synthesis.*

Peptide and polypeptide signalling molecules

In virtually all metazoans examined to date, the peptide class of signalling molecules include the largest number of different factors. Peptide hormones are synthesized directly from gene transcription and subsequent translation, with only a minimal amount of biosynthetic modification in the form of post-translational modification, relative to the non-peptide ligands described in the previous section. Depending upon the size of the peptide, they have particular chemical and biological properties and, therefore, it is convenient to group them in approximate size categories.

Amino acids, as we have discussed in Chapter 2, may be classified on their ability to partition themselves in either an aqueous (water-like) or lipid-like environment. Amino acids that possess an ionic group as part of their side chain will favour an aqueous environment, whereas amino acids without such groups and having longer side chains will partition selectively in a more lipid-rich environment. Amino acids such as glutamic acid and lysine, for example, are hydrophilic, whereas amino acids such as leucine or phenylalanine are comparatively more hydrophobic. Because the amino and carboxylic acid groups of amino acids are tied up in the peptide bonds that link amino acids, the bioactive character of peptides is associated with the combined nature of the side chains for each of the amino acids (or residues) that make up the peptide (Fig. 5.13).

All peptides consist of a number of small motifs of short sequences of amino acids that possess different functional attributes. For example, one motif may be responsible for recognition by degrading enzymes, other motifs may be used for receptor binding, or activation. Each of these motifs will evolve at different rates depending upon how the various interacting proteins have changed in a given species. It is not unusual for a peptide from one species to be inactive in another species. This may be due because it has poor affinity for the receptor. It may also be because, although it binds well to the receptor, it cannot activate the receptor. Alternatively, it may be degraded more rapidly by peptidases that have particularly high affinity for the peptide. It is usually, of course, a combination of all these reasons. Physiologically, it can be almost impossible to determine the differences between these effects. For example, a peptide that has low affinity for the receptor but is

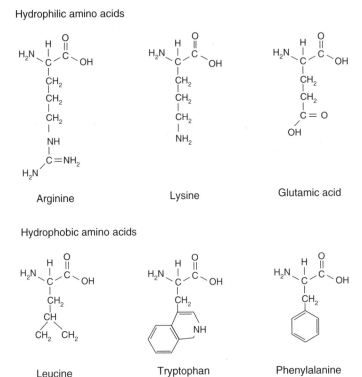

Figure 5.13   *Examples of hydrophilic and hydrophobic amino acids.*

resistant to degrading peptidases may appear to possess similar *in vivo* potency to a peptide that has high affinity for the receptor but is degraded very rapidly by peptidases.

Another element of peptide structure is its overall level of hydrophilicity or hydrophobicity. For example, blood serum or CSF is more hydrophilic relative to the tissues. Within a tissue, the extracellular matrix is hydrophilic relative to the plasma membranes of cells. A peptide that is particularly hydrophilic may tend to partition itself in the plasma preferentially, whereas a more hydrophobic peptide may remain bound to plasma or extracellular matrix proteins. Thus, the relative mobility of a peptide in a biological system will also affect its potency.

This section is not intended to be a complete analysis of all orthologues and paralogues of all neuropeptide families. It is, rather, a description of several of the neuropeptide families and examples of paralogues found in each group.

Small amphiphilic peptides

Peptides are generally classified as amphiphilic in that they possess a combination of both hydrophobic and hydrophilic regions and can, therefore, interact to a certain degree in both environments. Plasma and tissue interstices tend to be more hydrophilic than the interface at the plasma membrane and extracellular region. Small peptides might be classified as

Gonadotropin-releasing hormone (GnRH)

pEHWSYGLRPG—NH$_2$

Thyrotrophin-releasing hormone

pEHP—NH$_2$

Somatostatin

A G C K N F F W K T F T S C

Figure 5.14 *Examples of some small peptide hormones.*

those that have no defined tertiary structure. They tend to be short sequences of 2 to about 15 residues and are highly mobile in tissues. These peptides include most of the FMRFamide-related peptides that are found in many homologous forms in invertebrates and to a limited degree in vertebrates. Some of the more highly conserved neuropeptide hormones found in vertebrates include gonadotropin-releasing factor (GnRH), thryrotrophin-releasing factor (TRF), somatostatin, urotensin-II, enkephalins and cholecystokinin, to name a few (Fig. 5.14). The vasotocin family of peptides, which also includes vasopressin and oxytocin, are unusual in that they are constrained by the presence of the disulphide bonds resulting from two cysteine residues. In phylogenetically younger metazoans such as chordates and perhaps arthropods, the majority of these peptides interact with G-protein-coupled receptors. In diploblastic organisms such as in the cnidarians, for example, there are few G-protein-coupled receptors. Thus, many of the small peptide ligands appear to interact with other receptor systems such as the heptahelical plasma membrane receptors that do not interact with G-proteins such as the receptors for wnt and hedgehog (Chapter 3), receptor kinases and perhaps low density lipid (LDL) related receptors.

Peptides possessing a secondary structure

In longer peptides, a secondary structure is imposed upon the peptide chain by the interactions of the amino acid side chains with each other and molecular components in their environment (Fig. 5.15). These peptides tend also to be flexible and amphiphilic, but will

Vasoactive intestinal peptide (VIP)

HSDAVFTDNYTRLRKQMAVKKYLNSILN—NH$_2$

Galanin

GWTLNSAGYLLGPHAVGNHRSFSDKNGLTS—NH$_2$

Neuropeptide γ

YPSKPDNPGEDAPAEDLARYYSALRHYINLITRQRY—NH$_2$

Corticotrophin-releasing factor

SEEPPISLDLTFHLLREVLEMARAEQLAQQAHSNRKLMEII—NH$_2$

Figure 5.15 *Peptides with defined secondary structure.*

possess some form of secondary structures such as α helices or β turns, for example. Their size typically ranges from about 15 or 20 residues to about 40 or 50 residues. Examples of these peptides include adrenocorticotropic hormone (ACTH), growth hormone releasing hormone (GHRH), corticotrophin-releasing factor (CRF) and neuropeptide Y (NPY). Some of these peptides such as calcitonin also possess disulphide bonds that act to constrain part of the peptide into a particular orientation. These peptide ligands appear to interact almost entirely with G-protein-coupled receptors.

Polypeptides with a defined tertiary structure

This group of peptides, which are classified more accurately as polypeptides, resembles proteins more than peptides. Because of their large size, they begin to take on more of a globular structure where hydrophobic residues tend to be oriented towards the middle with other similar residues, whereas the hydrophilic residues are more likely to be found in regions more accessible to the ambient environment. Such polypeptides are frequently constrained by one or more sets of disulphide bonds. Examples of these peptides are growth hormone and its homologues, prolactin and somatolactin, leptin, growth factors and a number of the larger cytokines (Fig. 5.16). This class of ligands typically interacts

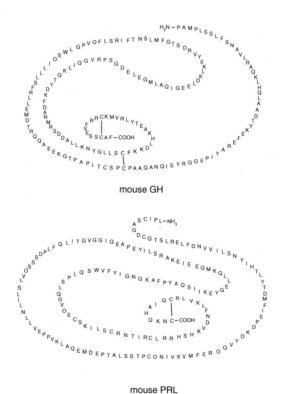

mouse GH

mouse PRL

Figure 5.16 *Peptides with tertiary structure. Reprinted from Manzon (2002) by the permission of Elsevier Science (USA).*

with receptor tyrosine kinases. Related to this class are a group of ligands that possess subunits that are held together by the cysteine bridges. There are several examples of these ligands. Glycoprotein peptide hormones, which are post-translationally modified with saccharide groups, include follicle-stimulating hormone (FSH), luteinizing hormone (LH) and thyroxine-stimulating hormone (TSH) and interact with G-protein-coupled receptors. Most of the ligands in this class are not glycosylated, however. Hormones such as insulin, relaxin, activin and inhibin all activate receptor kinases.

Peptide processing

Eukaryotic cells specialized for secretions possess at least two different pathways for secretion. These are the constitutive pathway, that is typically utilized by growth factors, cytokines and blood coagulating factors, and the regulated pathway, that is used by peptide hormones and neuropeptides (Fig. 5.17). A certain small proportion of neuropeptides are released via the constitutive pathway as well, however. Peptidergic neurons and endocrine cells have both pathways where the sorting of the constitutive and regulated pathway occurs in the trans-Golgi network (TGN).

Peptide hormones and neuropeptides are processed via the proteolytic conversion of prohormones in the regulated pathway in the acidic environment of the TGN and secretory granules (Fig. 5.18). Post-translational modifications may include endoproteolytic cleavages, glycosylation, sulphation, exoproteolytic cleavage, amidation and acetylation. Mature secretory granules remain in the cytoplasm until released by the appropriate stimulus. Proteins released by the constitutive pathway, on the other hand, are not concentrated in secretory granules and are constantly secreted. Stimulation by a secretogogue

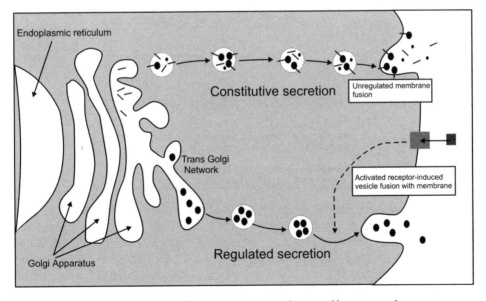

Figure 5.17 *Regulated and constitutive pathways of hormone release.*

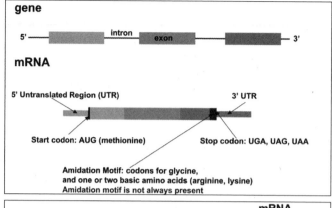

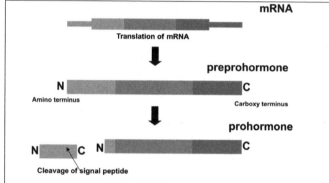

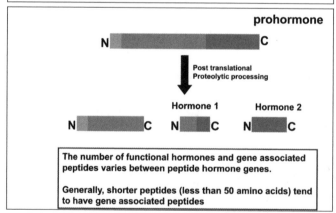

Figure 5.18   Peptide processing and post-translational modifications.

is not required. Secretory granules and synaptic vesicles appear to make use of similar molecular mechanisms to achieve docking with the plasma membrane for exocytosis. Prohormone convertases (PC) belong to the subtilisin family of enzymes and include at least seven enzymes. PC1 and PC2 are exclusively expressed in endocrine and neuroendocrine cells and play a fundamental role in the cleavage of neuropeptide precursors.

Structure and classes of receptors

A receptor can be any molecule, usually a protein, that acts to transduce a response once it has been bound by another molecule (ligand). Theoretically, any class of protein can act as a receptor, and novel classes are being recognized on a frequent basis. However, we shall only consider a number of the classes associated with the hormones discussed in this book.

G-protein-coupled receptors

The G-protein-coupled receptors are proteins with seven α-helical transmembrane domains (Fig. 5.19). They form one of the largest families in the mammalian genome. Most of the heptahelical transmembrane receptors signal through G-proteins; however, this has not been established for all members of the class, especially for newly cloned members or orphan receptors. Through interactions with G-proteins, G-protein-coupled receptors convey signals to control a multitude of physiological processes from metabolic to behavioural functions. This class of receptor may constitute 2% of the genes in the human genome. Well over 800 G-protein-coupled receptor-like genes have been identified so far, of which about 350 appear to be non-olfactory receptors. Different classification systems have been derived to organize them into families. The most common system classifies the G-protein-coupled receptors into clans based on sequence similarities. The six clans are (A) rhodopsin-like proteins which contains the majority of G-protein-coupled receptors; (B) the secretin-like receptors; (C) metabotropic glutamate receptor-like receptors;

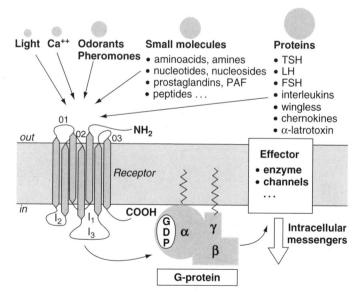

Figure 5.19 *G-protein-coupled Receptors. The G-protein-coupled receptors include the largest class of receptors and bind several classes of ligands. Reprinted from Bockaert and Pin (1999) with permission from the Nature Publishing Group.*

(D) fungal pheromone P and α-factor receptors; (E) fungal pheromone A- and M-factor receptors; and finally (F) cAMP-type receptors.

There are numerous investigations indicating that G-protein-coupled receptors, such as the D3 dopamine receptors, can form stable dimers or oligomers as part of the signal transduction process. Receptor dimerization was reported under basal conditions such as in the β-adrenergic receptor and agonist-induced conditions such as in B2 bradykinin receptor. Evidence also suggests that G-protein-coupled receptors can form heterodimeric complexes with other G-protein-coupled receptors such as the dimer formed between μ- and δ-opioid receptors which has different properties from each of its subunits alone.

G-proteins are heterotrimeric guanine nucleotide binding proteins that transduce a signal derived from a transmembrane receptor such as a G-protein-coupled receptor (Fig. 5.20). The trimeric subunits also form two complexes: G_α and $G_{\beta\gamma}$. Under the resting state, the G_α unit is bound to GTP and the $G_{\beta\gamma}$ complex. The trimeric units couple to a GPCR. Upon ligand binding of the receptor, GTP replaces GDP, G_α loses its affinity and dissociates from $G_{\beta\gamma}$, thereby forming the active state. The $G_{\beta\gamma}$ subsequently interacts with effector molecules. As the GTP is being hydrolysed, G_α regains its affinity to the other complex and binds $G_{\beta\gamma}$ again. The G-proteins bind G-protein-coupled receptors at the cytoplasmic region. Many regions of the G_α contribute towards association with the G-protein-coupled receptor. The C-terminus as well as several loops adjacent to both termini of G_α are important in defining receptor coupling of G-proteins. Different parts of the N-terminus of G_α are also involved in receptor specificity. The $G_{\beta\gamma}$ complex is thought to play a minor role in determining G-protein-receptor specificity. Some G-protein-coupled receptors are unfaithful to G-proteins and interact directly, via their C-terminal domain, with scaffolding proteins such as those containing PDZ domains.

There are many proteins involved in regulating the activation of G-proteins by G-protein-coupled receptors. Three important families involved in negative regulation are the Regulators of G-protein signalling (RGS), G-protein-coupled receptor kinases (GRKs) and the arrestins. RGS play several roles in negatively regulating the activation of G-proteins. RGS accelerate GTP hydrolysis of G_α and thereby rapidly turn off the signalling pathways initiated by means of the GTPase activating protein (GAP). RGS can

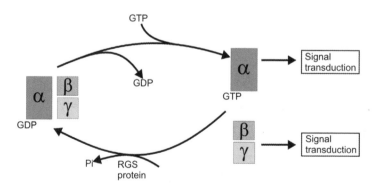

Figure 5.20   *G-proteins. G-proteins are a trimeric complex consisting of α, β and γ subunits. The there are several subtypes of each subunit. Both G_α and $G_{\beta\gamma}$ subunits can act to transduce distinct intracellular signalling pathways.*

also physically block the interaction between G-proteins and the receptor. In another way, they alter the number of free $G_{\beta\gamma}$ subunits available to interact with their effectors by enhancing the affinity of G_{α} subunits for $\beta\gamma$ subunits after GTP hydrolysis, thus accelerating reformation of the heterotrimer. More than 20 RGS proteins specific to different G-protein-coupled receptor pathways have been isolated. This specificity is achieved through many mechanisms like differential cell and tissue expression and post-translational modifications of RGS.

Two families of proteins, the GRKs and the arrestins, assist in deactivating and desensitizing the GPCR. GRKs phosphorylate the receptor, which then allows arrestins to bind and prevent further interaction between G-proteins and the receptor. Some of the arrestin-bound receptors are removed from the plasma membranes via clathrin-mediated endocytosis. In the endosomes, receptor dephosphorylation occurs and the receptor is recycled to the plasma membranes. It should be noted that G-proteins have also been found on intracellular membranes such as Golgi membranes, and the regulation of G-proteins on intracellular membranes might be different from the classical G-protein paradigm at the plasma membrane.

G_{α} subunits share primary structural similarity with other GTP-hydrolysing proteins such as p21 Ras, especially in the guanine-binding pocket. In general, the G_{α} subunit has two domains: a helical domain with seven α helices and a GTPase domain with five α helices and six β strands. The GTP bound G_{α} has a more compact structure to bury the GTP in the cleft between the helical and GTPase domain. The G_{β} and G_{γ} units are always associated together. The β unit comprises of two domains: the N-terminal helix, which is 20 residues long, and the core domain with antiparallel β strands arranged in seven tryptophan-aspartic acid (WD) repeats. The γ unit is comprised of two α helices with a disordered C-terminal tail. The entire γ unit interacts with G_{β} therefore making it impossible to separate them and preventing the γ unit from coming in contact with G_{α}.

There are specific combinations of G_{β} and G_{γ} units to form different $G_{\beta\gamma}$ complexes. This specificity is determined mostly by 14 residues lying in the middle of G_{γ} subunit. The $G_{\beta\gamma}$ complex exists in two forms: relaxed and tense states. In the relaxed state a hydrophobic farnesyl moiety of the G_{γ} is exposed mediating membrane association in the trimeric structure with G_{α}; however, in the tense state the farnesyl moiety is buried in a cavity formed in the G_{β} subunit. This conformation causes the sequestration of the $G_{\beta\gamma}$ complex from the membrane to the cytosol and turns off the signal-transduction cascade.

The G_{α} subunits are classified into at least five types based on sequence identity and functional specialization: Gi, s, q, 12 and h. The $G_{\alpha}i$ is an inhibitory regulator of adenylyl cyclase (AC). This class contains three main subtypes $G_{\alpha}i$ 1, 2 and 3. Recently, the $G_{\alpha}z$ unit, a G_{α}, found in neuronal tissues, has emerged as an alternative to $G_{\alpha}i$ by coupling to most G-protein-coupled receptors and inhibiting AC. The Gs class of G_{α} stimulate adenylyl cyclase and can positively regulate ion channels as well by interacting with tyrosine kinases, thereby allowing interaction between G-protein-coupled receptors and growth factors. $G_{\alpha}s$ exists in many alternatively spliced variants such as the long and short form. The Gq class contain proteins such as $G_{\alpha}q$ and $G_{\alpha}11$. They regulate phosphatidylinositol-specific phospholipase C-β (PLCβ) isoforms in response to mitogenic signals such as bombesin. Two second messengers employed are the diacylglycerol (DAG) and inositol-(1,4,5)-triphosphate (IP$_3$). Members of this class possess great functional redundancy. The G12 class are the smallest subfamily with only two members: $G_{\alpha}12$ and

$G_\alpha 13$. They share diverse signalling characteristics from c-Jun N-terminal Kinase (JNK) activation to GAP (GTPase-activation protein of RAS). They can also regulate cadherins and β-catenin signalling events. One final subfamily is the atypical Gh family with one member, named also tissue transglutaminase (TGII). This $G_\alpha h$ shares very low sequence homology with the other units. However, it activates PLCδ following activation by α-adrenoreceptor subtypes and causes intracellular calcium release. Gh is ubiquitously expressed in mammalian tissues.

Although there has been a tendency to think that only the G-protein-coupled receptors are capable of stimulating cAMP, in fact, several classes of ligand receptor pairs may do so. For example, adhesion proteins such as the integrins can stimulate cAMP by direct interaction via the heterotrimeric G-protein complex. Additionally, cAMP-dependent pathways can be modulated by a number of neurotransmitters and neuromodulators, adhesion molecules and calcium ions. The cells can separate these different actions of cAMP in part by the location where the cAMP response is initiated. It is, therefore, necessary that once a cAMP response is initiated in a particular part of a cell, it is inhibited shortly after initiation so that the cAMP cascade does not overwhelm the cell to initiate a number of non-specific signal transduction pathways not associated with the ligand in question. Similar situations occur for other signal transduction pathways.

Receptor kinases

The receptor kinases are classified on the basis of which residue is phosphorylated. Three main families are recognized: tyrosine kinases serine/threonine kinases and histidine kinases. The latter appears not to be major signalling system in the metazoans and, therefore, will not be discussed.

Protein tyrosine kinases include a large family of plasma membrane receptors that are characterized by a single hydrophobic core that acts as a membrane spanning region, and a highly conserved catalytic kinase domain (Fig. 5.21). Gene splice variants of these receptors, which include primarily the extracellular region, may be present as soluble binding proteins for their ligands. The high number of protein tyrosine kinase receptors in vertebrates appears to be associated with the genomic duplication events that occurred during the early evolution of this group of species. The ligands for these receptors are all peptide or polypeptide signalling molecules and include growth hormone, erythropoietin, several of the interleukins, interferon, leptin and most, if not all, of their structural homologues.

The initial transducing event for most of these receptors is the activation of one or more of the Janus kinase (JAK) family of tyrosine kinases. The JAK kinases, which form a complex with the receptor act to autophosphorylate themselves as well as phosphorylate the receptor. The phosphorylated tyrosines act as binding sites for a number of co-signal transducing molecules that include the signal transducers and activators of transcription (STATs) which can regulate transcription, the Shc proteins which act to bind Grb2-SOS protein complexes and initiate an Ras-MAP kinase pathway. In addition, the insulin receptor substrate (IRS) proteins may also be activated to subsequently regulate a number of metabolic functions within the cell.

The majority of sequence similarity between class I cytokine receptors occurs in the extracellular domain. Typically the extracellular domain consists of approximately 200aa.

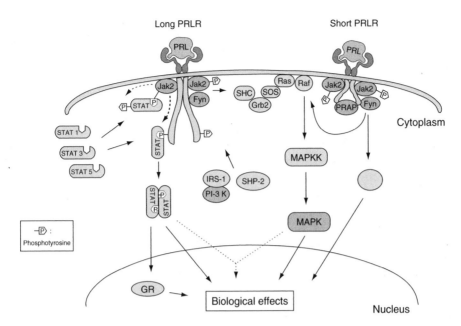

Figure 5.21 *Intracellular signalling pathways induced by the activated prolactin receptor. Reprinted with permission from Bole-Feysot* et al. *(1998), Endocrine Society.*

The cytokine receptor homologies are usually divided into two divisions of approximately 100aa and are referred to as D1 and D2. The conserved fibronectin-like domains primarily drive ligand interactions. There are five extracellular cysteines, the first four of which are located near the N-terminal region and the fifth near the transmembrane domain. Three N-linked glycosylation sites are present.

Serine/threonine kinase-based receptors are activated with the interaction of a number of peptide ligands including transforming growth factor (TGF) β, bone morphogenic protein (BMP), activin and inhibin, and anti-Mullerian hormone. Homologues of these peptides are found throughout the vertebrates and also the Ecdysozoa and possibly the Lophotrochozoa. The receptors have been associated with a variety of cell functions including differentiation, migration, adhesion and apoptosis.

Activation of the serine/threonine receptor kinases is initiated when the ligand binds the Type II receptor which facilitates heterodimerization between the Type I and Type II receptors. The Type II receptor activates the Type I receptor via phosphorylation. Associated with the receptor–ligand interaction are a group of accessory proteins. For example, a membrane-anchored proteoglycan betaglycan, also known as the TGF β Type III receptor, binds TGF β and increases its affinity for the signalling receptor. The Smad anchor for receptor activation (SARA) protein binds Smad 2 and 3 to enhance their interaction with the TGF β receptors. In addition, there are a host of proteins that interact with the ligand or the receptor to inhibit receptor activation.

The downstream effects of the activated receptor complex are mediated by the receptor-activated Smads (R-Smads). Smads 2 and 3 are recognized by TGF β and activin receptors, and Smads 1, 5 and 8 are recognized by BMP receptors, for example. Activation of the R-Smads leads to an association of the R-Smads with the co-Smads (i.e. Smad 4). This activated Smad heterodimer is translocated to the nucleus where it can interact with various DNA-binding cofactors, coactivators or corepressors to influence transcriptional activity.

Nuclear receptors

The nuclear receptor class of receptors acts functionally as transcription factors. Because they are located in the cytoplasm or in the nucleus, their ligands are lipophilic and pass easily through the membrane barriers of a cell. This is a large class of receptors that include steroid, thyroid and retinoic acid receptors. The thyroid and retinoid receptors along with the vitamin D receptor form a sister lineage to the steroid and retinoic acid orphan receptors (Fig. 5.22). The thyroid and retinoic acid receptor gene appears to have split off from the gene encoding a protosteroid receptor early in metazoan evolution likely before the origin of triploblastic and bilateral forms. The gene encoding this ancestral steroid-like receptor appears to have been lost in arthropods, whereas in molluscs it has taken on functions independent of hormone regulation. Thus, only in the deuterostomes has this receptor system been vastly expanded to act as receptors for a large family of diverse ligands. In insects, the ecdysteroid receptor complexes with the USP receptor which is an orthologue of the RXR retinoic acid receptor. One possibility is that the two receptor systems had a common origin early in arthropod evolution, and have taken on different functions during arthropod evolution.

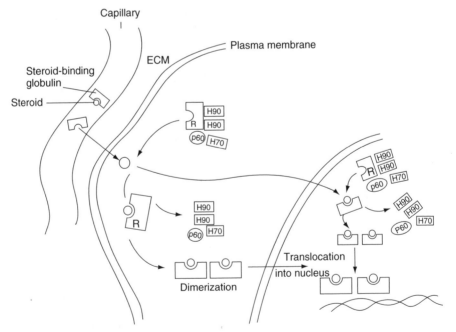

Figure 5.22 *Scheme for steroid ligand, receptor interaction in the cell.*

The nuclear receptors in their unliganded state are complexed with a number of chaperone proteins including some of the heat shock proteins (e.g. hsp90). These chaperones act as stabilizing factors and maintain the receptor in a form that allows interaction with its ligand. Upon binding the ligand, the chaperone proteins are displaced, allowing the receptor to either homodimerize or heterodimerize with other nuclear receptors or transcription factors that possess the appropriate interacting domain. Once dimerized, the cytosolic complex is translocated to the nucleus. In the nucleus, the complex acts to enhance or repress transcription of a given gene by direct interaction with a steroid responsive element of the gene promoter.

Nuclear receptors share a number of features including a DNA-binding domain composed of two zinc-fingers at the amino terminus, a nuclear localization signal in the middle portion of the protein and a hormone-binding region at the carboxy terminus. Depending upon the presence and sequence of the nuclear localization signal, the unliganded receptor may be found predominantly in either the cytoplasm or the nucleus. Three functional classes of receptors can therefore be recognized. The first class, exemplified by glucocorticoid receptors, is predominantly cytoplasmic that requires ligand binding for most of its actions such as nuclear translocation, specific DNA binding and transcriptional regulatory activity. The second class, for example, oestrogen and progesterone receptors, is capable of nuclear translocation, but the ability to bind their cognate DNA sequences is ligand dependent. The thyroid receptor is a model for the third class of receptor. It is localized primarily in the nucleus and binds to its specific DNA sequences with high affinity and generally represses transcription. The action of ligand-binding inhibits the repression.

Ionotropic receptors

The ligand-gated ion channel receptors act to mediate fast synaptic neurotransmission. Ligands for these receptors include acetylcholine, 5-HT, GABA, glutamate and glycine. This group of receptors form a superfamily that is characterized by the presence of an ion channel through the plasma membrane, formed from five subunits (Fig. 5.23). These channels may be selective for anions as in the case of $GABA_A$, glycine and the invertebrate glutamate-binding ion channels, or cations such as the 5-HT and acetylcholine receptors.

We might predict that ion channels represent among the oldest types of intracellular proteins that play a role with cell signalling. Ligand-gated channels may, therefore, represent the earliest type of hormone receptors. It is of interest that channel receptors being predicted to be one of the oldest classes of receptors are dedicated glutamate, GABA and glycine. As we saw in an earlier section, glutamate and glycine are amino acids that are not only easily synthesized by prebiotic conditions, but have also been found in meteorites suggesting that these amino acids were present at the beginning of the early development of life. Glutamate receptor-like ion channels are found in plants although appear not to be gated by glutamate. Thus, these proteins in metazoans may have begun initially as ion channels and after the divergence of the animals and plants they became associated with glutamate.

Ionotropic GABA receptors possess a heteromeric structure composed of three different genes. However, the GABA receptor in *C. elegans* required for locomotion requires

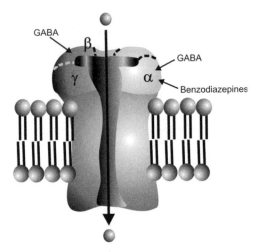

Figure 5.23   *Ionotropic receptors. (a) GABA receptor; (b) Position of glutamate ionotropic receptors in the post-synaptic membrane relative to positions of glutamate metabotropic receptors.*

only the UNC-49 gene. This gene contains one copy of the GABA receptor N-terminus, but three copies of the C-terminus. Thus three variants of the GABA receptor can be encoded by a single gene by the splicing of the N-terminus with each of the three different C-terminal regions.

As with most ligand-gated channels, the conductance is voltage insensitive for the GABA, AMPA and kainate receptors. In the GABA receptors, the amount of Cl^- introduced into the cell is dependent upon the membrane potential. The driving force of the Cl^- flow is the difference between the membrane potential and the chloride equilibrium potential ($-70\,mV$). If the membrane potential is substantially less than that of the Cl^- equilibrium potential, Cl^- will flow into the cell. When the membrane potential is equal to the Cl^- equilibrium potential, then there will be no net change on Cl^- flux. If, however, the membrane potential is substantially greater than the Cl^- equilibrium potential, then the Cl^- will leave the cytoplasm and pass to the extracellular spaces. A similar situation occurs in the AMPA and kainate receptors where the direction and magnitude of Na^+, K^+ and Cl^- flow is dependent upon the difference between the membrane potential and the equilibrium potential for each ion.

The mechanism of the NMDA receptor differs from that of the GABA, AMPA and Kainate receptors. NMDA receptors are voltage sensitive where the membrane potential affects their conductance. At the resting potential, the NMDA ion channel is blocked by Mg^{2+} ions. When the membrane becomes depolarized, the attractive forces on the Mg^{2+} ions weaken and diffuse away from the channel openings. Then K^+, Na^+, Cl^- and Ca^{2+} can all pass through. This ion flow tends to bring the membrane potential towards zero.

Receptor–ligand interactions

A receptor molecule as with any large protein is a highly dynamic structure. It is colliding, bumping and rotating constantly. The interaction and binding of a ligand with a receptor will act to stabilize its structure in a particular form such that it will increase the probability of interacting with the first proteins in the signal transduction cascade. However, given the dynamic nature of the receptor itself, it will to a limited degree interact with the transduction proteins without necessarily interacting with the ligand. The amount a receptor stimulates a given ligand is referred to as the constitutive activity of the receptor. Thus a ligand, instead of turning a ligand on or off is acting to increase or decrease the probability of action with its transduction proteins. Depending upon how a ligand interacts with a receptor it can have a different set of actions. Ligands can be classified as agonists or inverse agonists, antagonists or partial antagonists (Fig. 5.24).

Receptor–ligand matches

Until now, one might get the impression that ligand–receptor interactions follow a fairly organized pattern in that certain families of ligands only bind certain classes of receptors. This may be an artefact, in part, due to how we discover ligands and receptors. So much of our discovery process is based on homology searches. Because it is routine now to sequence genes and genomes, new peptide ligands and their receptors are identified by virtue of their sequence identity to known ligands and receptors. The concept of a particular peptide binding to different classes of receptors, for example, a G-protein-coupled receptor ligand, also activating a receptor kinase is largely unexplored. The head activator

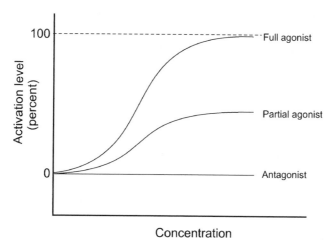

Figure 5.24 *Actions of agonistic and antagonistic ligands on a receptor response.*

peptide in hydra is required for normal development of the head region of hydra. It is synthesized and secreted by epithelial cells and appears to be under inhibitory regulation by the hydra nervous system. It is a small amphiphilic peptide similar to the type that typically binds G-protein-coupled receptors. Moreover, head activator peptide stimulates cAMP two-fold. CREB and PKA are also elevated. Surprisingly, no G-protein-coupled receptor has been identified. Instead, the head activator peptide binds to a member of the low-density lipoprotein receptor (LDLR) superfamily. It is a homologue of mammalian sorLA protein. Although this protein does not have an identified signal transduction system, other members of the LDLR superfamily do have. LRP6, a member of this superfamily, acts together with 'frizzled' as a core receptor for wnt. LRP6 is the receptor for the dickkopf family of wnt inhibitors.

In addition, T cell receptors known for their ability to bind antigens are also found in neurons where they also signal through a cAMP-mediated system. They may also bind to a variety of signalling molecules, although this concept has not been addressed. Steroid hormones on the other hand have been shown to bind G-protein-coupled receptors and ionotropic-type receptors as well as their own nuclear receptor.

Receptor–ligand co-evolution

The question of whether the ligand or the receptor evolved first for any given receptor–ligand system has occupied the thoughts of many evolutionary molecular biologists for a considerable period. As a result a number of models for receptor–ligand co-evolution have been developed.

Steroid receptor and ligand evolution

In the case of nuclear receptors, the position of a ligand-activated nuclear receptor in the phylogenetic tree is not related to the chemical nature of its ligand. Moreover, orphan receptors are present in most nuclear subfamilies. The ancestral nuclear receptor may have been an orphan receptor, in that it did not bind steroids, but later the various orphan receptors have acquired ligand-binding capability independently through evolution. It is possible that the original steroid receptors had a different function. In addition, although steroids have been identified in plants and fungi, receptors for these steroids are phylogenetically different from vertebrate nuclear receptors, suggesting that during evolution both the ligand and nuclear receptor coexisted before ligand-binding acquisition.

One possibility is that they simply acted as transcription factors that were independent of ligands, and evolved a ligand-binding ability after the rise of metazoans when it was necessary to coordinate the actions of an individual cell with the physiological needs of the organism. This may have also been the situation for some of the bioamine binding G-protein-coupled receptors and perhaps the ligand-gated ion channel receptors. Alternatively, the ancestral steroid receptors may have evolved as receptors for hydrophobic xenobiotic compounds synthesized by other organisms and released into the environment

(Chapter 13). An alternative hypothesis proposes that orphan receptors have evolved as liganded molecules, and that the ligand and its receptor have co-evolved over time. Gene duplication and divergence would have given rise to the present day diversity of nuclear receptors. This model, however, assumes that the nuclear receptors and their ligands co-evolve. However, because the ligand is not a protein, and has limited ability to change, as its structure is the end product of a suite of synthesizing enzymes, this scenario seems less likely. As such, slight modifications in sequence would be uncommon, which makes it unlikely that the receptor could change its specificity following duplication to bind a different ligand over time. It is difficult to conceive of what the ligand for the non-duplicated ancestor of the thyroid receptor and retinoic acid receptor would be, given the difference in structures of thyroid hormones and retinoic acid. Therefore, it appears as though the subfamilies of nuclear receptors were derived from ancestral orphan receptors, which acquired ligand-binding capacity independently through evolution, and that the present-day diversity of nuclear receptors can be attributed to two waves of gene duplication.

Peptide and receptor evolution

Peptides and proteins accrue a number of amino acid changes through mutation events. However, they may be lengthened or shorted by duplication or deletion of short strands of DNA. Orthologous peptides resident in different species will tend to retain many of the conserved motifs due to the similarity in the physiological and molecular constraints such as receptors, processing enzymes and binding proteins acting upon the peptide. The nature and type of change that occurs within a peptide is due to the more specialized niche adaption and the amount of physiological specialization occurs in such situations. For example, in artiodactyl ruminants, such as cattle and sheep, the evolutionary rate of corticotrophin-releasing factor, calcitonin and growth hormone has increased considerably. This change may have been due to the physiological and behavioural adaption of eating silicaceous grasses.

The structure of two sister paralogues at the point of gene duplication should be identical. If the gene duplication is due to a complete genome duplication, then the sister paralogues will behave in a similar physiological manner to each other, freely interacting with both of their associated receptors, processing enzymes and other associated molecules. Subgenomic duplication events may only allow for the duplication of the peptide, peptide and receptor, or any other combination depending upon how they are clustered on the genome. Theoretically, one of these paralogues is free to change while the other is not. However, several situations can occur as these peptides begin their movement towards separate identities. Initially they may be transcribed, translated and processed together and secreted in the same secretory vesicles. Binding and activation regions of a peptide are not necessarily the same, but the efficacy of both peptides could change as long as the peptides were released together. Thus, one might imagine where there is a change in a binding motif leading to a reduced affinity but similar activation ability once it does bind. In the other paralogue, activation ability may become compromised by the accrual of mutations in the relevant regions, whereas affinity does not change. If these changes confer a survival advantage to the organism, they will be selected for. If the changes are neutral they will remain in the gene pool.

Alternatively, one ligand may remain essentially the same depending upon the necessity of the motifs in the peptide required to interact with all other proteins. The other paralogue is, therefore, not under any such constraints and can accrue mutations and change in structure. Similar actions will be occurring at the receptor level and, indeed, all of the associated binding proteins and processing enzymes. We might imagine this as sort of a molecular ecosystem. Eventually changes will occur through the peptide genes such that its tissue and cellular-specific expression may change through mutations in the promoter or its function and ability to bind receptors will change. Once this begins to happen then the selective pressure on the two paralogous systems will begin a semi-independent evolution course. Thus, initially, after paralogues are initially formed they will go through a period where they accrue mutations at a relatively high rate. Once a new function of the peptide and receptor paralogue has developed, the pace of mutation accrual will slow down. Because both peptides may be interacting with both receptors, the system begins to co-evolve.

Chapter summary

The molecular basis of neuroendocrinology resides in a complex interaction of chemical messengers from distinct structural classes. The chemical nature of hormones has a bearing on the nature of receptor and other proteins they bind to, how they partition into tissues and ultimately how they are degraded. Most hormones are peptide- or protein-derived and comprise the largest group of hormones. Because of their relatively large size and amphiphilic nature, they cannot pass across the plasma membrane, and therefore bind and activate plasma membrane receptors primarily in the form of G-protein-coupled receptors and receptor kinases. Non-peptide hormones may be classified as lipophilic such as steroids, thyroid hormones and retinoids. These hormones pass across membranes and bind to nuclear receptors that are essentially ligand-activated transcription factors. A diverse group of hydrophilic hormones, derived biosynthetically from amino acids include monoamines, catecholamines, glutamic acid and GABA, activate G-protein-coupled receptors and ion channel receptors. The function of hormones and their receptors can vary among species (orthologues) and among genetic copies (paralogues). Several theories have been proposed for the co-evolution of ligands and their receptors.

6

Osmoregulation, metabolism and energy production

Introduction

Osmoregulation, metabolism and energy production have two things in common. On one hand, organisms must take in substances in the form of ions, water and nutrients for the processes to occur. On the other hand, these physiological processes are the most basic to the survival of the organism. All other systems are dependent upon the fulfilment of these basic needs. For this reason, all have been grouped in one chapter.

If the primary goal of a species is to reproduce, then the foremost goal of an individual organism is to survive long enough until the opportunity to reproduce arises. As we have seen in Chapter 1, the first step towards the definition of life was to partition life from non-life in the form of a plasma membrane. To ensure continued survival, the normal operation of the metabolic functions inside the cell must be protected. Among the most basic of these mechanisms is the regulation of water and ions transport across the membrane. The ionic character of the cell and tissues creates the appropriate environment for the various biochemical processes. Further, maintaining the ionic differential across the membrane creates an energy source that can be utilized by various reactions. Osmoregulation is the most basic of the cell's regulatory needs. Once this requirement is fulfilled, energy production via the various metabolic pathways can be achieved. Osmoregulation likely represents the phylogenetically oldest endocrine system, though not necessarily the oldest neuroendocrine system. The basic osmotic requirements of

Neuroendocrinology: An Integrated Approach   David A. Lovejoy
© 2005 John Wiley & Sons, Ltd

a cell have not changed appreciably since the evolution of the first eukaryotic cell. The signalling system for the control of osmoregulation, however, appears to have evolved after the first triploblastic animals evolved and is more or less intact in most triploblastic organisms.

If osmoregulation constitutes the primary and most important physiological need for organisms, then procurement of energy in the form of nutrients and its subsequent breakdown and distribution comprise, arguably, the second most important group of signalling systems in an organism. In an organism, feeding and osmoregulation are inter-related as food ingestion introduces water, salt and other essential ions into the organism. Because of this, many neurohormones regulate both processes.

Osmoregulation

Osmoregulation is the homeostatic regulation of dissolved ions and water balance to related but distinct physiological mechanisms. In one respect, there must be the maintenance of a constant volume of internal fluids in the face of changing ion concentrations. On the other hand, there must be the regulation of optimum ion concentrations during changing body fluid levels. The regulation of these activities occurs at both the cellular and organismal levels. Osmoregulation at the cellular level may involve changes in the permeability of membranes, active transport across membranes and passive movement of materials across membranes. Cellular dehydration results when the amount of dissolved ions (osmolality) in the extracellular fluid is greater than intracellular osmolality. As a result, water in the cells rushes down its concentration gradient, leaving the cells, and triggers dehydration and cell shrinkage. This occurs if the organism has not ingested enough water to keep up with metabolic demands. On the other hand, decreased extracellular volume may occur without accompanying osmolality changes. Such a situation occurs during injury with subsequent blood or body fluid loss. In vertebrates, this will be associated with a drop in blood pressure. In any organism, there are a number of physiological processes that are indirectly involved in the production and loss of water and ions. These are referred to as obligatory osmoregulatory mechanisms and involve passive diffusion across epithelial tissues, ingestion and defecation, and the production of metabolic water. The organism has no direct control over these processes. The organism must, therefore, compensate for the actions of the obligatory mechanisms and also for water and ion demand associated with particular environmental situations and the associated behaviours. In this case, the organism can regulate a number of active transport mechanisms to maintain homeostasis.

The amount of osmoregulatory ability varies considerably among species. Because metazoans evolved in an aqueous environment, osmoregulation was and remains the most basic regulated system to ensure cellular integrity and survival. For simple non-vascular organisms that remain in an aqueous environment, osmoregulatory mechanisms can be achieved primarily at the cellular or tissue level, and, therefore, will not be discussed here. These include many of the lophotrochozoan species. If organisms that are large enough require a vascular system, then the focus of regulation then shifts to the maintenance of the internal body fluid composition. This is particularly important for terrestrial organisms that must take a physiological water supply with them. In physiologically complex organisms that do not have a constant source of water, the regulation of behaviour associated with water ingestion also becomes an important regulatory mechanism. As a result, comparatively more regulation occurs at the central nervous system level.

Environment and osmoregulation

Depending upon the species and the environment it lives in, osmoregulatory pressures can vary considerably. Marine teleost fish, for example, are hypo-osmotic relative to the ambient seawater and, therefore, must protect against water loss. They can compensate by drinking seawater, and then secreting the excess salt via transporter systems in the gills. The cartilaginous fish, on the other hand, are slightly hyperosmotic relative to seawater, due to their ability to retain urea in their tissues as a compensating mechanism. Coelacanths have this ability as well. Thus, both groups need to protect against water entering the organism. These species, as a result, do not drink salt water and, in the case of elasmobranch fishes, will secrete excess salt via a rectal salt gland. Freshwater teleosts are in a physiologically similar situation in that they are also hyperosmotic to their ambient environment. These species do not ingest water, but also actively import salt across the gills. Once terrestrial chordates evolved, they were faced with the new challenge of taking a water and salt supply with them during their time on land. In aquatic species, water and ions can be easily obtained from the environment at any time. However, in terrestrial species, a number of new behaviours needed to evolve to be associated with the ingestion and retention of water and salt.

Renin-angiotensin system

Sodium, as the predominant cation, is required for extracellular fluid balance. Since the turn of the century, it has been known that the loss of extracellular fluid can generate thirst. However, sodium appetite is also increased under these circumstances. Sodium craving is present throughout a number of omnivorous and herbivorous terrestrial vertebrates, though the phenomenon is most studied in mammals and birds. Some species will travel great distances to ingest salt at mineral lick sites and other sources of salt when the sodium content of their diet is reduced. Sodium homeostasis is intimately tied to cardiovascular regulation and gustatory sensory input is the specific sensory system for identifying sodium in the environment. In mammals, females generally ingest greater amounts of sodium and water than males do, and can have greater concentrations of aldosterone circulating systemically.

The renin-angiotensin system (Fig. 6.1) is involved in the mediation of sodium regulation. Stimuli to the system include changes in blood pressure and blood osmolality. Although much of the initial regulation of this system occurs outside the brain, there are a number of important feedback mechanisms that modulate neural function and behaviour. The renin-angiotensin system can be activated during blood loss or by water and Na^+ deprivation.

Circulating angiotensin-II induces vasoconstriction, aldosterone release, augments the actions of the sympathetic nervous system and renal conservation of sodium and water. In vertebrates, this mechanism is initiated by the sodium sensors in the macula densa of the distal convoluted tubule of the nephron. The pathway continues to the juxtaglomerular granular cells found in the efferent arterioles of the nephron. These cells, when stimulated,

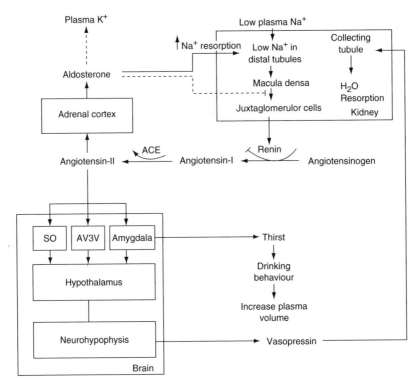

Figure 6.1 *Renin-Angiotensin System. Solid lines indicate stimulatory pathways, dashed lines indicated inhibitory pathways. ACE – angiotensin converting enzyme; AV3V – anteroventral tip of the third ventricle; SO – subfornical organ.*

secrete the enzyme renin in the blood stream where it actively converts angiotensinogen, an inactive plasma protein, into angiotensin-I. Angiotensin-I subsequently interacts with the carboxydipeptidase, angiotensin-converting enzyme (ACE), thereby converting angiotensin-I into angiotensin-II (Fig. 6.2). It was originally thought that ACE was limited to lung tissue; however, recent studies have shown that this enzyme is found in the

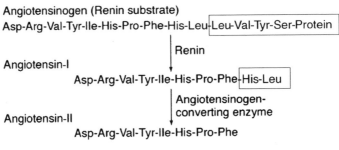

Figure 6.2 *Angiotensin-II processing.*

endothelium of blood vessels throughout the body. ACE possesses a number of substrates including bradykinin, tachykinins and substance P and, therefore, plays a much more widespread role in the processing of peptide hormones than originally thought. Liberated angiotensin-II has a direct effect on the adrenal cortex to stimulate the synthesis and release of the mineralocorticoid, aldosterone. Aldosterone acts on the kidney to increase sodium readsorption from the distal convoluted tubule.

Angiotensin-II also acts as a vasoconstrictor that elevates blood pressure by increasing blood volume and peripheral vascular resistance. Furthermore, angiotensin receptors found in the cardiovascular control centres can stimulate sympathetic output to heart and blood vessels thus increasing pressure by raising cardiac output. Once blood pressure has been restored and the retention of sodium has reached a threshold level, a feedback signal is sent to juxtaglomerular cells, which inhibits the release of renin thus maintaining homeostasis.

In the mammal brain, there are two types of angiotensin-II receptors – AT_1 and AT_2. The dipsogenic response to angiotensin-II is mediated by AT_1, whereas sodium appetite is mediated by both receptors. AT_1 receptors appear to be coupled to the phospholipase C/IP_3 system and a cGMP-mediated system where cGMP formation may be stimulated by nitric oxide. Peripherally, AT_1 receptors are located on pre- and post-capillaries on vascular smooth muscles and in the zona glomerulosa cells of the adrenal cortex. AT_2 receptors are located in the uterus and foetal tissue. When angiotensin-II reaches the adrenal glands AT_1 stimulates the synthesis and release of aldosterone.

The renin-angiotensin system is established in sarcopterygians and throughout the actinopterygians. It appears to be well developed in elasmobranchs and has recently been shown to be active in lampreys. A renin-angiotensin system has not been identified in hagfish, though this may reflect the technical difficulty of purification and characterization rather than the lack of such a system. The release of renin from the kidneys of fish can occur, like tetrapods, in response to a decline in blood pressure. In mammals, release of renin is also promoted by low plasma sodium concentrations, but this response is lacking in fish. Exogenously administered angiotensin-II has a vasoconstrictor action and increased blood pressure in teleosts, lungfish, elasmobranchs and in holosteans (bowfin). Injection of angiotensin or renin can promote the release of glucocorticoids in teleosts and elasmobranchs, and aldosterone and corticosterone in the Australian lungfish. Angiotensin-II can promote drinking in mammals, birds and reptiles (i.e. amniotes), and in amphibians it can stimulate water intake across the integument. Thus, this mechanism appears to have evolved as a function of terrestrial existence and a need to coordinate drinking behaviour with water sources, when they are available. This has also been observed in many teleosts and in some elasmobranchs but not agnathans. The teleosts that respond this way to angiotensin-II are usually species that may experience increases in the salinity of the water in which they live. The response may, therefore, represent an emergency one for promoting rehydration in such fishes.

Central actions of angiotensin-II

Although the peripheral renin-angiotensin system has been relatively well described in a number of species, local systems also appear to be present and active in the brain, heart, kidney, gonads and pancreas. In the brain, angiotensin-II may act as a paracrine neuromodulatory agent associated with a number of satiety, stress and behavioural neural circuits. In many cases it is not clear whether a neurological response is due to activation of the brain's renin-angiotensin system, or uptake of peripheral angiotensin-II into the brain.

Direct administration of angiotensin-II into the brain promotes the ingestion of water and sodium in a number of avian and mammalian species. Angiotensin-II-induced increase in water intake has been reported in amniotes, as well as amphibians and teleosts. However, some studies indicate that angiotensin-II may not have direct control of sodium intake in some teleost and lungfish species. The neural control of sodium ingestion by angiotensin-II may have evolved as part of the adaptations required for the terrestrial colonization by vertebrates.

When angiotensin-II is injected into the brain, mammals immediately begin to drink followed by a latency period before they are motivated to ingest sodium. Aldosterone and angiotensin-II can increase the sodium appetite in the brain of a sodium-depleted rat. Both are elevated during sodium depletion. The angiotensin-II system in the brain is widespread where it is acting as a central neuromodulator as well as in response to peripheral angiotensin-II and other signals. Angiotensin-II receptors and cell bodies are localized in the circumventricular organs, subfornical organ and organum vasculosum of the lateral terminalis (OVLT), and also the medial preoptic area (mPOA), magnocellular cells of the paraventricular nucleus (PVN), supraoptic nucleus (SON), zona incerta, lateral hypothalamus, parabrachial nucleus and solitary nucleus (Fig. 6.3). This pattern of expression reflects the role angiotensin-II has – ingestion and osmoregulatory activity. However, angiotensin-II infusion activates neurons in the central nucleus of the amygdala (CeA), anteroventral tip of the third ventricle (AV3V), subfornical organ, bed nucleus of the stria terminalis (BNST), PVN and SON. Thus, angiotensin-II also has a significant role in regulating the limbic system, and plays a role in the onset of some anxiogenic behaviours.

The blood–brain barrier restricts angiotensin-II entry into the brain. However, acting at circumventricular sites, particularly the subfornical organ and OVLT, peripheral angiotensin-II can regulate pituitary function, stimulate central pressor responses and elicit thirst. Subfornical neurons are responsive to changes in blood pressure; and in addition, osmoreceptors are located in the OVLT and AV3V. Systemic angiotensin-II acts on the

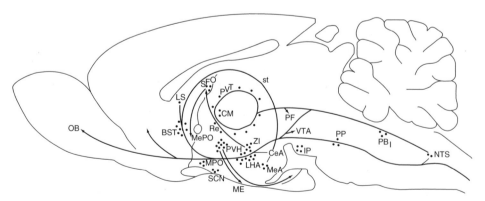

Figure 6.3 *Angiotensin-II in the brain. Reprinted with permission from Lind* et al. *(1985), Karger AG.*

subfornical organ to elicit the ingestion of water. Small amounts of angiotensin-II when ingested will elicit thirst. The subfornical organ is the most sensitive site in the brain for dipsogenic responses. Stimulation of these receptor systems, presumably by plasma angiotensin-II, then acts to stimulate vasopressin release from the neurohypophysis. Vasopressin increases water readsorption from the renal collecting tubule back into the blood (Fig. 6.1).

Angiotensin-II-induced thirst will occur if it is injected into the BNST and POA. Through subfornical connections to the anterior third ventricular regions that include the mPOA and OVLT, the two sites regulate the ingestion of water to angiotensinergic signals. Angiotensin injection into the BNST elicits thirst. The medial and central nuclei of the amygdala are functionally coupled to the BNST. The central nucleus of the amygdala receives the most projections from the brainstem gustatory sites and more general visceral information. It is rich in angiotensin nerve terminals. Thirst and sodium appetite, induced by central administration of renin or angiotensin-II and mineralocorticoid, are abolished in the central nucleus of the amygdala lesions through angiotensin-II-induced thirst.

Caudal neurosecretory system

Aquatic species utilize a second system to regulate ion balance. As discussed in Chapter 4, the urophysis is a neurohaemal organ in the caudal region of the spinal cord of most fishes. It possesses a structural similarity to the neurophysis in that the neurosecretory cells are found in the spinal cord and their axons terminate on fenestrated capillaries. The two principal hormones, urotensin-I and urotensin-II, are synthesized in these neurosecretory cells and released into the systemic blood supply. The urophysis also appears to contain significant amounts of acetylcholine, and in a few species, arginine-vasotocin may also be stored and released. Urotensin-I is a 41-amino acid peptide that is paralogous to CRF and the piscine orthologue of mammalian urocortin. Urotensin-II is a 12-residue cysteine-bridged peptide that some researchers suggested a structural similarity to somatostatin (Chapters 5 and 7) although the evolutionary origins of urotensin-II and somatostatin do not support a genetic commonality. There is also no structural similarity between urotensin-I and urotensin-II. They are named on the basis of the organ where they were found. Two populations of cells can be discerned. One group of cells expresses only urotensin-I, whereas the other expressed both urotensins. This arrangement is similar to that of the CRF- and vasopressin-expressing cells of the paraventricular nucleus (Chapter 9). Neurosecretory cells containing these hormones appear to exist in the caudal spinal cord regions of cartilaginous fish, non-teleost ray-finned fishes, lungfish and possibly lampreys. However, a discrete neurohaemal organ is not present in these species, only a region of diffuse neurosecretory tissue is present. There is no evidence of either hormone, or the presence of a caudal neurosecretory system present in hagfish. In teleosts, the urophysis receives rich aminergic, and to a limited extent, cholinergic and peptidergic innervation from the brain.

Urotensin-I in plasma has a number of apparent functions. It increases blood pressure and decreases chloride transport across gills. It also increases sodium transport across urinary bladder and intestine and may act on pituitary and adrenal glands. Urotensin-I likely acts directly on the pituitary gland to release ACTH (Chapter 9) and may also act directly on the interrenal tissue to stimulate the release of glucocorticoids. Urotensin-I

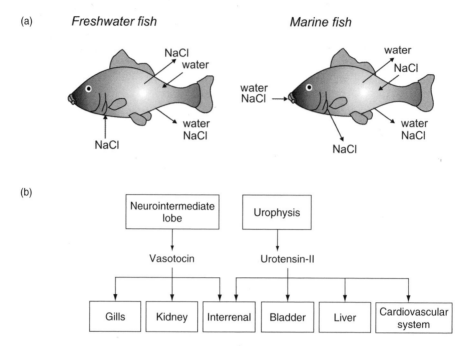

Figure 6.4 *Synergism between vasotocin and urotensin-II in teleost osmoregulation: (a) physiological challenges in fish depending on salinity conditions; (b) interaction between vasotocin and urotensin-II.*

also has a number of cardiovascular actions. In fish, urotensin-II has been linked with increased blood pressure, decreased chloride transport across the gills and increased sodium transport across the urinary bladder and intestine. The urophysis appears to play an essential role in fishes to deal with changes in ambient salinity conditions. Salinity conditions vary as a result of runoff, rainwater, evaporation and currents and so most fishes experience changing salinity conditions frequently. The urophysis may then offer a secondary neurohaemal mechanism to deal with osmoregulatory stress (Fig. 6.4). In terrestrial vertebrates, variants of urotensin-I and urotensin-II are produced in the brain and appear to have similar functional actions as those in fishes.

Neurohypophysial hormones

The principal neurohypophysial hormones consist of a single superfamily of cysteine-bridged nonapeptides (Fig. 6.5). They are classified as vasotocin (vasopressin)-like or oxytocin-like. Most chordates possess both variants, with the possible exceptions of hagfish and lampreys where only a vasotocin-like peptide has been identified. In vertebrates, the primary neurohypophysial hormone associated with the regulation of diuresis is [Arg8]-vasotocin, with the exception of mammals, which use the orthologous [Arg8] or [Lys8]-vasopressin. The peptide system appears to have evolved before the presence of triploblastic organisms as indicated by the presence of the related conopressins in gastropod molluscs (*Conus geographus*, *C. striatus*, *Lymnaea stagnalis*), cephalotocin

Oxytocin-like peptides

	1	2	3	4	5	6	7	8	9	
Oxytocin	Cys-Tyr-I1e-Gln-Asn-Cys-Pro-Leu-Gly(NH₂)									Placentals Some marsupials Ratfish
Mesotocin	---	---	---	---	---	---	---	Ile	---	Non-mammalian Tetrapods Marsupials Lungfishes
Isotocin	---	---	---	Ser	---	---	---	Ile	---	Bony fishes
Glumitocin	---	---	---	Ser	---	---	---	Gln	---	Rays
Valitocin	---	---	---	---	---	---	---	Val	---	} Spiny dogfish
Aspargtocin	---	---	---	Asn	---	---	---	---	---	
Asvatocin	---	---	---	Asn	---	---	---	Val	---	} Spotted dogfish
Phasvatocin	---	---	Phe-Asn		---	---	---	Val	---	

Vasopressin-like peptides

	1	2	3	4	5	6	7	8	9	
Vasopressin	Cys-Tyr-Phe-Gln-Asn-Cys-Pro-Arg-Gly(NH₂)									Mammals
Lysipressin	---	---	---	---	---	---	---	Lys	---	Pig Macropodids Didelphids Peramelids
Phenypressin	---	Phe	---	---	---	---	---	---	---	Macropodids
Vasotocin	---	---	Ile	---	---	---	---	---	---	Non-mammalian vertebrates

Figure 6.5 *Vasopressin superfamily of peptides. (*Residues identical with those of oxytocin or vasopressin are indicated by dashes.) After Acher (1999).*

in cephalopod molluscs (*Octopus vulgaris*) and [Leu², Thr⁴]-vasotocin in the suboesophageal and thoracic ganglia of the locust, *Locusta migratoria*. Like vasopressin in mammals, vasotocin has antidiuretic activity in birds and amphibians but has diuretic effects in fish. Vasopressin can increase the permeability of water in *Amoeba*. It appears to achieve this by direct interaction with the plasma membrane forming a local disruption through which water can pass. This can also occur with other amphiphilic peptides. Early in eukaryote evolution, membrane permeability may have occurred by a direct action of the peptide with the membrane and only later became to be mediated by a receptor system.

The vasotocin- and oxytocin-like peptides mediate their actions via at least four different receptor systems depending upon the species. The V1a receptor is associated with the vascular smooth muscle contraction and liver glycogenolysis, whereas the V1b receptor is implicated with ACTH release (Chapter 9). The V2 receptor on the other hand is required for the regulation of water permeability in the renal tubules and generally mediates the antidiuretic effects of vasotocin. The OT receptor mediates both the central and peripheral actions of oxytocin. The V1 and OT receptors utilize inositol triphosphate and Ca^{2+}-mediated signalling systems, whereas the V2 receptors primarily couple to a Gs protein that regulates cAMP. Two vasotocin-like/oxytocin-like receptors have been found in the snail *L. stagnalis*. The LSCPR2 does not discriminate between Lys-conopressin and oxytocin-like peptides. The LSCPR1, on the other hand, is relatively specific for Lys-conopressin. The vasotocin- and oxytocin-like receptors likely evolved from a relatively promiscuous receptor perhaps similar to the LSCPR2 receptor.

Amphibians' successful colonization of terrestrial habitats approximately 200–300 million years ago may be attributed, in part, to their regulation of total body water balance by vasotocin. Amphibians utilize a dual strategy depending upon their stage of development. In tadpoles, osmoregulation and volemia is based on the gut, kidney and gills, as in fresh-water fishes. In the adult, however, the gut, kidney, urinary bladder and skin are utilized. Much water is lost across the integument. Although vasotocin regulates the water permeability in the former three organs, it is less effective in skin. Anurans utilize a downstream post-translational to process vasotocin into vasotocinyl-Gly or hydrin-2. In *Xenopus laevis*, vasotocin is processed into vasotocinyl-Gly-Lys-Arg or hydrin-1. The hydrins are more active on the water permeability of skin and bladder but lack antidiuretic activity. Amphibians have two types of vasotocin receptors, V1 and V2, that are homologous to the vascular hepatic V1 and renal V2 vasopressin receptors respectively of mammals. Amphibians appear to possess two types of V2 receptors: a renal subtype that mediates the readsorption of water in renal tubules by vasotocin, and the skin/bladder subtype that is relatively specific for the hydrins.

Oxytocin acts as an inhibitory signal on ingestive behaviours. In mammals central oxytocin injections inhibit both hypovolemic and angiotensin-II–induced sodium appetite while also promoting sodium excretion. Oxytocin inhibition of this system may occur via the BNST. Oxytocin can function physiologically as an antidiuretic hormone. In a study done on the urinary bladders of toads, effects of vasotocin and oxytocin were compared. Vasotocin does not play a significant role in the overall regulation of water balance when the species was in a well-hydrated state. The plasma concentrations of vasotocin appeared to increase during periods of dehydration and reduced kidney glomerular filtration rate, as well increased the apical membrane permeability of distal tubules. Oxytocin has also been shown to increase water permeability in the urinary bladders of toads. In a study performed in Brattleboro, the strain of rats, which have a lack of vasopressin and excrete copious quantities of urine oxytocin, can function as an antidiuretic hormone although it is less potent than vasopressin with regard to its hydro-osmotic effect.

The peripheral role of the vasotocin-like peptides has changed throughout the various vertebrate classes. The ancestral actions of vasotocin may have been primarily a vascular response mediated by V1 receptors. In most vertebrates, vasotocin influences the contractility of vascular smooth muscle. In fish, however, it does not influence water readsorption across the renal tubules, in contrast to terrestrial vertebrates, although it does play a role in water movement across the gills. In some amphibians (notably anurans), birds and reptiles, vasotocin generally acts to increase water readsorption and decrease glomerular filtration rate. In mammals, however, vasopressin acts to decrease urinary water loss primarily by the increased readsorption of water across the renal tubules. It does not have the vasotocin-like effects on non-vascular smooth muscle contraction.

Diuretic systems

A number of hormonal systems act antagonistically to the renin-angiotensin-I system to decrease water and salt load if either increase beyond homeostatic limits. Cells in the atria of the heart resemble endocrine cells; the number of the cells can be increased by sodium loading and decreased by Na^+ restriction. Cardiac volume receptors are coupled to the endocrine function of the atria. The natriuretic peptides form a family of structurally related peptides including atrial (ANP), brain (BNP) and C-type (CNP) natriuretic peptides (Fig. 6.6). Elements of this system are present in the basal chordates and in invertebrates. In vertebrates, increased plasma volume stimulates atrial receptors by distention, in addition to the increased sodium concentration–releasing ANP. ANP is antagonistic to the renin-angiotensin system. ANP inhibits renin release by a direct action on the juxta-glomerular cells (Fig. 6.7). In fishes, the ANP system may be more acutely tuned to changes in ambient salinity and act as part of the renin-angiotensin-urophyseal osmoregulatory system. In the eel, *Anguilla anguilla*, ANP is secreted when blood plasma osmolality increases as it stimulates the excretion of Na^+ to promote saltwater adaptation.

These peptides have been classified into three or four groups based on several factors such as their structure on the organization of their separate encoding genes. The first group is found mostly in the atrial heart muscle and is called Type A natriuretic peptide or ANP-28. ANP has been identified in fish, amphibians and reptiles. When precursor ANP is cleaved its products exhibit biological activity in mammals. Examples include a sodium-stimulating peptide (proANP 31–67) as well as a vessel dilator peptide (proANP 79–98) and a kaliuretic stimulator peptide (proANP 79–98). The kaliuretic peptide promotes renal potassium excretion. Present in the heart and brain is the Type B natriuretic peptide known as BNP. BNP maintains the same ring structure as ANP; however, the N terminal amino acid chain is extended. There are a number of amino acid substitutions among BNP orthologues in mammals, unlike ANP, which is relatively conserved. Type C natriuretic

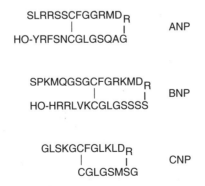

Figure 6.6 *Human peptide sequences of the ANP superfamily members.*

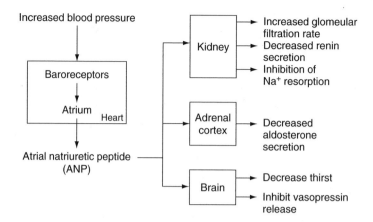

Figure 6.7   *Actions of ANP in mammals.*

peptide (CNP) is mainly found in the brain but have been found in the heart of some fish. CNPs lack the C-terminal amino acid tail that is characteristic in types A and B and it contains 22 residues. There is a high conservation of CNPs. The 17 residue rings of the CNP in pigs and killifish are identical. In the ventricles of teleosts, a fourth type of natriuretic peptide is found and is termed 'VNP'. It contains 36 residues and has greater similarity to ANP than to BNP. Natriuretic peptide can decrease the response of vasopressin, renin, aldosterone and CRF. There are three types of membrane receptors. Two of which are linked with the activation of guanylate cyclase and are called GC-A or ANP A and GC-B or ANP B. GC-A has the most affinity for ANP and BNP and GC-B for CNP. Other receptors are called C type or clearance receptors.

Atrial natriuretic peptide is expressed in BNST, central and medial nuclei of amygdala, AV3V, PVN, lateral hypothalamic regions, parabranchial and solitary nuclei in the brainstem (Fig. 6.8). Receptors are present in a number of regions including circumventricular organs and brainstem sites such as the solitary nucleus. ANP infused into the subfornical organ reduces angiotensin-induced water drinking. Centrally administered ANP decreases

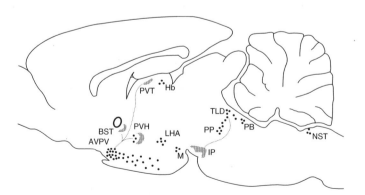

Figure 6.8   *ANP expressing sites in the rat brain. Reprinted from Standaert* et al. *(1985) by the permission of Elsevier Science Ltd.*

sodium appetite in sodium-depleted rats. Peripheral ANP shows no such effects. ANP reduces the motivated behaviour of the sodium-hungry rats. Thirst and sodium appetite induced by central administration of AII are also inhibited by ANP. However, ANP does not have an effect on other forms of ingestive behaviour such as sucrose intake. This it appears to be specific for sodium. In mammals, ANP is diuretic, natriuretic and vasodilatory and acts to reduce aldosterone and vasopressin secretion.

Role of prolactin

In fishes and amphibians, prolactin plays a major osmoregulatory role. All teleost prolactins lack the presence of an N-terminal disulphide bond due to the apparent deletion of several amino acids at the N-terminus, relative to the prolactins of the sarcopterygian and tetrapod lineages. This modification may be responsible in part for the increased osmoregulatory role of prolactin in teleosts. The majority of prolactin-secreting cells of the pituitary are found primarily in a cluster in the rostral pars distalis (Chapter 4). Prolactin can increase plasma Na^+ and Cl^- concentrations by reducing the rate of sodium chloride secretion from the branchial chloride-secreting cells. A number of studies suggest that prolactin can decrease the permeability of osmoregulatory organs such as gill, kidney, intestine, bladder and the integument to water and appears to be important for supporting survival in freshwater (see section on Metamorphosis in Chapter 7). However, there are considerable species differences with respect to the actions of prolactin on the various organs. There are over 24 000 species of teleosts occupying a wide range of salinities, temperatures and other conditions, and the synthesis and release of prolactin varies considerably with respect to these conditions. In amphibians, prolactin appears to have a similar action on the gills of the tadpole stage and may act to inhibit sodium loss in the adult by down-regulating sodium channels in the integument of adults.

As noted in Chapter 5, prolactin and growth hormone are paralogous. Functional evidence of this paralogy is apparent in teleosts where growth hormone also plays a role with osmoregulation. In salmonids, for example, Na^+/K^+ ATPase activity in the gill is enhanced in response to growth hormone. Both growth hormone and prolactin play key roles in freshwater-to-saltwater adaptation.

Osmoregulation in non-chordates

Several elements of the renin-angiotensin system are well established in both ecdysozoan and lophotrochozoan lineages suggesting that this osmoregulatory system evolved early in bilaterians, and well before the Precambrian explosion. Among lophotrochozoan species, annelids and molluscs have been comparatively well studied. Angiotensin-II orthologues are present in both the brain and segmental ganglia of the leech, *Theromyzon tessulatum*, and in the brain and ventral nerve cord of the polychaete, *Nereis diversicolor*. In leeches, there is a truncated and amidated version of angiotensin-II as well as the intact angiotensin-II peptides. Angiotensin-II amide may be as much as 100 times more potent than the untruncated variant at eliciting a diuretic response (Fig. 6.9).

Glial cells in leeches express immunoreactive forms of ACE, renin and angiotensin-II. Among ecdysozoan taxa, most of the investigations have been associated with arthropod

(a)

Amino acid sequences of AngI or AngII from various vertebrate and invertebrate species

		1				5					10
Mammals											
Human**		D	R	V	Y	I	H	P	F	H	L
Ox, Sheep		D	R	V	Y	V	H	P	F	H	L
Birds											
Fowl, Quail		D	R	V	Y	V	H	P	F	S	L
Reptiles											
Snake		Acyl.Asx	R	V	Y	V	H	P	F	Y	L
Turtle		D	R	V	Y	V	H	P	F	H	L
Alligator		D	R	V	Y	V	H	P	F	A	L
Amphibians											
Bullfrog		D	R	V	Y	V	H	P	F	N	L
Frog skin	A-P-G	D	R	I	Y	V	H	P	F		
Fishes											
Teleost											
Goosefish		N	R	V	Y	V	H	P	F	H	L
Salmon		N/D	R	V	Y	V	H	P	F	N	L
Eel		N/D	R	V	Y	V	H	P	F	G	L
Elasmobranch											
Dogfish		N	R	P	Y	I	H	P	F	E	L
Holostean		D	R	V	Y	V	H	P	F	N	L
Annelids											
Hirudinae											
T. tessulatum*		D	R	V	Y	I	H	P	F	H	L
E. octoculata*		D	R	V	Y	I	H	P	F-amide		

Acyl-AsX indicates that the N-terminal D or N is acylated. For further references regarding each AI (see Refs. [6–11]). **Pig, rat, horse and sheep AI have the same sequence. Underlined amino acid residues are those that differ from Human or leech AI. *Our data.

(b)

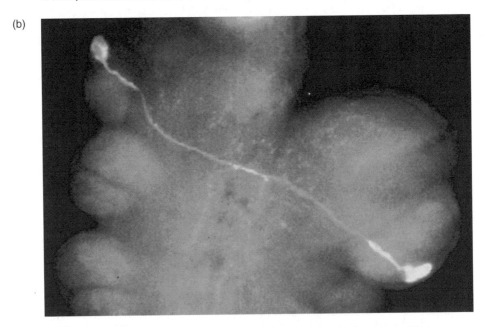

Figure 6.9 *Angiotensin-II in leech: (a) comparison of angiotensin-II sequences; (b) immunoreactive angiotensin-II in the brain of a leech. Reprinted from Salzet et al. (2001) by the permission of Elsevier Science B.V.*

species. Both angiotensin-II and ACE immunoreactivity have been detected in the central nervous system of the African locust, *L. migratoria*, where some of the cells also co-express variants of the FXPRL-NH2 (locustomyotropins) family. These cells project into the nervi corpori cardiaci which then lead to the neurohaemal region of the corpus cardiacum (Chapter 4). The crab, *Chasmagnathus granulatus*, possesses both angiotensin-II and ACE immunoreactivity in the thoracic and supraoesophageal ganglia. The enzyme, ACE, has been isolated and structurally characterized from a number of arthropods. Despite having a similar activity profile to mammalian ACE, it is structurally quite different. Little is known about the angiotensin receptors in invertebrates, as presently none have been structurally characterized.

In insects after feeding, or following adult eclosion, a number of hormones are released to stimulate urine production and to increase water loss via the excretory system. In *Rhodnius prolixus*, for example, ingestion of a blood meal induces an intense bout of diuresis that involves the crop, Malpighian tubules and hindgut and is under neuroendo-crine control. Urine production is achieved by secretion in the Malpighian tubules and is under active hormonal control but does not utilize the ultrafiltrate that is typical of the vertebrate mechanism as insects possess an open circulatory system and may not have the pressure requirements. The diuretic peptides, such as myokinins, cardioaccelatory peptide, 2b (CAP 2b), and the indoleamine hormone, 5-HT, all appear to play a role in diuresis. The diuretic peptides, which share structural similarity to the CRF peptides and play similar functional roles, stimulate the active transport of Na^+ and K^+ via a cAMP-mediated mechanism. Myokinins and CAP 2b utilize a Ca^{2+}-mediated pathway to increase passive Cl^- influx into the Malpighian tubule lumen. These hormones, therefore, act synergistically to promote urine production. A new variant of the diuretic hormone from the cockroach, *Diploptera punctata*, and the fruit fly, *D. melanogaster*, has structural similarity to both the vertebrate calcitonin peptides and the vertebrate CRF paralogues, urocortin II and III. Chicken calcitonin can stimulate fluid flow in *D. punctata*. Thus CRF peptides and calcitonin peptides may have arisen from the same ancestral gene in early metazoans and therefore both may have overlapping functions. This will be discussed in more detail in Chapter 9.

Calcium regulation

Calcium is essential for life in all organisms. Chemically, it can exist as a highly soluble ion, or as an insoluble mineral. Calcium can, therefore, possess both signalling and structural functions. Indeed, it was probably utilized early in cellular evolution as a signalling molecule. The concentration of calcium in vertebrates is similar to that in brackish water and may reflect the ancient ambient conditions of calcium when the first cells evolved. In organisms, it possesses a number of functions. It stabilizes biological membranes, and is also involved with calcium-mediated nerve impulse transmission. It is also essential for muscle contraction and cytoskeletal function, cellular and vesicle transport. It plays a major role in the secondary messenger system in cells. In vertebrates, it is required for the formation of bones and eggshells.

However, depending on the habitat of the species, the mechanisms of calcium homeostasis vary. Marine animals, for example, possess an unlimited store of calcium in the form of the sea around them but all other organisms must maintain an internal store of calcium and obtain it through their diet. Calcium equilibrium between the bones and the plasma can be maintained in two different ways. On the one hand, there exists a chemical equilibrium between the minerals of the bones and that in the plasma. Mineral ions are adsorbed or lost by bone via ionic interaction between the constituents of bone and plasma. On the other hand, a biological equilibrium exists in species that possess cells in their bones. Here, cells under organismal control actively secrete substances to promote or inhibit bone calcium. Lower teleosts and tetrapods possess cellular bone and therefore have active (biological) and dynamic equilibrium between calcium in bone and in other tissues. Higher teleosts possess acellular bone and, therefore, only possess a static equilibrium between bone and tissues and is under less active regulation.

Several organ systems are responsible for the regulation of calcium homeostasis in vertebrates. In the intestine, the control of calcium adsorption is regulated. In the kidney, calcium concentrations may be regulated via reabsorption from glomerular filtrate. In fishes, active efflux and influx of calcium ions are utilized. Species that possess cellular bone regulate the calcium storage or its readsorption. A number of hormones including parathyroid hormone, calcitonin, vitamin D and prolactin in terrestrial vertebrates all play a role in calcium homeostasis. In fishes, stanniocalcin is also utilized. The sex steroid, oestradiol and testosterone also play modulatory roles in the regulation of calcium.

Because calcium is so essential to the normal function of all tissues, like sodium regulation, much of calcium regulation occurs outside the nervous system. The concentration of calcium is determined in a variety of tissues by the calcium-sensing receptor, a G-protein-coupled receptor structurally homologous to the metabotropic glutamate receptor. It appears to be found in all calcium-regulating tissues in the body and is also present in the brain. Systemically, in mammals, a decrease in plasma calcium will act upon the chief cells of the parathyroid gland to increase synthesis and release of parathyroid hormone (PTH) into the blood (Fig. 6.10). PTH will act on the proximal convoluted

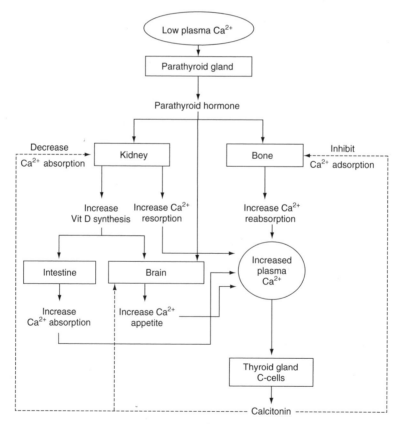

Figure 6.10 *Neuroendocrine control of calcium ingestion. The solid lines are positive, and the dotted lines are inhibitory pathways.*

tubules in the kidney to increase the synthesis and release of the active metabolite of vitamin D, 1,25-dihydroxycholecalciferol, that subsequently acts upon the intestine to regulate Ca^{2+} readsorption. PTH also induces the activity of renal Ca^{2+} transporter systems to increase the readsorption of Ca^{2+} from the glomerular filtrate. PTH also acts directly on the osteoclasts and osteoblasts in bone to increase Ca^{2+} readsorption into the blood. These mechanisms act synergistically to bring about an increase in plasma calcium concentrations. PTH and parathyroid glands are not present in the fish. However, parathyroid hormone-related peptide (PTHrP) is present in the brain and pituitary of all jawed vertebrates. The peptide can be post-translationally processed to produce different molecular forms. In fishes, the peptide expression, processing and release are modulated by the ambient salinity and, therefore, may play a role in the transition between different salinity conditions.

Vitamin D acts to conserve and redistribute sources of calcium and is analogous to aldosterone's role in sodium balance. Under normal circumstances, in mammals, increased production of the active vitamin D metabolite from the kidney will act to inhibit PTH release from the parathyroid glands. However, vitamin D receptors are localized in the same regions of the brain as aldosterone receptors, such as the medial amygdala that underlie sodium appetite and that also may be associated with calcium appetite. Vitamin D and calcium deficiency can activate calcium-binding proteins in a number of tissues. UV light, which increases the dermal production of vitamin D, also appears to induce Ca^{2+} ingestion. Calcium sensor systems in the limbic system may also play a role at stimulating calcium appetite if plasma levels of calcium fall too low.

Calcitonin acts antagonistically to parathyroid hormone to decrease plasma calcium concentrations if they rise above the homeostatic optimum. In mammals, calcitonin is released by the parafollicular or c-cells of the thyroid gland in response to high calcium concentrations. Plasma calcitonin acts to inhibit calcium readsorption in bone and from the glomerular filtrate in the kidney. Calcitonin also appears to cross the blood–brain barrier to gain access to the brain. Although the role of calcitonin in the brain is not well understood, it has been associated with neural function in mammals, including humans. The calcitonin-like peptides have been implicated in the origin of major depression and bipolar disorder. The calcitonin receptors form a sister lineage to that of the CRF receptors suggesting a functional overlap between the two peptide systems (p. 256). Cerebrospinal fluid concentrations of calcitonin are lower in patients with major depression than normal individuals. Recently, a 16-bp microdeletion polymorphism of the calcitonin/calcitonin gene-related peptide (CGRPα) gene was found in one family with multiple cases of unipolar or bipolar depression. Calcitonin injections into the midbrain can impair fear conditioning in rats. CT-binding sites are highly concentrated in regions of the brain associated with anxiety-related behaviours. Patients with bipolar disorder respond to 5-HT treatment by having higher intracellular calcium concentrations than control individuals. Moreover, the neuronal calcium sensor-1 protein gene is upregulated in the prefrontal cortex of patients with bipolar disorder. Thus, some mood disorders may be associated with an aberrant regulation of intracellular calcium.

Stanniocalcin, a homodimeric glycoprotein originally identified as a protein secreted from the corpuscles of Stannius in fishes, is now recognized as a major hypocalcaemic factor in all vertebrates. At least two forms of the protein appear to exist, and in some primitive bony fish, such as the osteoglossiformes, it may exist in the monomer form. It is present in a variety of tissues including the brain, heart, kidney, gill, gut, gonads, liver and pancreas. Moreover, recent evidence indicates that at least two immunoreactive forms of stanniocalcin are present in annelids, suggesting that the protein may play a much more fundamental role in calcium metabolism than previous thought. In mammals, stanniocalcin stimulates bone mineralization by increasing phosphate uptake in osteoblasts via a Na^{2+}-dependent phosphate transporter. In the kidney and intestine, stanniocalcin modulates calcium and phosphate excretion in most vertebrates. Recent studies have implicated stanniocalcin receptors on the mitochondria of hepatocytes and nephron cells where they may play a role in the regulation of cell metabolism. In the brain, stanniocalcin may act to protect neurons from an influx of calcium following ischaemia.

Feeding and appetite regulation

As western society continues to struggle with the growing obesity problem of its population, resources will continue to pour into understanding the physiological mechanism by which this occurs. In the last five to ten years, more has been learned about the mechanisms of appetite and metabolism than in the history of humans on this planet. Consequently, we have developed a long list of hormones, neuromodulators and transmitters that have been implicated in appetite regulation (Table 6.1). However considering the probability that only a few of the peptide hormones have been identified, we may expect the number of hormones associated with appetite regulation to double over the next five years as we learn more.

Why should there be so many modulators of appetite, ingestion and metabolism? As we have discussed in Chapter 1, these mechanisms are essential to survival and therefore the first to evolve. Moreover, these systems have co-evolved with sensory systems,

Table 6.1   *Hormones with feeding- and appetite-modifying properties*

Adrenocorticotropic hormone (ACTH)	Insulin
Agouti-related protein (AgRP)	Leptin
Calcitonin	Melanin-concentrating hormone (MCH)
Cholecystokinin (CCK)	Melanocyte-stimulating hormone (MSH)
Corticotrophin-releasing factor (CRF)	Neuropeptide Y
Cortisol/corticosterone	Norepinephrine
β-Endorphin	Parathyroid hormone (PTH)
Galanin	Prolactin
Gastrin	Secretin
Gastrin-releasing peptide (GRP)	Testosterone
Ghrelin	Thyroxine-stimulating hormone (TSH)
Glucagon	TSH-releasing factor (TRF)
Growth hormone	Urocortin/Urotensin-I
Growth hormone-releasing hormone (GHRH)	Vasoactive intestinal peptide (VIP)
Hypocretin/orexin	

locomotion, energy metabolism and as species become more advanced then psychosocial elements become associated with food intake and digestion. Consider that an organism must first be aware that it is becoming depleted of essential nutrients, then it must subsequently begin to search for food, a mechanism that involves the coordination of sensory systems and locomotory systems. Thus, we could consider that specific neurohormone systems exist for the anticipation of food, the stereotypical foraging of food, the perception of food and perhaps the orientation of the head and body towards the food source. Such systems may likely play a facilitatory effect with the interaction of the systems associated with hunting and capture of food. Subsequent to this will be locomotory systems associated with ingesting the prey, then the various systems associated with the digestions, absorption and excretion of food. Likely then, any one of these systems if inhibited will inhibit appetite and food ingestion. In addition to this, there will be of course all the stress-related neurohormonal systems that act to inhibit feeding (Chapter 9).

Energy production and utilization

Metazoans require a continuous supply of energy that is derived from the anaerobic process of glycolysis and the aerobic breakdown of primarily glucose and free fatty acids (Fig. 6.11). Recall from Chapter 2 that the earliest cells only possessed the anaerobic process of glycolysis, until they became symbiotic with an aerobic organism. In mammals, amino acids appear to account for less than 5% of the energy utilization. During increased activity, the enhanced production of glucose and free fatty acids is achieved primarily by an increase in sympathetic nervous system activation. In the rat, during moderate exercise, the adrenal medulla releases epinephrine with little or no norepinephrine being produced.

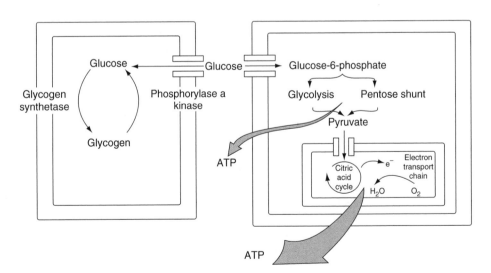

Figure 6.11 *Storage and breakdown of glucose.*

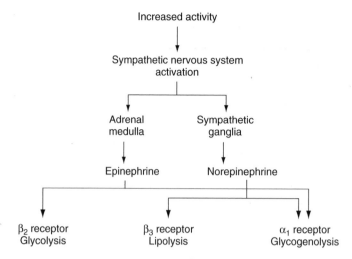

Figure 6.12   *Respective roles of epinephrine and norepinephrine during exercise.*

Circulating norepinephrine at this time is derived mostly from sympathetic nerve endings innervating the cardiovascular system.

Epinephrine has much higher affinity for β_2-adrenergic receptors than norepinephrine; thus under normal conditions, circulating levels of norepinephrine are insufficient to stimulate the β_2-receptors. The metabolic actions of the catecholamines are, therefore, mediated primarily by epinephrine. The other adrenergic receptors bind the ligands with more or less the equal affinity. Both epinephrine and norepinephrine stimulate glycogenolysis directly by an α_1-adrenergic-mediated activation of the liver parenchymal cells and indirectly by α_1-adrenergic-mediated release of prostaglandin synthesis in non-parenchymal cells. Lipolysis, on the other hand, is stimulated by β_3-adrenergic receptors. Norepinephrine has higher affinity than epinephrine for β_3-adrenergic receptors. Thus, epinephrine tends to mediate glycogenolysis and increased plasma glucose levels, whereas norepinephrine is responsible for the plasma-free fatty acid rise due to the lipolysis in the adipocytes (Fig. 6.12).

HPT axis and evolution

The hypothalamus–pituitary–thyroid axis is regulated centrally by a thyrotrophin-releasing factor in the hypothalamus (Fig. 6.13). Thyrotrophin-releasing hormone (TRH) is a tripeptide produced and secreted into the vasculature at the median eminence, in mammals, by the paraventricular cells in the hypothalamus and acts as the chief regulatory peptide to induce the release of thyroid hormone-stimulating hormone (TSH; thyrotrophin) from the pituitary gland. In a number of non-mammalian vertebrates, corticotrophin-releasing factor (CRF) appears to also play a significant role in stimulating TSH release from the pituitary. In phylogenetically older lineages of vertebrates, CRF may act as the primary TSH-releasing factor of the hypothalamus. In mammals some studies indicate that both CRF

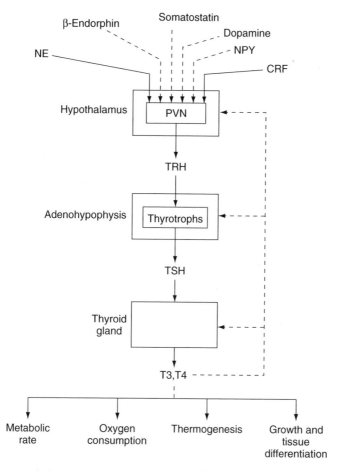

Figure 6.13 *Hypothalamus–pituitary–thyroid axis. Solid lines indicate stimulatory pathways whereas dashed lines indicate inhibitory pathways.*

and TRH have positive and reciprocal actions on the release of each other and can act in a synergistic manner (Fig. 6.14).

The release of TSH into the blood stream from the anterior pituitary stimulates the thyroid glands into releasing thyroid hormones into the blood stream. Thyroid hormones are biosynthetically derived from tyrosine and include two principle products: thyroxine (T4) and triiodothyronine (T3) (Chapter 5). These hormones differ in the number of iodine atoms attached to the phenyl ring of the hormone. The thyroid hormones are degraded in the liver and other tissues by deiodinase enzymes. Thyroid hormones have a number of functions. Generally they have modulatory effects on other hormones. They are associated with increased consumption of oxygen and the modulation of metabolic enzymes. They synergize with growth factors to establish adequate growth and tissue differentiation, and they facilitate thermogenesis. Thyroid hormones are highly hydrophobic and, therefore,

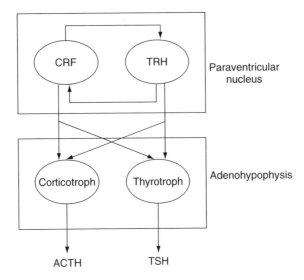

Figure 6.14   *Interaction between CRF and TRH.*

require a transport protein in the plasma to ensure that once released into the systemic circulation will remain there until they reach their target tissues.

The transthyretin proteins act as thyroid hormone distributor proteins in vertebrates and have been identified in all major gnathostome lineages. The transthyretins are synthesized and released by the choroid plexus from reptiles, birds and all mammal groups. It acts as the primary thyroid-distributing protein in the brain. The choroid synthesis of this protein may have first occurred in the stem reptile that was the common ancestors of modern reptiles, birds and mammals. The cortex as a region of the brain first occurs in this clade of vertebrates. Mammalian transthyretins bind T4 with higher affinity than T3 whereas avian transthyretins bind T3 with higher affinity than T4.

Larval lampreys have an endostyle like that of ascidian tunicate larva and *amphioxus*. It has the ability to bind iodide and synthesize thyroid hormones in addition to its function as a feeding apparatus. At metamorphosis the endostyle transforms into a thyroid gland with follicles. The thyroid gland may have evolved as organisms moved from an iodine-rich marine environment to the low-iodine concentration environment found in freshwater. Thus, it was necessary for these species to develop a mechanism to concentrate and store iodine.

Feeding and satiety in invertebrates

The allatostatins may play a role in feeding and digestion in the arthropods and other invertebrate species. The allatostatins are a large multifunctional family of peptides identified in the arthropods, primarily in insects and crustaceans, but also appear to be present in platyhelminthes and molluscs. In cockroaches and crickets, where they have probably been the most studied, they are released by the corpora allata and act to modulate, the synthesis of juvenile hormone (JH). They are distributed in a number of tissues but particularly in the brain. However, their function has not been established in other insect

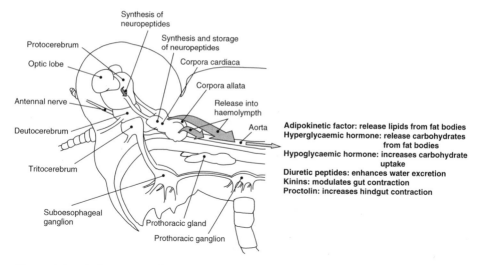

Figure 6.15 *Release sites of some key neuropeptides associated with ingestion in insects.*

orders or in other invertebrates and therefore these peptides may have been initially utilized as modulators of gut contractility, then utilized by the orthopteran species as neuroendocrine regulators of JH synthesis (Fig. 6.15).

The insect diuretic hormones, in addition to their role in osmoregulation, also appear to be involved in satiety and feeding. The *Locusta* diuretic hormone (DH) injected into food-deprived locusts will act to close the apical pores of the taste sensilla on the maxillary palps. Closure of these pores appears to indicate satiety in the insects as they typically close after feeding. This suggests that diuretic peptides may function in a similar manner as CRF in vertebrates to regulate feeding.

A number of other invertebrate peptides may be involved in feeding and satiety. For example, a family of related nonapeptides and decapeptides, the enterins, is present in the CNS and gut of *Aplysia*. The structure of the enterin precursor predicts 35 copies of 20 different enterins. Immunoreactive enterin neurons and processes are found in the gut. Enterins can inhibit contractions of the gut. Enterins are found in the cerebral and buccal ganglia. Another group of peptides synthesized in the corpora allata, the allatotropins, have been implicated in midgut ion transport, and the upregulation of acid and alkaline phosphatases in the gut.

Feeding and satiety in vertebrates

In vertebrates, gustatory sensory systems suggest development over a long phylogenetic history. The anterior part of the tongue is maximally responsive to sweet and salty tastes and initiates the acceptance of food. The front is innervated by the seventh cranial nerve and is linked to the perception of sweet taste. The back of the tongue is responsive to bitter tastes and it initiates rejections. The back is innervated by the ninth and tenth cranial nerves. The ninth cranial nerve is linked to bitter tastes. All three nerves project to the anterior portion of the solitary nucleus. The gustatory region of the nucleus of the solitary tract in the brainstem integrates internal signals (i.e. sickness) with external events such as the ingestion of food. This system appears to be preserved in both fish and mammalian lineages. Gustatory afferents follow two ascending paths from the parabranchial nucleus through the ventral posterior region of the thalamus to the insular cortex. A second route courses through the lateral hypothalamus and connects to the central nucleus of the amygdala and the bed nucleus of the stria terminalis (Fig. 6.16).

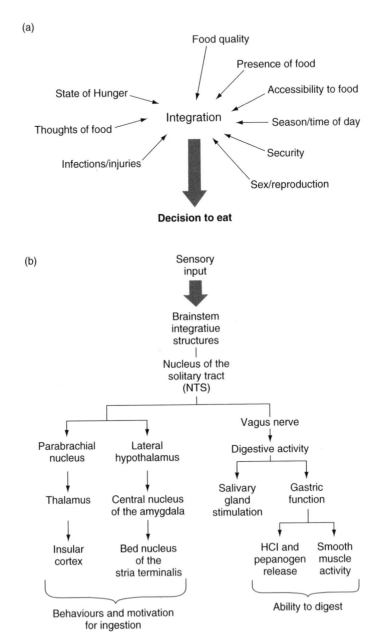

Figure 6.16   *Integration and circuits associated with feeding. (a) Decision making; (b) stimulatory circuits.*

Both the anticipation and the perception of food will stimulate the parasympathetic nervous system to prepare the animal for feeding. Parasympathetic nerves to salivary glands cause release of vasoactive intestinal peptide (VIP) to activate salivary stimulation. Parasympathetic stimulation via the vagus nerve centrally by neuropeptide Y stimulates gastric activity initially by stimulating HCl and pepsinogen secretion in the fundal part of the stomach. There is also an upregulation of gastrin receptors to increase the sensitivity to local secretion of gastrin. HCl acts to cleave the pepsinogen proprotein to pepsin. Further parasympathetic stimulation via the vagus nerve stimulates gastrin production and release and pancreatic exocrine release of salts, bicarbonate and digestive enzymes. Paracrine gastrin release further stimulates pepsinogen and HCl release. Introduction of food into the stomach will further stimulate these substances until one of a number of events occur. The distention of stomach from continued feeding acts as a negative feedback to the feeding and satiety centres of the brain. Plasma levels of glucose and other substances also feed back to brain. In addition, ingestion is complete and there is no more gustatory or olfactory stimulation.

A number of local paracrine and endocrine actions continue in the gut to complete the digestive process. As the food mass increases and moves towards the pyloric region of the stomach and into the small intestine (duodenum), several events occur. Secretin is released to further stimulate the exocrine actions of the pancreas. Gastrin inhibitory peptide (GIP) is released to inhibit further release of gastrin. Cholecystokinin is released to stimulate the release of bile juices, and increase stimulation of exocrine components of pancreas. The gut is highly vascularized to allow efficient uptake of nutrients from the gut into the blood stream. In addition, it picks up all the endocrine and paracrine secretions of the gut. Many of these, such as insulin and glucagon, act as endocrine agents for the rest of the body. Some of these hormones, such as somatostatin and cholecystokinin, are identical in structure to neuromodulators in the brain and so there may be secondary modulation of neurological activity by gut hormones via interaction at the circumventricular organs or specific transporter systems.

Neural circuitry associated with feeding

In mammals, a number of hypothalamic sites, such as the ventromedial nucleus (VMN), dorsal medial nucleus (DMN), paraventricular nucleus (PVN) and lateral hypothalamus, play pivotal roles in the regulation of feeding and satiety. In the lateral hypothalamus, neuropeptides, such as melanin-concentrating hormone (MCH) and orexin (hypocretin), play major signalling roles associated with appetite stimulation. These neuropeptide systems also target a number of regions in the hypothalamus including the arcuate nucleus, suprachiasmatic nucleus and supraoptic nucleus. They also influence midbrain sites such as the central grey and dorsal raphe nuclei (a major 5-HT producing region), and in the brainstem, the locus coeruleus, a major norepinephrine-producing site. In fishes, considerably less is known about the circuitry but the general mechanism appears to be present, although many of the nuclei are not as differentiated as they are in the brains of mammals. Historically, the olfactory lobes, inferior lobes of the hypothalamus and optic lobes have been implicated in the regulation of feeding. Most fishes appear to possess the same complement of neurohormones as mammals. Presumably, cartilaginous fishes also possess a similar set of signals as virtually all of the relevant hormone systems evolved well before the evolution of the sharks and the subsequent phylogenetically younger groups of vertebrates.

Neurohormones that stimulate feeding

As alluded to in the previous section, the number of neurohormones associated with the regulation of feeding and digestion is large, and their interactions complex. However, a number of key regulatory systems offer a model to the basic mechanism of feeding. A set of these neurohormones acts to initiate or facilitate the onset of feeding (Fig. 6.17).

Neuropeptide Y is a 36-amino acid peptide belonging to the pancreatic polypeptide family and is the most abundant neuropeptide in the vertebrate CNS. NPY appears to play a pivotal role in stimulating the onset of feeding behaviour. NPY is present in the arcuate nucleus, central nucleus of the amygdala and bed nucleus of the stria terminalis. These regions project to the dorsal vagal complex and parabranchial and solitary nucleus. NPY efferents project from ventral lateral medulla to the amygdala. The stimulation of feeding by NPY appears to be entirely a central nervous system-mediated event as systemically administered NPY does not elicit food intake. NPY appears to stimulate appetite with a preference for carbohydrate-rich food sources. NPY concentrations will increase in the PVN in anticipation of food reward following food deprivation. NPY appears to elevate the motivation to gain access to food but does not elicit changes to ingestion of food sources.

Galanin was originally isolated from the small intestine and is widespread throughout the brain. Pharmacological studies provided the first evidence that galanin has a role in energy and nutrient balance. Injections of galanin into the hypothalamus stimulate feeding behaviour and specifically the consumption of fat. The major site yielding the strongest action of galanin on feeding is the PVN. Additional sites at which galanin significantly increases consumption include the dorsomedial nucleus of the hypothalamus, the ventromedial

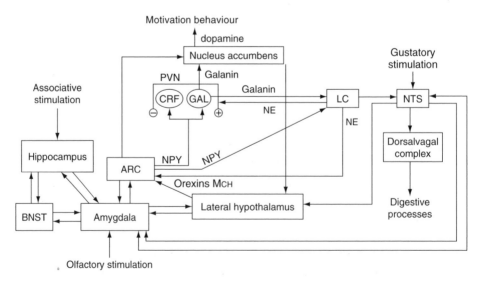

Figure 6.17 *A model of some of the neurological circuits associated with feeding. Note that many of the interactions are modulatory in a concentration dependent manner, where high and low concentrations may have opposite effects.*

nucleus of the hypothalamus, the amygdala, and the area postrema/nucleus of the solitary tract. Furthermore, galanin levels and mRNA concentrations in the PVN were significantly higher in Sprague-Dawley and obese Zucker rats that consumed high quantities of fat, in several different dietary regimens including access to pure fat, to a high-fat diet, to a cafeteria diet, and to neonatal overfeeding. Galanin could conceivably exert its action via stimulation or inhibition of another major neurotransmitter. Pre-treatment with antagonists of α_2-adrenergic receptors blocks galanin-induced feeding in rats and goldfish. Further, galanin microinjected into the paraventricular nucleus of the hypothalamus increases extracellular norepinephrine levels in the hypothalamus. These experiments suggest that galanin induces feeding by releasing hypothalamic norepinephrine. Also, some other experiments revealed that microinjection of galanin into the PVN increased extracellular dopamine and decreased extracellular acetylcholine in the nucleus accumbens of high food consumption rats. The nucleus accumbens has been associated with physiological reward. Galanin may activate neurons in the hypothalamus, which project to regions of the nucleus accumbens that mediate the rewarding properties of food consumption. Galanin action may be mediated, in part, by endogenous opioid peptides that promote feeding. In addition, leptin can partially inhibit galanin-induced food intake, suggesting a possible modulation by leptin of postsynaptic actions of galanin.

Neurohormonal systems that inhibit feeding

Essentially there are two main groups of hormonal signals that will inhibit appetite (Fig. 6.18). These include a series of factors produced by the gut, liver and adipose tissue, which

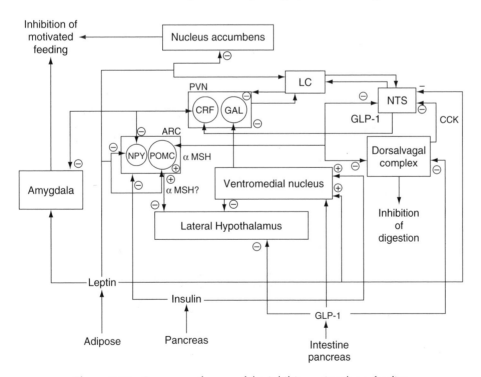

Figure 6.18 *Summary of some of the inhibitory signals on feeding.*

indicate satiety. They may also include neurohormones associated with habituation. A second group of hormones and neurohormones include those associated with sympathetic nervous system activation, indicating that when there is a homeostatic challenge event, the feeding process becomes interrupted to focus on these other events. This includes both environmental stimuli such as the presence of predators, potential mates or disease and injury. Corticotrophin-releasing factor (Fig. 6.19), the pivotal neurohormone that regulates the peripheral response to stress (Chapter 9), plays a major regulatory role in feeding. Since their discovery in the late 1970s and early 1980s CRF-related peptides were known to have significant affects on feeding and weight regulation. The discovery of additional CRF peptides – urocortin, urocortin II and urocortin III – has introduced new neurohormones that appear to have an inhibitory effect on feeding and appetite in most vertebrates.

Glucagon-like peptide GLP-1 (7–36) amide (Fig. 6.20) is a potent regulator of glucose homeostasis and is also produced in the brain where it has been implicated as a regulator

Perciformes

tilapia   SEDPPISLDLTFHLLREMMEMSRAEQLAQQAQNNRRMMELF

Salmoniformes

rainbow trout   SDDPPISLDLTFHMLRQMMEMSRAEQLQQQAHSNRKMMEIF
Sockeye salmon   SDDPPISLDLTFHMLRQMMEMSRAEQLQQQAHSNRKMMEIF
arctic char   SDDPPISLDLTFHMLRQMMEMSRAEQLQQQAHSNRKMMEIF

Siluriformes

bullhead   SEDPPISLDLTFHLLREMMEMSRAEQLAQQAQNNRRMMELF

Cypriniformes

sucker 1   SEEPPISLDLTFHLLREVLEMARAEQL AQQAHSNRKMMEIF
sucker   SEEPPISLDLTFHLLREVLEMARAEQL VQQAHSNRKMMEIF
carp   SEEAPISLDLTFHLLREVLEMARAEQMAQQAHSNRKMMEIF
goldfish   SEEPPISLDLTFHLLREVLEMARAEQMAQQAHSNRKMMEIF

Amphibia

African clawed frog   AEEPPISLDLTFHLLREVLEMARAEQIAQQAHSNRKLMDII
western spadefoot   AEEPPISLDLTFHLLREVLEMARAEQIAQQAHSNRKLMDII
toad

Mammalia

Sheep   SQEPPISLDLTFHLLREVLEMTKADQLAQQAHSNRKLLDIA
cow   SQEPPISLDLTFHLLREVLEMTKADQLAQQAHNNRKLLDIA
pig   SEEPPISLDLTFHLLREVLEMARAEQLAQQAHSNRKLMEII
Human   SEEPPISLDLTFHLLREVLEMARAEQLAQQAHSNRKLMEII
dog   SEEPPISLDLTFHLLREVLEMPGAEQLAQQAHSNRKLMEII
rat   SEEPPISLDLTFHLLREVLEMARAEQLAQQAHSNRKLMEII

Figure 6.19 *CRF orthologue sequence variability amongst actinopterygian (top) and tetrapod species (bottom). Conserved sequences are shown in grey.*

Members of the super family of Glucagon-related peptides

(a)

```
                    5           10          15          20          25          30          35          40          45
GLUCAGON      H S Q G T F T S D Y S K Y L D S R R A Q D F V Q W L M N T
GLP-1(7-37)   H A E G T F T S D V S S Y L E G Q A A K E F I A W L V K G R G
GLP-1(7-36)NH2 H A E G T F T S D V S S Y L E G Q A A K E F I A W L V K G R NH2
GIP           Y A E G T F I S D Y S I A M D K I H Q Q D F V N W L L A Q K G K K N D W K H N I T Q
EXENDIN-3     H S D G T F T S D L S K Q M E E E A V R L F I E W L K N G G P S S G A P P P S NH2
EXENDIN-4     H G E G T F T S D L S K Q M E E E A V R L F I E W L K N G G P S S G A P P P S NH2
SECRETIN      H S D G T F T S E L S R L R E G A R L Q R L L Q G L V NH2
PHM           H A D G V F T S D F S K L L G Q L S A K K Y L E S L M NH2
GLP-2         H A D G S F S D E M N T I L D N L A A R D F I N W L I Q T K I T D
HELOSPECTIN-1 H S D A T F T A E Y S K L L A K L A L Q K Y L E S I L G S S T S P R P P S
HELOSPECTIN-2 H S D A T F T A E Y S K L L A K L A L Q K Y L E S I L G S S P R P P S
HELODERMIN    H S D A I F T E E Y S K L L A K L A L Q K Y L A S I L G S R T S P P NH2
PACAP-38      H S D G I F T D S Y S R Y R K Q M A V K K Y L A A V L G K R Y K Q R V K N K NH2
PACAP-27      H S D G I F T D S Y S R Y R K Q M A V K K Y L Q S L L A NH2
PRP           D V A H G I L N E A Y R K V L D Q L S A G K H L Q D I M S R Q Q G E S N Q E R G A R A R L NH2
GRF           Y A D A I P T N S Y R K V L G Q L S A R K L L Q D I L N
VIP           H S D A V F T D N Y T R L R K Q M A V K K Y L N S I L N NH2
```

Figure 6.20 GLP-1 superfamily and its actions: (a) alignment of the glucagon-like peptides with related peptides; (b) endocrine and neuroendocrine actions of GLP-1. Reprinted with permission from Kieffer and Habener (1999), Endocrine Society.

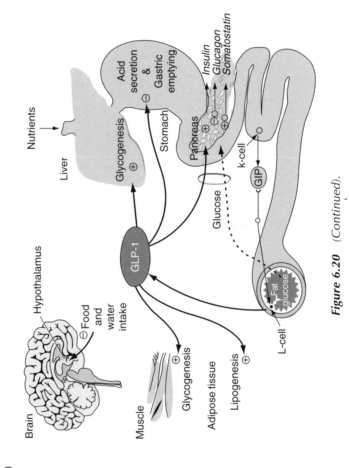

(b)

Figure 6.20 (Continued).

$$Q\,G\,P\,W\,L\,Q\,E\,E\,E\,E\,A\,Y\,\boxed{G\,W\,M\,D\,F-NH_2}\quad \text{Gastrin}$$
$$D\,Y\,M\,\boxed{G\,W\,M\,D\,F-NH_2}\quad \text{CCK-8}$$

Figure 6.21   *Comparison of human gastrin and cholecystokinin-8 amino acid sequences.*

of food intake. GLP-1 fibres and terminals are found in the septum, hypothalamus, thalamus and brainstem and appear to originate from GLP-1 neuronal cell bodies in the solitary nucleus. Central administration of GLP-1 increases plasma corticosterone levels and activates the CRF neurons of the PVN. GLP-1 fibres and nerve terminals are found in the parvocellular regions of the PVN with highest concentrations in the anterior and medial parvocellular subdivision where they are juxtaposed to many of the CRF neurons and establish synapses on both perikarya and dendrites of CRF neurons. The magnocellular division of the PVN has moderate numbers of GLP-1 nerve fibres. GLP-1 neurons contain leptin receptors indicating they are a site for feedback mechanisms.

Cholecystokinin (CCK) (Fig. 6.21) has been implicated with a number of inhibitory effects on feeding. Systemic injection of CCK will decrease food intake in rats dependent upon CCK_A receptors. CCK may decrease the incentive value of food sources. This food intake suppressive effect has also been shown in the white-crowned sparrow and goldfish. It may be associated with afferents issuing from the vagus nerve, as transection of this nerve abolishes the CCK-mediated cessation of food intake. CCK may also play a role in the integration of the response associated with the cessation of feeding that occurs during the end of a meal. CCK can activate regions of area postrema, solitary nucleus and dorsal motor nucleus of the vagal nerve. Regions of the PVN, central nucleus of the amygdala and BNST are also activated. Some of CCK's inhibitory effects may be due to the stimulation of an oxytocin-mediated mechanism. CCK can activate oxytocin neurons in the PVN. Oxytocin is generally inhibitory to ingestive behaviours.

Central oxytocin projects to the area postrema, solitary nucleus and dorsal motor nucleus of the vagus. Oxytocin influences ingestive behaviour and may contribute to the reduction of food intake that follows the administration of CRF. Bombesin will also decrease food intake but not water intake. Bombesin is found in the brain and in the stomach. In the brain, it is present in the solitary nucleus and area postrema, parabranchial nucleus and also the PVN, ventromedial hypothalamus and central nucleus of the amygdala. Bombesin in the solitary nucleus and area postrema will reduce food intake. Bombesin infusion into the fourth ventricle but not third ventricle will abolish sucrose and NaCl intake, indicating that it has a non-specific effect on ingestive behaviours and its action is mediated via brainstem sites.

Cytokines act on the brain to induce fever and behavioural depression after infections. This may be due to mediation by the vagus nerve activating limbic structures, whereas fever may be primarily due to hormonal mechanisms affecting the preoptic area including interleukin-6 action on the OVLT with subsequent induction of prostaglandins. In rats, vagotomy can block behavioural depression after an injection of $IL1\beta$ or lipopolysaccharide and activation of limbic structures and ventromedial POA but not in the OVLT.

Satiety feedback mechanisms

Many of the investigations that have examined the physiology of feedback signals indicating satiety in an animal have tended to focus on glucose, insulin and, now recently,

Insulin

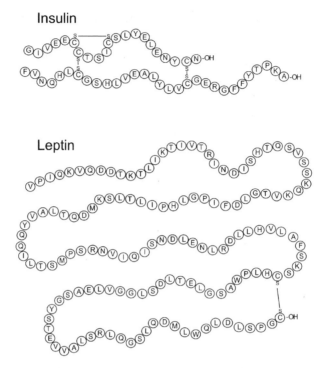

Leptin

Figure 6.22   *Structures of Leptin and Insulin.*

leptin (Fig. 6.22). However, there are likely a number of feedback signals in the form of nutrients, and a suite of gut hormones associated with the regulation of digestion.

The discovery of leptin in the mid-1990s provided researchers with a novel set of molecular tools and a new mechanism upon which to investigate feeding homeostasis and the associated feedback mechanisms. In mammals, leptin is produced and secreted mainly by adipocytes but is also present in other tissues such as placenta, brain, mammary glands and the pituitary gland. The gastric epithelium also expresses leptin. Plasma leptin concentrations increase with adiposity and are reduced during food deprivation. There are numerous regions of the brain than express leptin receptors but evidence showing the expression of the leptin gene in the brain is not strong.

Entry of leptin into the brain has two main effects: it decreases appetite and increases energy expenditure. The physiological goal is to reduce adipose loads. The increase in energy expenditure is associated with the neural branch of the sympathetic nervous system, stimulating the release of norepinephrine that activates the β_3 receptors on the adipocytes resulting in increased lipolysis and thereby reducing triglyceride stores. The decrease in triglycerides yields a decrease in leptin secretion.

Leptin-like peptides appear to be present throughout the jawed vertebrates, but differences in their mode of action among species is not understood. The published sequence for chicken leptin shows a surprisingly high level of identity to the mammalian leptin, much more so than what would be predicted phylogenetically. Its highest level of expression occurs in the liver and adipose tissue. The hepatic expression may be associated with the primary role that the liver plays in the lipogenic activity in avian species. Similar to mammalian leptin, expression in chickens is regulated by both hormonal and nutritional status. The highest sensitivity occurs in the liver in comparison to adipose tissue. Recombinant chicken leptin inhibits food intake and may do so via hypothalamic leptin receptors. The chicken leptin receptor possesses the same functional motifs that have been identified in the mammalian receptor. The chicken leptin receptor is expressed in the hypothalamus and also in the pancreas, where leptin can inhibit insulin secretion. In birds, therefore, leptin may play a major role in regulating nutrient utilization. Immunoreactive leptin has also been found in the oxyntic-peptic cells of the frog and reptiles but has not been found in the trout. In trout, frog and snake, immunoreactive leptin was found in elements of the enteric nervous system that were also positive for VIP.

Peripheral administration of leptin can induce phosphorylated STAT3 in the arcuate nucleus, VMH, lateral hypothalamic area of the hypothalamus, nucleus of the solitary tract, dorsal motor nucleus of the vagus nerve, lateral parabranchial nucleus and central grey of the brainstem. In mammals, leptin may exert its effects, in part, through a POMC-melanocortin-mediated event. In this model, leptin activates OB-Rb receptors in POMC-expressing neurons of the arcuate nucleus where it acts to increase the synthesis of POMC mRNA and decrease the synthesis of agouti-related protein (AgRP) mRNA. α-MSH is a natural endogenous ligand for the melanocortin 3 and 4 receptors whereas AgRP is an endogenous antagonist of these receptors. The increased α-MSH and decreased AgRP released from the terminals of the POMC neurons act to stimulate α-MSH responsive neurons by direct activation of the receptors and also by the loss of inhibition induced by AgRP. Both the dorsal vagal complex (DVC) and nucleus of the solitary tract (NTS) of the brainstem are regions of MC3/4 receptors. Cells of the DVC give rise to preganglionic parasympathetic fibres of which a proportion is associated with gastric acid secretion. The rostral part of the NTS receives many of its inputs from taste fibres from the facial and glossopharyngeal nerves and has been referred to as the gustatory nucleus. Thus gustatory afferent signals entering the NTS may be inhibited by α-MSH (Fig. 6.23).

Injections of murine leptin into goldfish decrease food intake. NPY and orexin A increases food intake in goldfish but when co-injected with leptin induces a lower food intake than when not co-injected. Leptin treatment in goldfish increases hypothalamic CCK mRNA expression. Blockade of CCK receptors results in an inhibition of the leptin-induced decrease in food intake and an attenuation of the inhibition action of leptin on both NPY- and orexin A-induced feeding. Fasting has no effects on brain expression of CCK but increases brain expression of NPY and decreases the expression of CART. In goldfish, leptin influences food intake in part by modulating the orexigenic effects of NPY and orexin and that its actions are mediated in part by CCK.

Insulin is a protein hormone produced and stored in the beta cells of the islets of Langerhans in the pancreas. It is released into the circulation in response to raised blood glucose levels and facilitates transport of glucose and other metabolites into cells. The structure of insulin consists of two polypeptide chains (A and B chains) that are linked by two disulphide bonds. Insulin-like peptides and receptors are present in all three major clades of metazoans – ecdysozoans, lophotrochozoans and deuterostomes. However, this

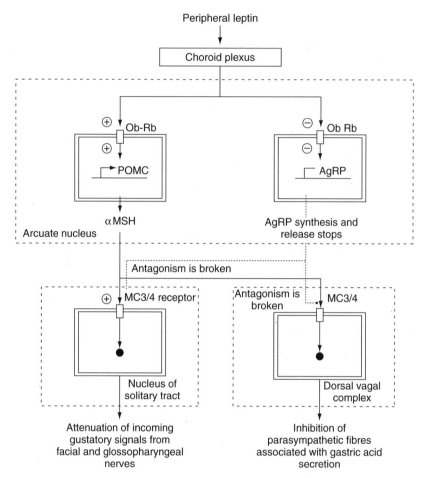

Figure 6.23 *Interaction of α-MSH and Agouti-related peptide (AgRP) to suppress the feeding response in mammals.*

gene appears to exist as a single conserved copy in most invertebrates. Related peptides that have been sequenced are bombyxin, found in the silkworm, *Bombyx*, and molluscan insulin-related peptide (MIP), found in the freshwater snail, *L. stagnalis*. The sequence similarity of the A chain is about 50% between bombyxin and human insulin and about 40% between MIP and human insulin. In the B chain the similarity is 25 and 20%, respectively. Three-dimensional models of bombyxin and MIP indicate that bombyxin and MIP do not form the dimers or hexamers characteristic of mammalian insulin.

Sweet tastes will induce an animal to secret insulin. Damage to the ventral medial hypothalamus increases insulin secretion whereas vagal damage reduces it. If food is anticipated, then insulin will be secreted in anticipation of the food. Injections of insulin will reduce food intake in many species but the extent of this effect depends on the diet that is offered. Like leptin, plasma insulin levels vary with adiposity. Direct administration into the brain can result in a decrease in food intake, and mice lacking insulin receptors are hyperphagic and obese. However, the adiposity feedback actions of insulin should not be confused with its role in blood glucose regulation. For example, a suppression of food intake will occur with high levels of insulin associated with increased adiposity, whereas increased appetite and food intake may occur as a secondary effect resulting from the hypoglycaemia induced by administration of a high concentration of insulin. Thus the actions of insulin in responsive regions of the brain may depend in part whether leptin levels are high or low. For example, in some cells of the ventromedial hypothalamus and the arcuate nucleus, insulin can only depolarize cells if the leptin receptor OB-Rb is present.

Chapter summary

The regulation of sodium and water in cells and tissues is the most primary endocrine system devoted to the survival of the individual. At the heart of osmoregulatory physiology is the renin-angiotensin system. Although primarily studied in vertebrates, elements of this system are found in both ecdysozoan and lophotrochozoan lineages. The key hormones associated with this system are angiotensin, aldosterone, and vasotocin-like peptides. Both central nervous system and peripheral renin-angiotensin systems exist. Fishes possess a caudal neurosecretory system in the caudal most segments of the spinal cord, plays a role in the adaptation to changes ambient salinity. Calcium regulation has been tied in part to sodium regulation since early stages of evolution. Calcitonin- and parathyroid hormone-like peptides are the primary calcium regulating systems although numerous other hormones will regulate calcium in different tissues. If osmoregulation represents the most essential system to maintain continued survival, then feeding and energy metabolism arguably represents the second most important set of systems. A vast array of neurohormones, notably neuropeptide Y, galanin, leptin and corticotrophin-releasing factor has been implicated in the regulation of feeding and appetite at the hypothalamic level. The neurohormones of feeding can be divided into those that regulate motivation, locomotion and digestion. The utilization and storage of nutrients incorporate yet a different set of hormones. Depending upon the physiological state of the animal and the environmental conditions, a number of additional pathways may be involved.

Allatotropin: A multifunctional insect neuropeptide
Frank M. Horodyski

Neuropeptides are an important class of regulatory compounds that control a wide variety of physiological processes either by acting at the site of their release from neurosecretory cells or by acting as a hormone following their release into the circulation. A neuropeptide is often initially characterized by its effect on a target tissue in a well-defined *in vitro* assay. While this reveals an important biological

---

(Continued)

function, it also limits our appreciation for the diverse functions that can be controlled by a single compound.

This diversity of function is illustrated by the neuropeptide allatotropin (Manse-AT) that was first isolated from the insect *Manduca sexta*. Manse-AT was first characterized by its ability to stimulate the synthesis of juvenile hormone (JH) by the adult corpora allata which is required for egg maturation and reproductive processes in adult insects. The availability of antisera to Manse-AT and the cloned gene to use as a probe for *in situ* hybridizations led to observations that Manse-AT is present in a defined and diverse population of neurons in the central and enteric nervous systems, consistent with multiple functions of Manse-AT. It has since been demonstrated that Manse-AT acts on muscles, the heart, the midgut, the ventral diaphragm, and the Malpighian tubules to regulate critical functions throughout the life of the insect.

An additional level of complexity has entered the picture with the discovery that the Manse-AT gene is expressed as at least three mRNAs that differ by alternative splicing, in which the longer mRNAs differ by the inclusion of one or two exons within the open reading frame. Manse-AT can be derived from each precursor protein, but each exon that is uniquely present in the longer mRNAs contains a sequence encoding a peptide that is structurally related to Manse-AT. These predicted peptides have been designated allatotropin-like (ATL) peptides and were shown to possess biological functions that overlap with those controlled by Manse-AT. Alternative splicing of Manse-AT mRNAs is regulated in a tissue- and stage-specific manner providing a mechanism for the regulated production of related neuropeptides to orchestrate diverse physiological actions during different life stages. The nutritional state of the insect also dramatically and specifically increases the levels of the longest Manse-AT mRNA, predicted to encode Manse-AT and two Manse-ATL peptides. This suggests that the complex response to starvation might be in part controlled by three structurally related peptides derived from an alternatively spliced mRNA. A major challenge now is to better understand the diversity of functions of Manse-AT and the Manse-ATL peptides through a combination of physiological, molecular biological and reverse genetic approaches.

References

Elekonich, M.M. and Horodyski, F.M. (2003) Insect allatotropins belong to a family of structurally-related myoactive peptides present in several invertebrate phyla. *Peptides* 24, 1623–1632.

Lee, K.-Y. and Horodyski, F.M. (2002) Restriction of nutrient intake results in the increase of a specific *Manduca sexta* allatotropin (Manse-AT) mRNA in the nerve cord. *Peptides* 23, 653–661.

Lee, K.-Y., Chamberlin, M.E. and Horodyski, F.M. (2002) Biological activity of *Manduca sexta* allatotropin-like peptides, predicted products of tissue-specific and developmentally-regulated alternatively spliced mRNAs. *Peptides* 23, 1933–1941.

Melanin-concentrating hormone
Jackson C. Bittencourt

The discovery of melanin-concentrating hormone (MCH) was due to the fact that some fishes change colour depending upon the background of river or sea. Initially the researchers had just a hint about the existence of the hormone responsible for turning the fish pale. However, they did know that there was a hormone that turned the fish dark, which was the alpha-melanocite-stimulating hormone (α-MSH). The theory of such control was called the 'dual hormone control' of the fish colour (Hogben and Slome 1936). The same mechanism works for other classes of animals, such as reptiles and amphibians.

After the characterization of MCH from the chum salmon hypophysis (Kawauchi *et al.* 1983) much has been done to study the actions of this hormone in the mammalian endocrine and nervous systems. The very first step taken was the mapping of this peptide in the fish and mammalian brains. One very interesting aspect of this hormone is that in fish, reptile and amphibian classes it was a neurohormone ruling the pigmentation, expressed in the hypothalamus and secreted in the blood stream by the hypophysis. Nevertheless, this way of acting is not present in mammals.

In fish MCH has 17 amino acids and in rat/human 19 amino acids with a cyclic structure. There is a prepro-melanin-concentrating hormone with 165 amino acids that encodes at least three putative neuropeptides, the MCH, neuropeptide E-1 (NEI) and neuropeptide G-E (NGE). In the rate central nervous system MCH is localized mainly in the lateral hypothalamic area, the rostromedial zona incerta and dorsomedial tuberomammilary nucleus. Some other places like olfactory tubercle and the paramedian pontine reticular formation also express the transcript and the MCH mRNA (Nahon *et al.* 1989; Bittencourt *et al.* 1982). MCH gene transcripts are also found in several organs of the rat and mouse alike – stomach, intestine, testis, lung, thyroid, heart and spleen (Nahon 1994).

Since 1995 the scientific community has given much attention to the orexigenic role (evokes hunger) of MCH in the feeding behaviour (Qu *et al.* 1996). The MCH effect is due to a huge amount of the transcript and MCH mRNA present in the LHA, which receives information from the arcuate nucleus of the hypothalamus, an area adjacent to the median eminence (a circum ventricular organ) that responds to leptin hormone levels. One should argue about the other rules of MCH by just paying attention to those regions densely innervate by MCH fibres, for instance, the medial septal nucleus, the *pars lateral* of the medial mammilary nucleus, the cerebral cortex, the hippocampus formation, the periaqueductal grey matter and the shell part of the nucleus accumbens (Bittencourt *et al.* 1992).

The described functions for these regions are compatible with the different actions of MCH, as following: sleep–wake cycle (Verret *et al.* 2003); exploratory behavior, locomotor activity and grooming behaviour (Sanchez, Baker and Celis 1997; Gonzalez *et al.* 1998); emotional and anxiety controls; control of the acoustic sensory gate (Miller *et al.* 1993); and learning and memory (Monzon and De Barioglio 1999). Therefore, we can assume that most of these functions are likely to work as the basis of a motivated behaviour, such as the search for food.

(Continued)

Two MCH receptors are described so far: the MCH-R1 and MCH-R2. Both MCH-Rs belong to the subfamily of G protein-coupled receptors and expressed in several brain regions. The MCH-R1 and MCH-R2 are found in primates and carnivores, whereas the MCH-R2 sequence was not found in rat, mouse and rabbit. There is a 92% identity between rat, mouse and human DNA sequence of MCH-R1, 98% identity of protein sequence between rat and mouse and 96% with human MCH-R1 (Eberle *et al.* 2004).

References

Hogben, L. and Slome, D. (1936) The pigmentary effector system. VI, the dual character of endocrine coordination in anphibian colour change. *Proc. R. Soc. Lond. B Biol. Sci.* 120, 158–173.

Kawauchi, H., Kawazoe, I., Tsubokawa, M., Kishida, M. and Baker, B.I. (1983) Characterization of melanin-concentrating hormone in chum salmon pituitaries. *Nature* 305, 321–323.

Bittencourt, J.C., Presse, F., Arias, C., Peto, C., Vaughan, J., Nahon, J.L., Vale, W. and Sawchenko, P.E. (1992) The melanin-concentrating hormone system of the rat brain: An immuno- and hybridization histochemical characterization. *J. Comp. Neurol.* 319, 218–245.

Nahon, J.L., Presse, F., Bittencourt, J.C., Sawchenko, P.E. and Vale, W. (1989) The rat melanin-concentrating hormone messenger ribonucleic acid encodes multiple putative neuropeptides coexpressed in the dorsolateral hypothalamus. *Endocrinology* 125, 2056–2065.

Nahon, J.L. (1994) The melanin-concentrating hormone: From the peptide to the gene. *Crit. Rev. Neurobiol.* 8, 221–262.

Qu, D., Ludwig, D.S., Gammeltoft, S., Piper, M., Pelleymounter, M.A., Cullen, M.J., Mathes, W.F., Przypek, J., Kanarek, R. and Maratos-Flier, E. (1996) A role for melanin-concentrating hormone in the central regulation of feeding behavior. *Nature* 380, 243–247.

Verret, L., Goutagny, R., Fort, P., Cagnon, L., Salvert, D., Leger, L., Boissard, R., Salin, P., Peyron, C. and Luppi, P.H. (2003) A role of melanin-concentrating hormone producing neurons in the central regulation of paradoxical sleep. *BMC Neurosci.* 4, 19.

Gonzalez, M.I., Baker, B.I., Hole, D.R. and Wilson, C.A. (1998) Behavioral effects of neuropeptide E-I(NEI) in the female rat: Interactions with alpha-MSH, MCH and dopamine. *Peptides* 19, 1007–1016.

Sanchez, M., Baker, B.I. and Celis, M. (1997) Melanin-concentrating hormone (MCH) antagonizes the effects of alpha- MSH and neuropeptide E-I on grooming and locomotor activities in the rat. *Peptides* 18, 393–396.

Kela, J., Salmi, P., Rimondini-Giorgini, R., Heilig, M. and Wahlestedt, C. (2003) Behavioural analysis of melanin-concentrating hormone in rats: Evidence for orexigenic and anxiolytic properties. *Regul. Pept.* 114, 109–114.

Miller, C.L., Hruby, V.J., Matsunaga, T.O. and Bickford, P.C. (1993) Alpha-MSH and MCH are fuctional antagonists in a CNS auditory gating paradigm. *Peptides* 14, 431–440.

Monzon, M.E. and De Barioglio, S.R. (1999) Response to novelty after i.c.v. injection of melanin-concentrating hormone (mch) in rats. *Physiol. Behav.* 67, 813–817.

Eberle, A.N., Mild, G., Schlumberger, S., Drozdz, R., Hintermann, E. and Zumsteg, U. (2004) Expression and characterization of melanin-concentrating hormone receptors on mammalian cell lines. *Peptides* 25, 1585–1595.

Physiological role of Urotensin-II
Hubert Vaudry and Howard A. Bern

The caudal neurosecretory system of teleost fish, terminating in the urophysis, produces several regulatory factors including acetylcholine and two neuropeptides termed 'urotensin-I' and 'urotensin-II'. Urotensin-I is a C-terminally α-amidated peptide that exhibits significant sequence identity with CRF; three homologous peptides called urocortins have now been identified in mammals. Urotensin-II is a cyclic peptide that possesses some structural similarity to somatostatin (Pearson *et al.* 1980) (Fig. B6.1). Urotensin-II was long thought to be synthesized exclusively in the caudal neurosecretory system of fish. However, in 1992, characterization of urotensin-II from the brain of the European green frog *Rana ridibunda* provided evidence that the peptide was also produced in the brain of tetrapods (Conlon *et al.* 1992). Subsequently, the cDNA encoding the urotensin-II precursor has been characterized in frog, mouse, rat, pig and humans (Coulouarn *et al.* 1998, 1999). All isoforms of urotensin-II identified so far possess a C-terminal cyclic hexapeptide that has been strongly conserved from fish to mammals, whereas the sequence of the N-terminal region of the peptide is highly variable. Recently, a paralogous gene encoding a urotensin-II-related peptide (URP) has been characterized in mammals (Fig. B6.1). Structure–activity relationship studies have shown that the cyclic C-terminal heptapeptide common to urotensin-II and URP determines their biological activity (Chatenet *et al.* 2004). The urotensin-II and URP genes are primarily expressed in motoneurons located in brainstem nuclei and in the ventral horn of the spinal cord. Urotensin-II exerts its biological actions by interacting with a G-protein-coupled receptor (GPR), identified as the orphan receptor GPR14. The GPR14 gene is actively expressed in the heart and vascular smooth muscle, and urotensin-II has been found to modulate the vascular tone in representative species of several vertebrate classes. GPR14 mRNA is also abundant in the pancreas, where urotensin-II inhibits glucose-induced insulin secretion. The GPR14 gene is expressed in various brain regions, and central administration of urotensin-II to mammals has been found to increase locomotor activity, to induce anxiety, to stimulate prolactin and thyrotrophin secretion, and to control cardiovascular homeostasis. In addition, in teleosts, myotropic and osmoregulatory actions have been described (Bern 1990). It has been recently shown that GPR14 is expressed in rat astrocytes and that urotensin-II activates astroglial cell proliferation. Taken together, these observations indicate that the 'fish peptide' urotensin-II may have

Urotensin-II	Glu - Thr - Pro - Asp - **Cys - Phe - Trp - Lys - Tyr - Cys - Val**
URP	Ala - **Cys - Phe - Trp - Lys - Tyr - Cys - Val**
Somatostatin-14	Arg - Gly - **Cys** - Lys - Asn - **Phe - Trp - Lys** - Thr - Phe - Thr - Ser - **Cys**

Figure B6.1 *A comparison of the primary structure of human urotensin-II, human urotensin-II-related peptide (URP) and somatostatin-14. The conserved amino acids are in bold characters.*

(Continued)

a wide variety of endocrine, neuroendocrine and neurotransmitter/neuromodulator activities in vertebrates generally, including humans. They also suggest that urotensin-II antagonists may prove to have therapeutic value in the treatment of various diseases including hypertension, diabetes, cancer and psychiatric disorders.

References

Bern, H.A. (1990) The caudal neurosecretory system: Quest and bequest. In *Progress in Comparative Endocrinology*, Eds Epple, A. *et al.*, Wiley-Liss, New York, pp. 242–249.

Chatenet, D., Dubessy, C., Leprince, J., Boularan, C., Carlier, L., Ségalas-Milazzo, I., Guilhaudis, L., Oulyadi, H., Davoust, D., Scalbert, E., Pfeiffer, B., Renard, P., Tonon, M.C., Lihrmann, I., Pacaud, P. and Vaudry, H. (2004) Structure–activity relationships and structural conformation of a novel urotensin II-related peptide. *Peptides* 25, 1819–1830.

Conlon, J.M., O'Harte, F., Smith, D.D., Tonon, M.C. and Vaudry, H. (1992) Isolation and primary structure of urotensin II from the brain of a tetrapod, the frog *Rana ridibunda*. *Biochem. Biophys. Res. Commun*. 188, 578–583.

Coulouarn, Y., Lihrmann, I., Jégou, S., Anouar, Y., Tostivint, H., Beauvillain, J.C., Conlon, J.M., Bern, H.A. and Vaudry, H. (1998) Cloning of the cDNA encoding the urotensin II precursor in frog and human reveals intense expression of the urotensin II gene in motoneurons of the spinal cord. *Proc. Natl. Acad. Sci. USA*. 95, 15803–15808.

Coulouarn, Y., Jégou, S., Tostivint, H., Vaudry, H. and Lihrmann, I. (1999) Cloning, sequence analysis and tissue distribution of the mouse and rat urotensin II precursors. *FEBS Lett*. 457, 28–32.

Pearson, D., Shively, J.E., Clark, B.R., Geschwind, I.I., Barkley, M., Nishioka, R.S. and Bern, H.A. (1980) Urotensin II: A somatostatin-like peptide in the caudal neurosecretory system of fishes. *Proc. Natl. Acad. Sci. USA* 77, 5021–5024.

7

Growth and development

Introduction

As we alluded to in the last chapter, growth and differentiation occurs only when the osmoregulatory and energy needs of a cell or organism are met. Generally, if there is any homeostatic challenge or stress to an organism, then the pathways associated with growth and differentiation may be inhibited. Thus, growth and differentiation of an organism tend to occur during a period of quiescence. The life history of all organisms is characterized by a number of stages from conception to death. Often the same hormones will have different functions during different stages of development. The growth history may be characterized by a continual transition from immaturity to maturity, or may involve a number of periods punctuated by rapid change from one stage to another. Depending upon the life history of an organism, hormones may play significantly different roles. For example, growth in insects and other arthropods is intrinsically tied to moulting and metamorphic processes. It is therefore useful to place these topics together when discussing growth in arthropods.

The molecular pathways associated with growth, development and differentiation evolved well before the appearance of the radiate species (cnidarians and cteno-phores). Despite this, many of the hormone systems, such as growth hormone in chordates or juvenile hormone in insects, for example, are relatively recent hormone systems, in that they represent highly derived variants from a hormone lineage that is much older.

Neuroendocrinology: An Integrated Approach   David A. Lovejoy
© 2005 John Wiley & Sons, Ltd

Growth and the growth hormone, prolactin, somatolactin superfamily

Much of the pituitary control of growth processes in vertebrates appears to be achieved via the combined actions of several pituitary hormones. Growth hormone, prolactin, somatolactin and placental lactogen form four paralogous lineages of related hormones. Structurally, all are classified as growth factors and activate receptor tyrosine kinases.

Growth hormone

Growth hormone or somatotropin is a single-chain polypeptide with approximately 190 residues. It is classified as a member of the helix bundle group of peptides as it shares the same three-dimensional structure consisting of four antiparallel a-helices connected by random coil segments. There are two cross-linking disulphide bridges that help stabilize this structure. Aside from the prolactin-like peptides discussed below, a number of cytokines such as interleukin 2–7, 9, 11 and 12, erythropoietin, macrophage colony-stimulating factor and also leptin have this basic structure (Chapter 6).

Growth hormone is released from the somatotropes of the pituitary gland and is under stimulatory control by growth hormone-releasing hormone (GHRH), and under inhibitory regulation by somatostatin (Fig. 7.1). Both neurohormones are synthesized in the arcuate nucleus of the hypothalamus and secreted into the portal system of the median eminence. The release of growth hormone from the pituitary follows a pulsatile pattern that reflects the pulsatile release of both GHRH and somatostatin. The release of GHRH and somatostatin follow a reciprocal pattern to each other such that when GHRH is at its maximal point of secretion, somatostatin is at its minimal level of secretion, and vice versa. The inhibitory aspects of high levels of somatostatin predominate over the release characteristics of GHRH. Thus at maximal levels of somatostatin, GHRH cannot induce growth hormone release (Fig. 7.2). Growth hormone release is also stimulated by both endogenous forms of pituitary adenylate cyclase activating peptide (PACAP): PACAP 27 and PACAP 38. PACAP is a structural paralogue to GHRH, and in a number of species, notably teleosts, it appears to act as the primary growth hormone secretagogue.

A number of studies have implicated galanin in the modulation of the GHRH–somatostatin growth system to regulate growth hormone secretion. A subset of galaninergic neurons in the arcuate nucleus contains GHRH, and in the periventricular nucleus, galaninergic neurons projecting from other hypothalamic nuclei synapse on neurons containing somatostatin. Moreover, studies showed that galanin gene expression and peptide content are dramatically increased in the anterior pituitary gland of the hGHRH-overexpressing mouse and that the increased levels of galanin peptide within the hyperplastic pituitaries of hGHRH transgenic mice are due to an increase in the population of cells containing galanin. Although galanin has stimulatory effects on growth hormone secretion, the exact mechanism of galanin-mediated GH secretion is not clear. Other peptides may modulate the feedback loop of galanin–GHRH–GH to manipulate the activity of galanin.

Growth hormone released into the blood stream, exerts its effects on a number of target organs including muscle, bone, adipose and liver. Growth hormone has a number of specific actions in the body and generally has actions opposite to that of insulin. Physiologically,

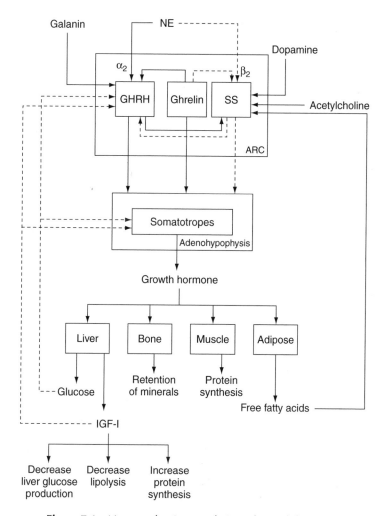

Figure 7.1   *Neuroendocrine regulation of growth hormone.*

bone and muscle growth is promoted at the expense of adipose stores. Thus, nitrogen retention in the body is promoted to allow for increased synthesis of amino acids. There is a stimulation of amino acid transport and protein and increased protein synthesis leading to increased growth of muscle and bone. Concomitantly, there is also atrophy of adipose tissue due to both decreased lipogenesis and increased lipolysis, and fatty acid oxidation. Growth hormone also acts to increase blood glucose, and stimulates the deposition of glycogen as well as stimulating the retention of minerals and incorporation of calcium and phosphate into bone.

In the liver, growth hormone stimulates the production of insulin-like growth factor-I (IGF-I). IGF-I promotes growth in a number of tissues including organs of the viscera, bones and gonads. IGF-I activates an RTK that is a structural paralogue of the insulin receptor. Growth hormone release can be inhibited by somatostatin or by

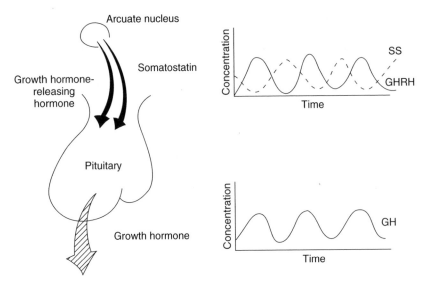

Figure 7.2 *Pulsatile release characteristics of growth hormone releasing hormone, somatostatin and growth hormone.*

feedback of IGF-I. However, the ability of IGF-I to suppress growth hormone declines with age.

Growth hormone causes the release of IGF-I and IGF-II from many tissues in the body (Fig. 7.3). Growth hormone also regulates the binding proteins specific to the IGFs. IGF-II is more potent and much more common than IGF-1 during embryonic development in mammals. In adult life IGF-II is much rarer. Production of three of the IGF-binding proteins – IGFBP 3, 5 and 6 – are upregulated by growth hormone, whereas the other three IGFBPs (1, 2 and 4) are downregulated. The latter IGFBPs are upregulated by stress, starvation and other catabolic events. The suppressing IGFBPs appear to sequester IGFs on cell membranes, preventing them from interacting with their target receptors, thus together they act to impart specificity to IGF. In mammals, IGFBP-3 is the most highly expressed compared to the other binding proteins, and is present in the blood at much higher concentrations than in fish, birds and amphibians. At neutral pH IGF-I and II are bound to IGFBP-3 in a trimeric complex that also includes an acid labile subunit. IGFBP-3 acts as a blood reservoir of IGFs, storing them until they are needed. This large complex is unable to cross capillary walls. It increases the half-life of IGFs in the blood stream from less than ten minutes (about the same half-life of insulin) to over 12 hours. Removing the acid labile subunit component allows the complex to pass through capillary walls. The high pH that occurs in regions of high metabolism is sufficient to induce the dissociation of the IGF from the bound complex. Other IGFBPs can cross capillary walls easily and even bind to cell membranes. The inhibitory IGFBP-2 is produced by cells throughout the body and binds to the membranes of the releasing cell and nearby cells. It acts as a mimic to the IGF-1 receptor and, in fact, has about ten times the affinity for IGF as the IGF-1 receptor. IGF molecules preferentially bind to the IGFBP-2, which disengages from the cell and floats away. Thus, the IGFBP-2 is a fairly short-term inhibitor of IGF for these

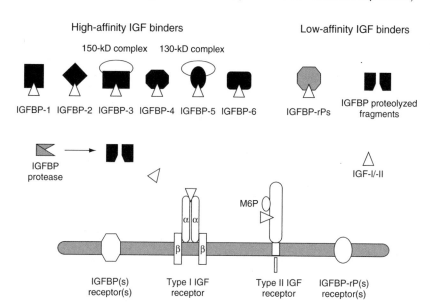

Figure 7.3 *IGF, binding proteins and their receptors. Reprinted with permission from Hwa* et al. *(1999), Endocrine Society.*

cells. The six main IGFBPs in mammals are paralogous. It is not clear when the gene evolved. Recently, piscine orthologues of IGFBP-3 have been found in Tilapia and zebrafish that are upregulated in response to growth hormone or IGF-1 injections.

The M6-P (mannose-6-phosphate)/ IGF-II receptor is unrelated to the IGF-I receptor, and only binds to IGF-II–it has very little binding affinity for IGF-I and undetectable binding with insulin. In mammals and brown trout, the M6-P receptor appears to sequester IGF-II for lysosomal destruction, but it does not carry out this purpose in birds and amphibians. In chickens, the circulating protein, vitronectin, binds IGF-II, but not IGF-I. Vitronectin is not related to any of the IGF-binding proteins. It has the same properties and function in humans and cattle. In birds, vitronectin levels are not affected by stress or starvation. The function of the M6-P receptor has not been well studied, and the mechanism of its action is still unknown but it may act as a sink for IGF-II to direct them to the lysosome for degradation. The function of the M6-P receptor may have changed during evolution. It has the IGF-II binding property in some fish such as the brown trout, as well as in mammals, but not amphibians. M6-P may not have been found in avians and amphibians because of its rarity. Avian and amphibians have lower levels of IGF-II, however, and may be able to use their IGFBPs to sequester excess IGF-II during embryonic development.

The growth hormone–IGF-I axis appears to be present throughout actinopterygian and sarcopterygian lineages of fishes. The neuroendocrine loop regulating growth appears to have evolved before the appearance of the vertebrates. Both growth hormone and IGF are present in the sea lamprey, *Petromyzon marinus*, where growth hormone has a stimulatory effect of IGF production. Two paralogous IGF peptides are found in gnathostome vertebrates, whereas only a single IGF peptide has been found in hagfish, *Amphioxus* and tunicates. Somatolactin is present in lamprey. IGF and insulin are found in tunicates and hagfish.

Despite the presence of a similar growth hormone regulatory system acting throughout vertebrates, poikilothermic animals may respond somewhat differently to the growth axis than homeothermic species. In the rainbow trout, growth hormone may or may not change with different environmental temperatures. In turbot, however, growth hormone levels appear to be directly related to temperature. Growth hormone may also vary inversely to fat body content. In hypoxic conditions, growth hormone decreases correlate with a decline in growth.

There may be a much closer relationship with the co-regulation of the growth axis and the reproductive axis. In goldfish, a number of studies have supported a direct regulation of growth hormone release by gonadotropin-releasing hormone (GnRH), the hypothalamic-releasing factor associated with the regulation of the reproductive system. The GnRH-induced release of growth hormone may be transduced by a nitric oxide and cGMP-mediated system.

Prolactin

Prolactin was originally discovered as a factor that stimulated milk secretion in rabbits and crop sac growth in pigeons in the first part of the 20th century (Fig. 7.4). It is part of a family of peptides that includes growth hormone, somatolactin and placental lactogen. There are two other proteins with structural similarity to prolactin. These are proliferin and proliferin-related protein and are expressed in a number of tissues including the placenta and brain. They have been associated with the regulation of angiogenesis. Prolactin has over 300 described functions and can be broadly classified into aspects of water and electrolyte balance, growth and development, endocrinology and metabolism, reproduction, brain and behaviour, reproduction, and immune regulation and protection (Fig. 7.5). Prolactin and its actions will be discussed in greater detail in Chapter 10. Prolactin is a 23-kD

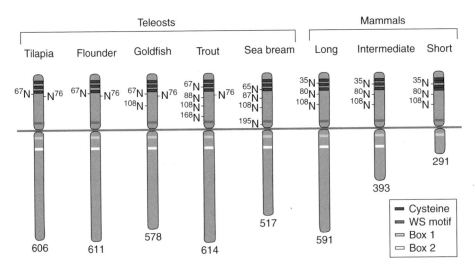

Figure 7.4 *Comparison of prolactin receptors in fish and mammal species. Reprinted with permission from Manzon (2002), Elsevier Science (USA).*

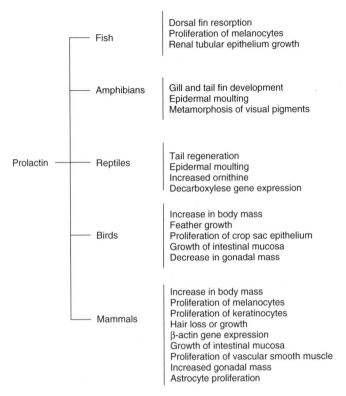

Figure 7.5 *Actions of prolactin on growth and differentiation. Adapted after Bole-Feysot* et al. *(1998).*

peptide, which is synthesized and secreted primarily from the lactotrophic cells of the anterior pituitary of all vertebrates. In addition, there is subpopulation of mammosomatotroph cells that secrete both growth hormone and prolactin. Prolactin is also produced and secreted from extra pituitary sites such as decidua, lymphoblastoid cell lines and lymphocytes.

Somatolactin

Somatolactin has a highly conserved amino acid sequence and is present throughout ray-finned fishes, including sturgeons (Chrondrostei), gar (Holostei) and teleosts. However, somatolactin is also present in the pituitary of lungfishes indicating that the hormone was present before the bifurcation of the actinopterygians and sarcopterygians. Somatolactin is structurally and sequentially similar to the growth hormone (GH) and prolactin (PRL) family. Somatolactin contains four of the seven conserved nucleotide clusters within the growth hormone and prolactin families that may be involved in receptor binding or hormone configuration. There is also a signal peptide present that is distinctive of secretory proteins. The presence of somatolactin among any tetrapods has not been shown. Because somatolactin may be glycosylated or non-glycosylated, detection of somatolactin using immunohistochemical analysis is not accurate. Antibodies derived from other teleost fishes used for analysis may not be suitable in detecting somatolactin in tetrapods due to the expression of different surface glycogens. Somatolactin has been implicated physiologically in growth regulation, reproduction, background adaptation and pH regulation.

Evolution of the growth hormone and IGF superfamilies

There is evidence that this group of hormones evolved well before the appearance of chordates. Both growth hormone and prolactin immunoreactivity have been found in a number of ecdysozoan, lophotrochozoan and invertebrate deuterostome species. In the insect *Leucophaea maderae*, two distinct forms of prolactin immunoreactivity have been found. In the tobacco hornworm, *Manduca sexta*, both interferon gamma-binding sites were found in particulates in the haemolymph. The interferon could be displaced by prolactin at these sites. Although presently no structures have been obtained from invertebrates, evidence suggests the presence of a variant that may be similar to an ancestor to the growth hormone–prolactin–cytokine family of peptides.

In vertebrates, growth hormone evolved at a comparatively slow rate with period intervals characterized by sudden changes in its structure when the rate of sequence evolution increased 25–50 above the basal rate. Mammalian growth hormone generally shows a slow rate of evolution with two bursts in the artiodactyl ungulates and primates. The burst in artiodactyls took place after the divergence of the cetartiodactyls but before ruminants diverged. The second burst took place in primates preceding the divergence of the new world monkeys, about 40 million years ago.

The insulin-like growth factor (IGF) I and II, insulin and relaxin in vertebrates, and several such invertebrate insulin-related peptides as insulin-like peptide (ILP) are members of the insulin-related gene family. The insulin family contains structurally related peptides that are essential for growth, development and metabolism in vertebrates and invertebrates. Insulin and IGF have been shown to share a very similar structure. The molecular cloning of cDNAs of insulin and IGF receptors has revealed that they are homologous structures with about 60% of identical amino acid sequences. In the early evolution of chordates, an ancestral gene is believed to have duplicated giving rise to the insulins and IGFs of today's vertebrates. In the cephalochordates, *Branchiostoma californiensis*, an insulin-like peptide (ILP) exists as a single gene product which is structurally related to both human insulin and IGF. In urochordates, *Chelyosoma productum* (tunicate), insulin-like molecules exist as two separate molecules. One molecule is similar to insulin and the other molecule is similar to the IGF molecule. The cloning of an IGF cDNA from the Atlantic hagfish revealed the presence of both insulin and a proto-IGF gene, hence demonstrating that the divergence of the IGF and insulin genes occurred prior to the separation of the Agnatha from the main line of vertebrate evolution. Insulin and IGF have maintained a separate gene lineage in both vertebrate and protochordate evolution. Later in vertebrate evolution, the IGF precursor gene duplicated giving rise to IGF-I and IGF-II. Distinct IGF-I and IGF-II cDNA have been cloned in teleostean fishes, amphibians, birds and mammals. In contrast to the aforementioned classes, agnathans represented by cyclostomes (the hagfish) have only one IGF that has characteristics of both IGF-I and IGF-II. The appearance of two genes encoding distinct IGF peptides in the cartilaginous fish may reflect that a partial chromosomal duplication occurred in the main chordate lineage prior to the divergence of the Chondrichthyes some 400 million years ago.

Aberrations and manipulations of the growth hormone axis

Selective breeding and pathological states have contributed much to our understanding of the physiological effects of growth hormone relative to the developmental state of the organism.

Dogs can be used as a model system to understand the genetics and ontogeny of growth hormone secretion. Compared to other mammals, there is a large difference in size between the largest and smallest dog. The largest adult dog can weigh up to one hundred times than that of the smallest. Plasma concentration of IGF-I appears to be correlated with body size. High plasma concentrations of both growth hormone and IGF-I occur during prepubertal growth in great danes as compared with miniature poodles. The mean body weight in great danes can increase by over 21 kg between week 6 and 24, whereas the mean body weight in beagles may only increase by a third of that over the same time period. In great danes, plasma growth hormone concentrations are much higher between weeks 6 and 24 in comparison to beagles. In addition, plasma GH concentration of great danes remain at high levels for almost 18 weeks, whereas in beagles the concentrations decrease after week 7. There were more growth hormone peaks in great danes that in beagles during weeks 19 and 23 although IGF-I and IGF-II concentrations do not differ between breeds. Great danes have higher levels of GH at a young age with both a higher pulse frequency and amplitude compared with beagles of the same age.

The term 'acromegaly' is derived from the Greek words for 'extremities' and 'enlargement'. It is a disorder that results from the prolonged secretion or excess GH by the pituitary gland. Acromegaly is often confused with a similar GH disorder known as Gigantism. Although they are both caused by the hypersecretion of GH, their physiological effects on an individual differ considerably. Gigantism begins in childhood before the epiphyseal plate closes and results in proportional growth throughout the body. Acromegaly on the other hand begins in adulthood and abnormal growth only affects certain parts of the body because the long bones can no longer be stimulated to grow. Acromegaly usually results in a shortened lifespan and can increase a patient's susceptibility to other detrimental conditions. It is most prevalent in people between the ages of 30 and 50 years. There are two main types of acromegaly, GRF-induced acromegaly and pituitary tumour acromegaly. About 90% of acromegalic patients have the latter type. In pituitary tumour acromegaly, a benign tumour, an adenoma, forms in the pituitary gland, which causes an abnormal high secretion of GH. The earliest signs of acromegaly are the swelling of soft tissues and hypertrophy of facial extremities. This is characterized by the lengthening of the jaw, enlargement of the lips, tongue and nose, and thickening of the brow ridge. Hands and feet become augmented and the digits become spade-like in appearance. Due to the rapid growth rate of skins cells, the texture of the skin all over the body becomes leathery. Sebaceous glands become overactive causing an oily complexion and sebaceous cysts. The parasinuses along with the vocal cord become enlarged causing a marked deepening of the voice. Severe headaches and delayed reaction rate are other indications of the condition due to the adenoma's compression on surrounding brain tissue. Due to compression of surrounding pituitary tissues that secrete other hormones, changes in menstruation and breast discharge in women, and impotence in men also occur.

Metamorphosis and development

A number of neuroendocrine systems are responsible for metamorphic development in vertebrates. The hypothalamus–pituitary–thyroid axis plays essential roles during larval growth in fish, metamorphosis in amphibians and embryonic and foetal development in birds and mammals (Fig. 7.6). However, growth hormone and prolactin also play essential roles.

Embryonic development

Several hypothalamus–pituitary systems have been implicated in vertebrate embryogenesis. Notable among these circuits are the thyrotrope-, corticotrope-, lactotrope- and somatotrope-associated systems. In bird embryos, for example, thyroid hormones increase towards hatching. In chickens, TRH acts as the principal thyrotrophin-releasing hormone and somatostatin acts in an inhibitory role. Both TRH and somatostatin hypothalamic levels rise towards hatching. After hatching, TRH levels continue to rise whereas somatostatin levels decrease towards adulthood. Plasma TSH levels drop towards hatching but then rise following hatching moving towards adulthood. CRF also has TSH-stimulating ability in the chicken embryo. The decrease in T3 activity prior to hatching is the result of a high activation rate in T4 but also a drop in the hepatic Type III deiodinase activity. This

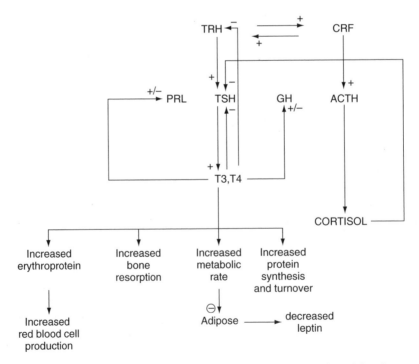

Figure 7.6 *Some of the functions of the thyroid actions in growth and development.*

transcription of this enzyme may be regulated in part by growth hormone and glucocorticoids. In human foetuses, the HPT axis becomes functional around week 11. Before this period, the foetal thyroid gland does not concentrate iodine. The placenta synthesizes a significant amount of type 3, 5′-deiodinase and therefore most maternal T3 and T4 is degraded by the placenta before it reaches foetal circulation. Thus, the foetus is dependent upon its own production of thyroid hormones for normal development. A lack of thyroid hormones in human foetuses has been associated with abnormal brain and skeletal development.

Although the role of prolactin in adult animals is relatively well understood, its roles in the growth and development of the foetus are poorly understood, although prolactin is implicated in most developmental processes. High levels of prolactin are generally found in foetuses in late gestation. In the rat, the biological actions of prolactin and placental lactogen are mediated through the PRL-R. Expression of PRL-R in the foetal olfactory epithelium and bulb is of particular interest because lactogenic hormones regulate food intake and maternal caretaking behaviour, both of which may be dependent on olfactory function. The PRL-R is expressed in low levels in the olfactory bulb, but in abundance in the olfactory epithelium and olfactory bulb of the foetal rat in late gestation. At mid-gestation mRNAs encoding the long and short isoforms of the rat PRL-R are found in the lateral nasal processes, the epithelial lining of the olfactory pit and the neuroepithelial lining of the cerebral ventricles in the region of the rhinencephalon. PRL-R mRNA has also been found in the rostral nasal mesenchyme and in the underlying mesenchymal tissue of the developing brain. With advancing gestation the PRL-R is expressed intensely – but discontinuously in the olfactory epithelium. PRL-R mRNA has also been detected in the olfactory bulb of the lactating rat. The expression of PRL-R in the olfactory system of the foetal and neonatal rat implicates novel roles for lactogenic hormones in olfactory differentiation and development and may provide new mechanisms by which the lactogens may regulate neonatal behaviour and mother–infant interactions.

Vertebrate metamorphosis

Most metazoans go through some stage of metamorphosis. The type of metamorphosis and therefore the physiological mechanisms that drive it vary considerably among metazoans. In comparison to the number of species that go through metamorphosis, only a few species have been studied in detail (Fig. 7.7).

The onset of metamorphosis is a mechanism transduced by the brain by integrating external information such as photoperiod and temperature with the developmental state of the organism. Metamorphosis evolved several times independently to solve different physiological and environmental constraints on the survivability of the species. Thus the physiological mechanisms can differ significantly among species. Also in many cases, it is likely that the metamorphosis has been lost or highly modified for the same reasons.

A delay in developmental timing or heterochrony likely played a significant role in the development and hence evolution of many metazoan groups. A delay or hastening of the timing of a key developmental event, such a metamorphosis, could alter the time when sexual development is initiated. In poikilothermic animals, of which the vast majority of metazoans belong to, mutations to a couple of codons that encode the binding site of the transcription factor or the sequence of the responsive element of the promoter may be enough to alter the thermodynamic range of this molecular interaction. Thus enhanced

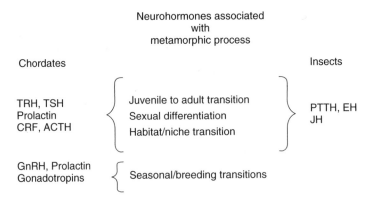

Figure 7.7   *Types of metamorphic transitions and neurohormones involved.*

activity or binding affinity may allow for the event to occur during cooler periods, say earlier in the spring, whereas less binding affinity may allow for the developmental event to occur later in the year. This may allow the mutated species the opportunity to go through a developmental state during a period relatively free from predators. This might be the case in which the species was part of a mature ecosystem where predator species were timed with the maturation of the metamorphosizing species.

Metamorphosis in amphibians has been comparatively well studied and acts a model system to understand metamorphosis in vertebrates. Amphibians show considerable variation in the duration of their larval periods and because of this plasticity, the larval period is regarded as a life history trait subject to natural selection. Both the external environment and genetic factors influence the function of several endocrine glands during development ultimately affecting rates of growth and differentiation. Biotic factors include food availability and quality intra- and inter-specific competition predation and density-dependent factors. Abiotic factors are temperature, photoperiod and hydric environment. Habitat desiccation is one of the most important environmental factors affecting metamorphosis in amphibians. Desert amphibians breed in ephemeral ponds that are sporadically filled with rain. Thus, metamorphosis needs to be synchronized to such events.

Differentiation and growth exhibit differential sensitivity to environmental factors and are controlled by antagonistic hormonal systems. During development larval phase tadpoles must make a switch from physiological processes that favour growth to physiological processes that favour differentiation. A threshold minimum body size may be required to be reached before metamorphosis is possible. Once it is reached, habit desiccation from decreased water volume and related processes such as temperature or density-dependent factors will affect biochemical processes that define morphogenesis. The timing of endocrine initiation of metamorphosis may depend on the recent growth history of the tadpole. As growth rate decreases due to reduced food availability and because of constant locomotion and foraging, a change in growth rate initiates the endocrine cascade leading to metamorphosis. From here, there are two main ways the environmental factors can affect the physiology and development of amphibians. It can either have a direct effect on tissue or work through the CNS. In the latter, sensory information is transduced by the neuroendocrine system to produce a response that will affect growth and differentiation.

Integral to the entire system are the thyroid hormones (Fig. 7.8). Thyroid hormones appear in early prometamorphosis when morphogenesis is increasing and continues until metamorphic climax is reached. At this point it then drops to normal adult levels. During development, the neuroendocrine centres of the brain begin to synthesize the neurohormones required to activate the thyroid axis and increase plasma thyroid hormone concentrations. T3 is essential for the development of the vertebrate brain by influencing neuronal migration, myelin formation, axonal maturation and dendritic outgrowth. The basic transcription element binding (BTEB) protein is upregulated by T3 in the premetamorphic tadpole brain and therefore T3-mediated effects could be through this transcription factor. However, CRF may also play a role in metamorphosis. CRF may act as a TRH allowing the thyroid axis to be associated with conditions of stress. TSH under the control of CRF stimulates the production of thyroid hormones. The plasma thyroid hormones are relatively low during premetamorphosis and early prometamorphosis and become elevated during late prometamorphosis and reach a maximum at early climax. There is a twin action of CRF on TSH and ACTH. The subsequent stimulation of glucocorticoids by ACTH has the effect of potentiating the actions of the thyroid hormones. The plasma glucocorticoid rise follows that of the plasma thyroid hormones. Although some studies have suggested that the rise in prolactin may act in part as a signal to inhibit thyroid hormone production, other studies indicate that the rise in prolactin may be associated with lung maturation. Metamorphosis is also a period when there is development and maturation of the reproductive system (Chapter 10). In *Rana esculenta*, FSH and LH increase during the metamorphic climax or immediately thereafter. Thyroid hormones may activate the development of the hypothalamic GnRH system to stimulate gonadotropins.

Lampreys, unlike hagfish, undergo metamorphosis as part of their lifestyle. Larval lampreys (ammocoetes) share a number of morphological characteristics with the ascidian larvae of tunicates and with *Amphioxus* (Branchiostoma). The spring rise in water temperature

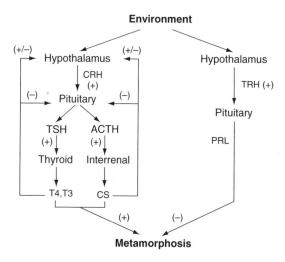

Figure 7.8 *Neuroendocrinology of metamorphosis in amphibians. Reprinted from Denver (1998) by the permission of Elsevier.*

is a cue for the initiation of metamorphosis. The first external morphological effects of metamorphosis coincide with a drop in serum thyroid hormones. The thyroid hormone profile in lampreys is, therefore, directly opposite to what is seen in anurans and teleosts. In non-parasitic lampreys sexual maturation occurs shortly after or immediately after metamorphosis. In parasitic lampreys there is usually a feeding period and continued somatic growth before sexual maturation.

The thyroid axis is also involved in the parr to smolt transition (smoltification) in anadromous salmonids. During smoltification, there are a number of morphological and physiological adaptations required for the transition from freshwater to seawater. There is a surge in plasma thyroid hormones during this transition that appears to mediate much of the differentiation of the tissues. The onset of smoltification may be induced in part by melatonin action (Chapter 8). Activation of the interrenal glucocorticoids is also required, and plasma cortisol peaks after the thyroid hormone peak.

The onset of metamorphosis is linked with the neuroendocrine systems regulating stress, osmoregulation and diuresis. Perhaps for this reason in some anurans, the loss of habitat by desiccation results in an increase of CRF. Metamorphosis in amphibians is controlled by TSH but appears to be stimulated by CRF. In the bullfrog, *Rana catesbeiana*, irCRF shows a marked increase in the median eminence during metamorphosis. Metamorphosis in the spadefoot toad, *Scaphiopus hammondii*, is accelerated when the tadpoles are subjected to habitat desiccation. In this species, acceleration of metamorphosis due to decreasing water levels appears not to be the result of population density, high concentrations of solutes or presence of pheromones, but rather the restriction of movement and perhaps the associated reduction in feeding. Indeed, CRF has been implicated in both the latter behaviours. Moreover, irCRF is elevated in the hypothalamus under conditions of habitat desiccation, and injections of sauvagine will advance metamorphosis in this species. Although growth hormone is clearly involved in the growth aspects of metamorphosis in anurans, it appears not to involve the induction of any metamorphic processes by itself. Transgenic *X. laevis* overexpressing growth hormone is much larger than the wildtype animals but shows normal metamorphic events (Fig. 7.9).

Moulting in birds utilizes a number of the same neurohormone mechanism as used in the metamorphic processes in other vertebrates. A number of hormones, such as progesterone, androgens, GnRH, prolactin and thyroid hormones, have been implicated; however, in direct manipulation of the moulting process, prolactin and thyroxine are among the more potent. In the brain, TRH is the primary factor responsible for stimulation of the thyroid axis, whereas vasoactive intestinal peptide (VIP) is required for prolactin release. A group of neurons in the avian forebrain analogous to the visceral forebrain system of mammals expresses VIP. This system appears to regulate the balance of the autonomic nervous system. The TRH-expressing neurons of the paraventricular nucleus are a key component of the visceral forebrain system. TRH appears to play a role in the activation of the sympathetic nervous system that is required as a prerequisite for moulting.

Metamorphosis in arthropods

Insect growth is discontinuous for the cuticular parts of the body because the cuticle limits the size the insect can attain. Thus size increase occurs by successive moults. The mechanisms associated with growth, moulting and metamorphosis are therefore closely integrated.

(a)   (b)

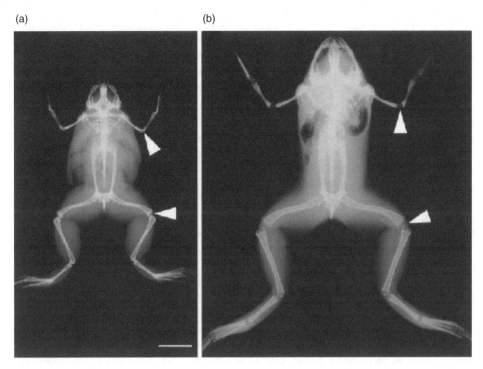

Figure 7.9 *(a) X-ray image of a wild-type Xenopus; and (b) a transgenic version of over-expressing growth hormone of the same age. Reprinted with permission from Huang and Brown (1999), National Academy of Sciences.*

There are two components to growth. The first is the moult increment and refers to the increment in size, which occurs during the period between two successive moults, or instar. The second component of growth is referred to as the intermoult period which is the time between two successive moults, known as the stadium or instar duration. Insects can be divided into those that do not undergo metamorphosis (ametaboly), those that undergo partial metamorphosis (hemimetaboly) and those that achieve complete metamorphosis (holometaboly). For most insects, a reduction in the amount of circulating juvenile hormone due to a decrease in corpora allata activity is required to initiate metamorphosis. Moulting involves hormonal, behavioural, epidermal and cuticular changes that lead to the shedding of the old cuticle. Both moulting and metamorphosis are controlled by three basic types of hormones. These include the neuropeptides, prothoracicotropic hormone (PTTH) and eclosion hormone (EH); juvenile hormone (JH); and the moult-regulating hormones, ecdysteroids. There are several variants of JH that are synthesized. All ecdysteroid receptors characterized so far require the heterodimerization to ultraspiracle (USP), the insect homologue of the vertebrate retinoid X receptor (RXR). This heterodimerization is required for the high affinity binding of their ligand and the subsequent binding to DNA. In crustaceans, methyl farnesoate (MF) is an unepoxiated form of insect JH and appears to be the crustacean version of JH.

During moulting, PTTH-synthesizing neurosecretory cells of the brain send their axons to the corpora allata where PTTH is stored in the nerve terminals in a manner analogous to the neurohypophysis in vertebrates (Fig. 7.10). PTTH is subsequently released into the haemolymph and acts to stimulate ecdysteroid synthesis and release by the prothoracic glands. The ecdysteroids initiate the changes in the epidermal cells that lead to the production of the new cuticle. JH inhibits the expression of adult features. A high haemolymph concentration of JH is associated with larva-larva moults, lower concentrations occur during larva-pupal moults, and a complete absence of JH is associated with pupa-adult moults. For most ecdysis events, EH appears to act upon the steroid-primed nervous system to induce the coordinated motor activity required to escape from the old cuticle.

In crustaceans, crustacean hyperglycaemic hormone (CHH), moult-inhibiting hormone (MIH) and gonad-inhibiting hormone (GIH) are structurally related neuropeptides that are predominantly produced in the X organ sinus gland neurosecretory system in the crustacean eyestalk. CHH-related peptides belong to one subfamily whereas MIH- and GIH-related peptides are associated with a second subfamily. Several paralogues of each peptide may exist within a single family. MIH acts to inhibit ecdysteroid synthesis. CHH is associated with MF synthesis.

Prothoraciotropic hormone release continues through development and is under circadian control. This rhythm acts on the prothoracic glands where it functions in the regulation of rhythmic steroidogenesis. There are two oscillators, the brain and prothoracic gland. They are synchronized by the ability of PTTH to entrain the prothoracic gland. Most cells in insects have ecdysone-responsive genes that are temporally expressed. Thus, the ecdysteroids may also be acting in part to provide time cues to developing cells to modulate gene expression in a circadian framework.

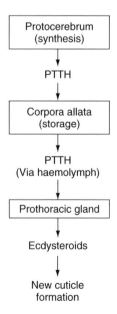

Figure 7.10   *Regulation of ecdysteroids by PTTH during the moulting process in insects.*

Paralysins may play a role in neurometamorphosis. These are small molecules that are toxic to mammalian cells possibly by interacting with glutamate receptors. In insects they act to constrain the movement of the insect as it prepares for the metamorphic process or subsequent moults.

Sexual differentiation

Gender-specific behaviours can be found throughout the animal kingdom and many of these have been shown to be under the direct regulatory effects of sex steroids during perinatal development. During this time, steroids such as testosterone and oestrogen exert an organizational effect on the brain that differs from their activation effects during adulthood (Fig. 7.11). Female rodents will fail to ovulate or display receptive behaviour in adulthood if they are exposed to androgens prenatally. Androgens act to masculinize the female brain during development so that even when administered oestrogen and progesterone as adults their hormones fail to activate parts of the brain that normally controls the female reproductive system. Among many species of songbirds it is the males that sing in order to attract mates, whereas the females normally do not sing. When a female

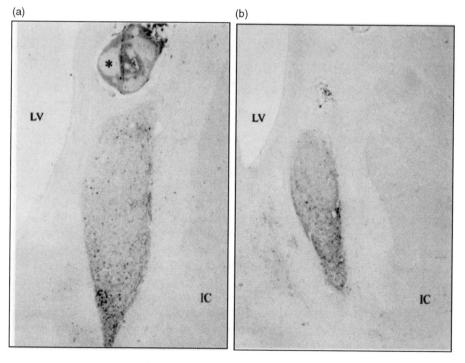

(a)   **(b)**

Figure 7.11 *Sexual dimorphism in the human bed nucleus of the stria terminalis (a) male; (b) female. Reprinted with permission from Kruijiver et al. (2000), Endocrine Society.*

songbird is administered oestrogen or testosterone during development it will also sing in adulthood. Similarly, males administered anti-aromatase or anti-oestrogen drugs during development will fail to sing as adults.

The sexually dimorphic nuclei of the medial preoptic area (SDN-MPOA) have been shown to be 2.5–5 times larger in males and this difference is dependent on testosterone converting to oestradiol because both castration or anti-oestrogen treatment during development results in the feminization of the male SDN-MPOA. Males who are insensitive to androgens due to a mutation of the androgen receptor gene also develop a normal male SDN-MPOA. The medial amygdala is also larger in males but seems to be under the direct influence of testosterone and not oestradiol. Male rats genetically altered to be insensitive to androgens failed to develop a masculine medial amygdala.

Another region which exhibits sexually dimorphic characteristics is the ventromedial hypothalamus (Fig. 7.12). This nucleus is interconnected with the arcuate and supraoptic

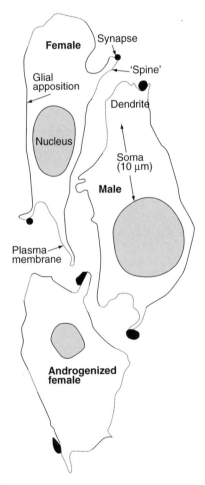

Figure 7.12 *Sexual dimorphism in GnRH neurons. Reprinted from Kim et al. (1999) by the permission of Biology of Reproduction.*

nuclei as well as the median eminence. It has been implicated in ingestive and motivational behaviours. The arcuate nucleus, in particular, contains neurons that secrete growth hormone-releasing hormone and somatostatin, both of which are involved in the modulation of growth hormone which exhibits a sexually dimorphic pattern of release. Castration of males during development has been shown to prevent the masculinization of the ventromedial hypothalamus. Preventing the masculinization of the VMH will also cause male rats to exhibit lordosis.

The dentate gyrus of the hippocampus is sexually dimorphic with male rats having both more neurons and more volume overall than females. Male rats also perform better on spatial tasks as in the Morris water maze that is dependent on the hippocampus. Females who were administered androgens during development, however, score equally well on this task as the male counterparts. Females who have two intrauterine male neighbours also perform as well as males on spatial tasks indicating that androgens from their male siblings can enter the amniotic fluid and have an effect on the developing female brain.

Perinatal sex steroids also regulate the neuroendocrine system. The secretory pattern of growth hormone is sexually dimorphic with males showing surges of larger amplitude and duration every three hours and decreased baseline levels. Male rats gonadectomized before birth displayed a female pattern whereas females treated with testosterone before birth displayed a male pattern. One factor which may play a role in the differential release of growth hormone between sexes is the structure of the arcuate nucleus which shows sexually dimorphic astrocyte morphology. Astrocytes in males exhibit a stellate morphology and ultrastructural neuron morphology. Females have twice as many axodentritic synapses both of which are dependent on the presence of sex steroids during perinatal development because females administered testosterone during development displayed a male morphology. GnRH neurons while similar in number and distribution receive greater synaptic input in females and this difference can be reversed in prenatal testosterone exposure (Fig. 7.13).

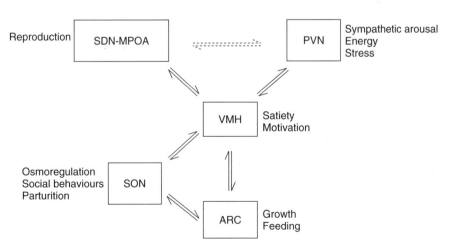

Figure 7.13 *Interactions of the sexually dimorphic nuclei in the medial preoptic area (SDN-mPOA) and ventromedial hypothalamus (VMH) with the arcuate nucleus (ARC), supraoptic nucleus (SON) and paraventricular nucleus (PVN). A small number of key sexually dimorphic nuclei have the ability to regulate a wide variety of physiological functions.*

Galanin is also expressed in GnRH neurons and its concentration and time of transcription is sexually dimorphic. Both oestradiol and progesterone effect the expression of galanin in adult rats. Neonatal exposure to testosterone abolishes the sexually dimorphic coexpression and regulation of galanin by oestrogen and progesterone.

Mechanisms of ageing

In western society our obsession to find an anti-ageing cure continues. Despite our growing scientific sophistication, over the last few years many hormones such as oestradiol, melatonin, dihydroxytestosterone and growth hormone have been touted as miracle cures for ageing. In the late 1800s and early 1900s, gonadal tissue from such species as ram, goat, deer, boar and monkey were transplanted into humans with the mistaken belief that it would increase strength, health and intellectual capacity.

Ageing is a consequence of life. DNA possesses a number of weak spots. Junctures between the purine bases and sugars are prone to split apart as the molecule jostles at normal temperatures. The bonds between nucleotides can split, the bases nitrogen rings can decompose by the actions of ultraviolet and ionizing radiation or alkylating agents in the DNA's own environment. Lifespans of multicellular organisms are extremely variable. Amongst mammals, for example, bowhead whales live for over 200 years whereas the rodent lifespan can be as short as 1–2 years. In the due course of evolution, selective pressure to adapt to a particular environment and occupy distinct ecological niche determined the development of reproductive and lifespan strategy. There is, however, considerable plasticity in the expectancy of life. It has been known for almost a century now that delay in reproduction and caloric restriction increases lifespan of rodents, primates and insects. The mechanism of this extension is being studied.

In rats, somatotrope subpopulations show age-related differences in their secretory response to GRF and somatostatin. The age-related decline in GH production that occurs in rats may be due to a reduction in both the proportion and sensitivity to GRF of the most highly responsive and secretory somatotropes that tend to occur during ageing.

Besides the determination of the lifespan by the ecological niche and reproductive strategy, the obvious questions are why and how senescence occurs. Evolutionarily it is advantageous to keep genomes adapting and changing which means old individuals die and new come in. So how is senescence regulated? One of the theories postulates that the accumulation of damage to cellular proteins and DNA by reactive oxygen species (ROS) is the main culprit. Most of the cellular ROS are generated during mitochondrial respiration. So higher mitochondrial metabolism results in more damage and more wear and tear to the cell.

A number of the key metabolic processes associated with ageing are controlled by various neuroendocrine systems. The first indication of neuroendocrine control of ageing was obtained from studying mutations that extend lifespan of model organisms, the nematode *Caenorhabditis elegans* and fruitfly *Drosophila melanogaster*. *C. elegans* mutants in the enzyme that is essential for 5-HT synthesis live twice as long as normal, wild-type worms. These 5-HT mutants also had decreased feeding rates and egg laying and increased their fat storage. Food and favourable temperature upregulate serotonin or the response to 5-HT to in turn regulate reproductive development and low fat storage. This is reminiscent of 5-HT receptor knockout mutant mice that exhibit hyperphagia and obesity. Possible 5-HT receptors in *C. elegans* reside in specific sensory neurons and are involved in insulin-like growth factor (IGF) and transforming growth factor β (TGFβ) signalling cascades. Insulin-like ligand binds to IGF receptor (daf-2) which leads to its activation and further signal transduction to protein kinase (age-1) and culminates at the transcription factor (daf16) mediated gene regulation. Mutations in age-1 and daf-2 result in lifespan increase up to 400% in *C. elegans* and *D. melanogaster*. Meanwhile, mutations in daf-16 transcription factor abolish increased longevity indicating that the activity of this transcription factor is necessary for lifespan extension. The heterozygous knockout of mouse IGF-II increases the lifespan of the animals by 25%. Thus, IGF is evolutionarily conserved longevity regulating system. Mammalian lifespan control is more complex as there are more factors influencing IGF. Growth hormone regulates the secretion of IGF. Mice mutants in pituitary developmental gene and in turn deficient for growth hormone, prolactin and TSH are long-lived, dwarf and mildly obese. The mutation in GH receptor results in the same phenotype that shows an essential role of GH signalling in these processes.

A number of systems have been implicated in the regulation of longevity. Experiments of restoration of the IGF cascade in different cells of *C. elegans* showed that in mutant background introduction of IGF signalling components in neurons results in normal lifespan, whereas restoration of the signalling in muscle rescued the metabolic phenotype such as increased fat accumulation. Thus, the sensory neurons of *C. elegans* represent the main hub that integrates incoming environmental information to regulate lifespan. The same IGF signal in the periphery regulates metabolic processes. Low periphery insulin-like signals act to suppress energy expenditure and stimulate eating; thus animals increase their fat storage. Abundant food signals insulin release, high periphery insulin and high insulin in hypothalamus or equivalent control centre where it is translated into inhibition of food intake. Thus, mutations in IGF create the situation where no high IGF is present even with abundant food leading to fat accumulation due to slower metabolism.

The determination of lifespan by the IGF pathway is not completely autonomous, but rather appears to be modulated by other neuroendocrine pathways. Signalling pathways associated with reproduction has been implicated. The ablation of germline cells in *C. elegans* or delayed reproduction in *Drosophila* increase life expectancy. This increase seems to be dependent on IGF signalling in the neuroendocrine system. This way the information from the gonads is integrated into the network of other signals to determine lifespan. Evolutionarily it is more important to reproduce than to extend life, although there may be periods of particular environmental austerity, which it becomes important to delay reproduction in favour of survival (Chapter 9). The nuclear hormone receptor, daf-12, mediates the signal from the *C. elegans* gonads to the longevity coordination centre. On the other hand, IGF regulates diapause, vitellogenesis and reproduction. This way, if there is no food; animals do not reproduce and enter diapause. *Drosophila* insulin receptor mutants have ovaries of non-reproductive animals and treatment with juvenile hormone (JH) rescues the reproduction and the lifespan. Reduction in JH in insects is associated with diapause, postponement of reproduction and stress resistance. Thus the IGF signalling affects the ability of the neurosecretory body corpora allata to secrete JH in *Drosophila*. In mammals, GnRH secretion is thought to be influenced by IGF-1 signals.

Mutations in the IGF pathway that result in lifespan extension also increase resistance to stress. Animals are more resistant to oxidative damage, elevated temperatures and heavy metal exposure. Higher levels of molecules protecting against these toxic insults, such as catalase, superoxide dismutase (SOD), heat shock proteins and metallothioneins, were found in the animals. This is in agreement with higher stress resistance in diapause animals and the fact that daf-16 transcription factor upregulates these protective factors. Interestingly, overexpression of SOD in motor neurons of *Drosophila* resulted in lifespan extension although to a smaller degree than IGF pathway mutations (50%). Could this indicate that IGF determines the amount of oxidative damage in neurons and that is the reason of senescence? At present this is still under intense investigation. However, it seems that the IGF signalling is part of the neuroendocrine system that integrates environmental information and sends signals for determining organismal size, metabolism, vitellogenesis, fat storage and acts as primary lifespan plasticity centre at least partially through sensitivity to ROS.

A number of neuroendocrine pathways change during ageing. Decreases associated with ageing are observed in the dopaminergic, serotonergic, noradrenergic, cholinergic systems and HPA axis in humans. IGF and growth hormone also display reduced levels during human senescence. How much it controls the rate of senescence is unclear but these decreases are associated with frailty, cardiovascular conditions and reduced muscle mass. Increased levels of IGF and growth hormone had been linked to diabetes and cancer. It is possible that decrease in IGF and growth hormone enable humans to live longer post-reproductive life. As the human society evolved there was selective advantage in having post-reproductive members. Alongside that, selection favours genotypes that can adapt to harsh environments like natural disasters, infection and starvation. Partial 'diapause' would be beneficial under these conditions. Genes determining fat accumulation, fasting survival and delayed reproduction are winners in these situations. In an affluent society, however, these genes are also implicated in obesity and type 2 diabetes.

Parkinson's disease is a neurodegenerative disorder resulting from the loss of striatal dopamine. The striatum is a major component of the basal ganglion in the brain and it uses dopamine to regulate movement. Movement is derived from the coordinated balance of cortical and thalamic excitation of the striatonigral and striatopallidal pathways that regulate the tonic activity of the substantia nigra pars reticulate neurons. Common symptoms of Parkinson's disease are progressive tremors, bradykinesia and rigidity, which are caused by the degeneration of the dopaminergic nigrostriatal pathways and subsequent loss of dopamine. Dopamine is essential in the treatment of Parkinson's disease because the degeneration of the nigrostriatal neurons result in the depletion of dopamine and one gets a reduction in the acquired sensory responsiveness of striatal neurons. A class of neurons in the striatum that are known as the tonically active neurons (TAN) can acquire responsiveness to sensory conditions stimulated during learning. Dopamine depletion results in a decrease in the acquired sensory response of TAN. The nigrostriatal dopamine system is necessary for the expression of response profiles acquired during the behavioural learning. Dopamine, therefore, acts as an enabling system that allows the expression of behaviourally released neuroplasticity in the striatum. Injection of D1 and D2 dopamine receptor agonists selectively reverses the effects of dopamine depletion because they cause the striatopallidal and striatonigral neurons to express D1 and D2 receptors.

Chapter summary

The hormones involved in growth processes relate to the life history and developmental stages of the animal. Thus, the neurohormones associated with growth may also be involved in energy metabolism, sexual differentiation, metamorphosis and the ageing process. In vertebrates, growth hormone and prolactin play fundamental roles in growth and development. The structure of these hormones is archetypal for the growth factor family of polypeptides. Included in this superfamily are the insulin-like peptides as well. The activation of the hypothalamus–pituitary–thyroid axis plays a significant role in the onset of the metamorphic process in a number of vertebrates. In insects, prothoracicotrophic hormone and eclosion hormone are involved in growth, moulting and metamorphosis. Growth and developmental physiology in most species is sexually dimorphic. Hormones regulating the structure and development of sexually dimorphic regions will modify the subsequent pattern of growth characteristics. In vertebrates growth and developmental processes change as a function of the age of the organism.

Evolution of pituitary adenylate cyclase-activating peptide (PACAP)
Nancy M. Sherwood

Human hormones are usually known by their structure and physiological effects, but the complexity of the human biological system often obscures the relationship of one hormone to another or to less obvious functions. Comparative neuroendocrinology probes the origin of hormones in animals that evolved earlier and examines functions in well-chosen model organisms where it is easier to study specific functions during early development or in adults.

Pituitary adenylate cyclase-activating polypeptide is a prime example of a neuropeptide that is related by structure to eight other hormones in humans, suggesting that this group may have evolved from a common ancestor. PACAP was discovered in sheep as a hormone (27 or 38 amino acids) made in nerve cells in the hypothalamus, but capable of stimulating an increase in cAMP in pituitary cells. Later, PACAP was shown to be more widely expressed in the nervous system and other tissues, and to have many functions in addition to an action on the pituitary.

A clue to the origin of PACAP and its relationship to other hormones came from the high conservation of the PACAP protein structure. In fairly rapid succession, the genes were isolated from sheep, humans, rat, salmon and other fish, mouse, chicken, reptiles and amphibians. Finally, the PACAP gene was isolated from a protochordate, the ancestors of the vertebrates. The result of gene and peptide analysis of PACAP revealed a number of important ideas. First, the N-terminal region provides the structural link between PACAP and the superfamily members, which include growth hormone-releasing hormone (GHRH), glucagon and its two related hormones (glucagon-like peptide 1 and 2), vasoactive intestinal peptide (VIP), peptide histidine methionine (PHM), glucose-dependent insulin-releasing polypeptide (GIP) and secretin. These nine hormones tend to be expressed in nerve cells and gut or its derivative, the pancreas. Second, several of the hormones are encoded in tandem in one gene: glucagon with GLP-1 and GLP-2, VIP with

(Continued)

PHM, and PACAP with GHRH (Fig. B7.1). However, PACAP and GHRH are in one gene only in animals that evolved before the mammals. Thereafter, the hormones are encoded in separate genes. Third, exon duplications appear to be the explanation for the presence of more than one hormone in a gene. Thus, the duplicated

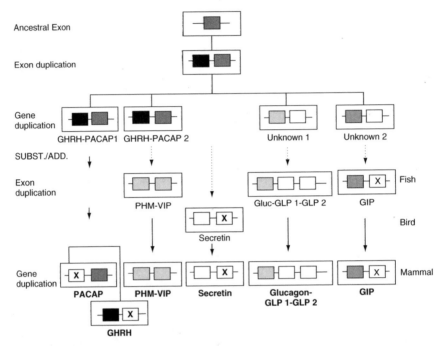

Figure B7.1 *Proposed evolution of the PACAP/glucagon superfamily. The larger open boxes represent genes, whereas the smaller boxes inside represent exons that encode hormones. The peptides found in mammals are shown along the bottom for the six known genes (9 hormones).*

hormones originally had identical, but later, overlapping functions; they probably shared the same receptor for at least a period of time. An example is PACAP, which shares two receptors with VIP, but in addition, PACAP has a third receptor that is specific. Fourth, the genes that encode only one hormone in this superfamily may have once encoded two hormones, but one hormone was lost by a substitution, deletion, unequal crossover or another mechanism. An example is the PACAP gene in mammals, which still encodes an altered GHRH region, but the product is not a functional peptide that binds to a receptor. Rather, GHRH now resides on its own gene in mammals with separate control compared with the PACAP gene.

The structure of PACAP is conserved more tightly than that of GHRH, which led us to speculate that PACAP is an important hormone in all vertebrates. We prepared a mouse with a disrupted (knocked out) PACAP gene. Mouse pups lacking PACAP die within two weeks after birth with a wasting syndrome and fatty liver, heart and skeletal muscles. The pups cannot defend their body temperature as well as being wild-type pups, and have problems with respiration, reproduction and maintenance of glucose levels under stress. The comparative study was the key to the importance of PACAP not only in mammals, but in all vertebrates.

References

Gray, S.L., Cummings, K.J., Jirik, F.R. and Sherwood, N.M. (2001) Targeted disruption of the pituitary adenylate cyclase-activating polypeptide gene results in early postnatal death associated with dysfunction of lipid and carbohydrate metabolism. Mol. Endocrinol. 15, 1739–1747.

Sherwood, N.M., Krueckl, S.L. and McRory, J.E. (2000) The origin and function of the pituitary adenylate cyclase-activating polypeptide (PACAP)/glucagon superfamily. Endocr. Rev. 21, 619–670.

Corticotrophin-releasing factor and animal development
Robert J. Denver

Members of the corticotrophin-releasing factor (CRF) family of peptides play central roles in the regulation of neuroendocrine, autonomic and behavioural responses to physical and emotional stress. Corticotrophin-releasing factor is a member of a family of related peptides in vertebrates that includes the fish urotensins-I and the tetrapod urocortins. Hypothalamic CRF is the principal regulator of pituitary adrenocorticotropic hormone (ACTH) secretion, and ACTH stimulates corticosteroid production by the adrenal cortex. CRF is also expressed in the brain outside of the hypothalamus, where it functions as a neurotransmitter/neuromodulator, and in peripheral tissues where it may have diverse actions, perhaps as a cell growth/survival factor.

CRF plays critical roles in animal and human development. For example, CRF injections can accelerate amphibian metamorphosis. Since the early 20th-century scientists have known that amphibian metamorphosis is controlled by thyroid hormone (T3) produced by the thyroid glands. Factors that control the production, metabolism and actions of T3 determine the timing of metamorphosis. The synthesis and secretion of T3 is controlled by pituitary thyroid-stimulating hormone (TSH), which is controlled by hypothalamic-releasing factors. Despite being named for its role as an ACTH-releasing factor, CRF is now known to be a potent stimulator of TSH secretion in amphibians and other non-mammalian species. Thus, the actions of CRF on metamorphosis are thought to be due in large part to the stimulation of thyroid activity.

CRF accelerates amphibian metamorphosis through its combined actions on T3 and corticosteroid production. Corticosteroids are known to synergize with T3 at

(Continued)

the level of target tissues (e.g., the tadpole tail) to promote metamorphosis. This synergy results from corticosteroids increasing the expression of T_3 receptor (TR) and the enzyme (Type II monodeiodinase) that converts the inactive form of thyroid hormone (thyroxine; T4) to the active form (T3). Thus, the thyroid and the adrenal axes interact at central and peripheral levels to influence the timing of metamorphosis. These findings led to the hypothesis that exposure to a stressful environment accelerates tadpole development through the activation of both the thyroid and the adrenal glands. This prediction is supported by the observations that pond drying accelerates metamorphosis of desert toad tadpoles, and this acceleration is accompanied by the precocious activation of their thyroid and adrenal axes. Furthermore, this metamorphic response can be blocked by treatment with CRF antagonists.

Recent findings in mammalian species including humans have shown that CRF is responsible for the timing of birth, and animal studies have shown that the foetus is responsible for establishing this timing. Furthermore, elevated CRF has been implicated in preterm birth in humans caused by intrauterine stress. Thus, environmental stress results in changes in hormone secretion and hormone action at both central and peripheral sites, with the result that the timing of development is altered. The basic signaling components of the endocrine stress system are evolutionarily conserved among vertebrates. The integrated neuroendocrine response to stress, and its role in timing critical life history transitions, likely arose early in the evolution of vertebrates.

References

Crespi, E.J. and Denver, R.J. (2004) Ancient origins of human developmental plasticity. Am. J. Hum. Biol. 17, 44–54.

Denver, R.J. (1997) Environmental stress as a developmental cue: Corticotropin-releasing hormone is a proximate mediator of adaptive phenotypic plasticity in amphibian metamorphosis. Horm. Behav. 31, 169–179.

Denver, R.J. (1999) Evolution of the corticotropin-releasing hormone signaling system and its role in stress-induced developmental plasticity. Ann. NY Acad. Sci. 897, 46–53.

Denver, R.J., Boorse, G.C. and Glennemeier, K.A. (2002) Endocrinology of complex life cycles: Amphibians. In Hormones, Brain and Behavior, Eds Pfaff, D., Arnold, A., Etgen, A., Fahrbach, S., Moss, R. and Rubin, R. Vol. 2, Academic Press, Inc., San Diego, pp. 469–513.

8

Biological rhythms

Introduction

Species are under intense selective pressure to adapt to their environment. Adaptation consists of a multitude of factors. For the most part of this book we have been discussing organismal adaptation to their environment with respect to physical attributes such as oxygen availability, temperature, salinity, pH and food sources. However, there is also a survival advantage if animals are temporally adapted to their environment. During the course of a 24-hour period, light intensity, temperature, humidity and composition of organismal interaction vary. Over the years, seasonal changes in the form of temperature, photoperiod and precipitation regulate food availability, predator–prey relationships and habitat availability. For many species, events such as migration, hibernation and reproduction are timed to particular periods in the season and require significant physiological preparations. Thus, the ability to anticipate changes in the environment provides a selective advantage over species that do not have this ability. Physical or temporal adaptation maximizes the efficiency by which animals maintain homeostatic mechanisms. Homeostasis may be classified as being reactive or predictive. Reactive homeostasis occurs in response to a homeostasis-challenging event. Predictive homeostasis, on the other hand, is anticipatory, for example when an animal forages for food and anticipates when a food source will become available.

Metazoans have evolved internal clocks in the form of molecular and physiological rhythms that allow the anticipation of temporal changes in the environment. The endogenous biological rhythms may be synchronized with one or more naturally occurring cycles,

Neuroendocrinology: An Integrated Approach   David A. Lovejoy
© 2005 John Wiley & Sons, Ltd

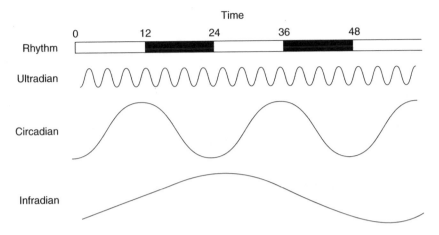

Figure 8.1   *Types of biological rhythms.*

such as the periodicity defined by diurnal, lunar, tidal or seasonal cycles. Three basic types of periodicity are recognized (Fig. 8.1). Circadian rhythms are those that are about a day in duration. Ultradian rhythms occur with a periodicity shorter than a day. These periods may be in the order of minutes to hours. Many of the pulse times of hypothalamic-releasing factors, pituitary hormones and the peripheral hormone systems they drive, fall into this category. Because these cycles have been discussed in the chapters specific to their physiological function, they will not be discussed in detail here. However, a number of species that follow tidal rhythms also fall into this category. Finally, rhythms with a periodicity of greater than a day are referred to as infradian rhythms. Examples of infradian rhythms include seasonal, annual and oestrous or menstrual cycles. For an apparent cycle to be deemed an endogenous rhythm, it must be shown to persist in the absence of cues associated with that rhythm. Moreover, it must be shown to have the capability to be entrained by the environmental cues. We might think of the entrainment of rhythms as the equivalent of resetting a watch periodically so that it remains in harmony with other clocks.

Origin of biological clocks

Biological clocks are ancient. They are found in all kingdoms of life. The most primitive organisms showing periodicity are the cyanobacteria. The presence of clock mechanisms in both prokaryote and eukaryote lineages attests to the physiological importance of these clocks in that they were among the first of the molecular pathways to evolve. We can only speculate what might have been the selection pressure leading to the evolution of the first molecular clocks. However, one possible theory for the evolution of periodicity holds that cells were selected to synchronize cell division with the night-time, when ultraviolet radiation levels were lower. As discussed in Chapter 2, atmospheric oxygen levels were low on Earth at that time. Consequently, there was little in the way of an ozone layer and the planet was subjected to considerably higher levels of ultraviolet and other forms of interstellar radiation than what is present now. In the simple organisms that populated earth at that time, evolving the ability to undergo DNA replication and division during the dark phase, when ultraviolet radiation levels were at a minimum, would have attenuated the mutation rate within the DNA and, hence, reproducibility of these organisms. Then, a couple of billion years later, when organisms were possessed the necessary cellular detoxification mechanisms and an ability to move, they did not necessarily need to have their growth phase in the dark hours, and instead could compensate in a behavioural manner, by locating in a protected spot during light hours, for example, when growth activities could be maximized.

Although biological clocks can regulate physiological events spanning a few minutes to about a year, there is a similar set of mechanisms common to all biological clocks. The most basic level of organization within these clocks lies at the molecular level. There is an inherent periodicity in molecular interactions. It takes a discrete amount of time to complete a particular reaction. If the composition and concentration of the reactants is similar in each reaction, then the completion time for each reaction will be the same. Recall the notion of the autocatalytic and amplifier circuits from Chapter 2. These early metabolic reactions were intrinsic to the earliest protocells and cells. Once particular circuits were selected as being essential for cellular survival, then they would have also imparted their intrinsic reaction times to the cell. Thus from the earliest cells, short or ultradian periodicity would have already been characteristic of these cells. The output of a photosensory organelle, once it evolved, then acted to link a series of ultradian molecular cycles into a circadian rhythm.

Circadian rhythms

Most organisms possess a biological clock mechanism that can become synchronized to daily events to allow the organism to prepare physiologically for the different requirements. Physiology and associated behaviours will alternate between active and quiescent states. And as we alluded to in Chapter 7, physiological activity such as growth and development tend to occur during the quiescent periods when the response to external or environmental events are at a minimum. Circadian rhythms are based on the 24-hour rotational period of the earth. The onset of a number of different behaviours and physiological cycles associated with a particular time of the day will persist even in the absence of time cues such as the exposure to environmental rhythms such as light–dark cycles or tidal cycles. This is due to a self-sustaining biological clock or oscillator, which causes the rhythm to 'free-run' with a period of about 24 hours. The rhythm is, therefore, termed 'circadian', meaning 'about a day'. This circadian period is referred to as Tau (τ) and has been shown to be genetically determined. In humans, for example, free-running periods can vary typically from 22 to 26 hours, although some individuals possess periods greater or less than this. The mean period is about 24 hours. Similarly, a wild-type hamster also has a circadian period about 24 hours. Then, a remarkable discovery of a Tau mutant hamster was made. Homozygous Tau mutant hamsters have a Tau of about 20 hours. Transplantation of the wild-type suprachiasmatic nucleus (SCN) tissue from the hypothalamus (p. 225) into a Tau mutant can restore the rhythm back to about 24 hours (see box 'Hamster Tau mutant'). The recent identification of casein kinase II as the Tau mutant gene has led to a better understanding of the molecular clock mechanism in cells.

Circadian rhythms affect virtually all behaviours and physiological mechanisms in one form or another. In most mammals this may include foraging behaviour and quiescence (sleep). It may also include body temperature, melatonin secretion, osmoregulatory mechanisms and/or cognitive performance in humans. Although there is a common set of neurological loci that act to drive and entrain the master clock mechanism, the manner in which various neuroendocrine circuits are integrated with this clock vary. As a result, the developmental stage of an organism, and particularly mammals, has an affect on clock-mediated circuits. For example, ageing can affect both the amplitude and the frequency of many circadian rhythms. The degradation of some rhythms vary more than others, hence there may be either a loss or disharmony of rhythms that are meant to act in tandem. Such an effect can attenuate the flexibility of the physiological or behavioural response to environmental events. For example, the maintenance of pituitary hormone secretion is related to several factors that involve the SCN. The brain and, in particular, the SCN must maintain a 24-hour rhythmicity (Fig. 8.2). However, the ability of the SCN to drive the outputs that

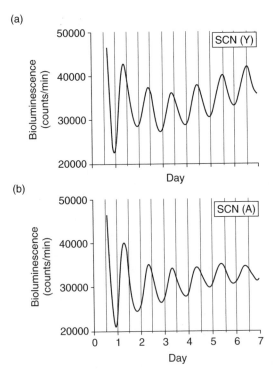

Figure 8.2 *Per2 expression in isolated SCN from (a) young rat and (b) aged rat. Circadian rhythm of the SCN persists after removal from the hypothalamus. Note the decreased amplitude in the aged animal. Reprinted from Yamazaki* et al. *(2002) by the permission of National Academy of Sciences.*

regulate hypothalamic-releasing hormone-secreting neurons, and the ability of these releasing factor neurons to respond to SCN efferents can be compromised to varying degrees. Other brain loci integrating the ability of stimuli such as sleep, light or locomotion to entrain the circadian aspects of neuroendocrine rhythms may also be differentially affected.

Circadian rhythms control a wide variety of behaviours and endocrine rhythms. In vertebrates, photoperiodic information is relayed via the retino-hypothalamic tract, to the SCN then to the pineal gland where it is converted from neural information to an endocrine signal, for example, the daily pattern of melatonin secretion (p. 226). Factors that can entrain of biological clocks include environmental factors such as photoperiod, temperature and social interactions, and physiological influences such as satiety, injury or sleep. Such entrainment factors may act to phase-shift the biological clock, such that the onset of the activity cycle is shifted either forwards or backwards relative to the quiescence cycle (Fig. 8.3).

Non-photic input such as locomotor behaviour, social stimulation and other kinds of arousal-inducing activity can influence phase-shifting activities in animals. Initially, it had been observed that the rate of adjustment to an advanced light–dark cycle could be significantly increased by placing hamsters in a novel running wheel for three hours in the middle of their subjective day. Since then, arousal-inducing situations such as sexual arousal, social interaction, novel running wheels, dark pulses, cage changes or the administration of the benzodiazepine, triazolam, which causes a paradoxical arousal in hamsters, could all act to reset the endogenous clock. However, not all apparently arousal-inducing events could achieve this, and it has been speculated that the arousal needs to be associated with a rewarding effect. Nevertheless, these effects appear to be mediated by a non-photic pathway. Two major non-photic neural inputs to the SCN, 5-HT input from the raphe nuclei of the midbrain, and NPY input from the intergeniculate leaflet of the thalamus, have been implicated in this phenomenon (Fig. 8.4). Although a number of studies implicating the role of 5-HT in the non-photic phase-shifting of the clock have been equivocal, at least as far as hamsters are concerned, the evidence supporting a role for NPY is stronger. Novelty-induced running behaviour in hamsters activates a subset of NPY neurons of the intergeniculate leaflet, as measured by *c-fos* expression. Moreover,

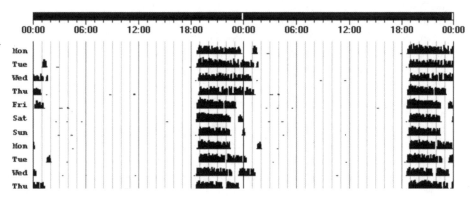

Figure 8.3 *Actogram showing hamster running behaviour at the same time during the subjective night. Image courtesy of Martin Ralph, University of Toronto.*

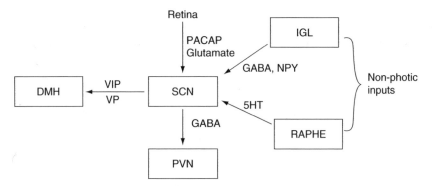

Figure 8.4   *Major input and output pathways associated with the suprachiasmatic nucleus.*

NPY antisera, delivered to or near the SCN by cannulae block the phase-advancing effect of novelty-induced wheel running.

Infradian rhythms

Reproduction, migration and hibernation require long periods of preparation. The fitness of an animal is improved if it is capable of obtaining predictive information confirming future environmental conditions. Like diurnal rhythms, seasonal rhythms may also be divided into alternating periods of activity and quiescence. Colder seasons are characterized by an inhibition of reproduction along with physiological adaptations associated with hibernation, migration or pelage changes. In each case, survival through the harsher conditions means a greater expenditure of energy. Metabolic rate, as a result, varies throughout the year. Seasonal variations of metabolic rate may manifest as variations in body weight, food intake, growth rate, milk production, fat storages and mobilization in different species. A number of mammalian species including rodents, ungulate carnivores and primate species show the presence of circannual rhythms. Among birds, the Peking duck is one of the best-studied species. When this animal is kept in constant darkness, it will show a mean rhythm of about 85% of a year for as long as five years. In humans, seasonal actions may appear in the form of seasonal affective disorder that may be characterized by depression, hypersomnia, carbohydrate craving and weight gain.

Effect of photoperiod on infradian rhythms

Photoperiod appears to be the main factor at regulating seasonal changes. However, there can be a latency of several weeks from time of exposure to different daylengths to the onset of the physiological changes. This onset is not dependent on the photoperiod length *per se*, but rather the direction of photoperiod change. Responses to photoperiod is an integrative phenomenon for many species in that the physiological changes is determined by the lengthening of photoperiod relative to the length of the photoperiod preceding it. Thus, a lengthening photoperiod will induce a set of changes associated with the coming of spring whereas the perception of a shortening photoperiod will induce an opposition set of changes. This system regulating seasonal changes must do so with respect to environmental conditions that may alter the perception of photoperiod, for example, long-term cloud cover. In addition, this mechanism must be relatively resistant to stochastic neuroendocrine events that may be induced by injury, disease or simply random fluctuations in hormonal release that could potentially act to modulate the seasonal clock mechanism. In other words, this ability to integrate changing photoperiod must be able to differentiate the change in environment from the ambient noise. This filtering effect is particularly important, for example, for migrating animals that must integrate seasonal changes with photoperiodic changes associated with the movement across lines of latitude. The sensitivity to photoperiodic change differs among species, populations and individuals. The rate of change can affect species differently. Among humans, the high rate of change of photoperiod during the autumn and spring months in regions near the poles has been linked to neurological problems, such as depression in some individuals. Thus, the integration rate may be epigenetically determined.

It is not the actual daylength or night length of the light cycle that is measured. Instead the phases when the light occurs within the circadian cycle is important for entrainment. Brief periods of light pulses can mimic a long photoperiod if it occurs at the appropriate phase in the circadian cycle. There are three components to photoperiod. This includes the length of photoperiod, intensity of light and the wavelength. Highly cloudy areas in temperate conditions, for example, in western Europe or the North American pacific northwest, may be highly variable between years; thus circannual rhythms may be advantageous.

The physiological mechanisms of a circannual oscillatory are not entirely understood, but a generally favoured model incorporates a series of different physiological states of which each have a discrete set of changes requiring a certain time. The completion of each stage leads to the onset of the next stage such that the series spans about a year. An analogy of this might be an oestrous or menstrual cycle (Chapter 10) where a series of endocrine events take place. A number of loci in the brain have been implicated in circannual rhythms. For example, in ewes, pinealectomy does not interfere with circannual rhythms in LH release. Similarly, in ground squirrels, disruption of the SCN and VMN do not appear to be critical for circannual rhythms. However, each of these sites can modify the characteristics of the cycle suggesting that several neurological loci are likely involved in the generation of such cycles. Several of these neurological loci, acting together can form a physiological hierarchy to regulate the onset of these rhythms. Depending upon the niche adaptation of the species, the organization of the hierarchy can vary. Laboratory rats, which are not generally periodic, will show an advancement of puberty if kept in short day conditions after removal of the olfactory lobes. In this species, social and pheromonal cues (Chapter 12) are incorporated at a higher hierarchical level and can attenuate the physiological effects of photoperiod.

Reproductive cycles

Reproductive timing mechanisms are under high selective pressures because relatively small temporal changes in the onset of parturition can drastically reduce survivability. Environmentally, organisms must coordinate reproductive activity with climatological changes in order that progeny are born under the most hospitable conditions as possible. Sources of food, scarcity of predators, temperature and precipitation must be optimal for this to occur. The coordination of reproductive events with environmental conditions is species-dependent and reflects the physiological capabilities and flexibility of the species, for example, metabolic rate, hibernation or torpor, gestation length or embryonic diapause.

Such environmental factors include dietary and climatic factors, particularly food availability, rainfall and temperatures, species competition and exposure to predators. Animals with short gestation periods, for example a ferret, or having a gestational period of about a year, such as a horse, tend to mate in spring or early summer. Animals with gestational periods of about six months, like sheep, tend to mate in the autumn. On the other hand, mating will tend to occur in the early summer in animals showing embryonic diapause, such as the roe deer, then be followed by five months of diapause, delaying implantation until December and birth in May.

In some anuran species, such as *Rana temporaria* and *Rana dybowskii*, spontaneous activation of the hypothalamus–pituitary–gonadal (HPG) axis appears to occur. In *R. temporaria*, pituitary LH increases in the second third of hibernation during mid-January around week 13. The regulation of this event may occur in part via the HPT axis. In this species, serum T3 and T4 significantly increases during about this time followed by a decrease in both free and bound forms of the thyroid hormones. This low level of serum T3 and T4 remains low until the end of hibernation; however, the thyroid content of free T3 and T4 increases and reaches a peak about mid-February.

Hormonal systems involved in circannual and seasonal rhythms

Many of the same hormonal systems utilized in metamorphosis are also utilized to regulate the onset of seasonal rhythms (Fig. 8.5). In Chapter 7, we discussed the synergism between the hypothalamus–pituitary–thyroid (HPT) axis and the hypothalamus–pituitary–adrenal (HPA) axis in regard to metamorphosis. In some cases, both axes may be mediated by CRF or by a reciprocal positive relationship between CRF and TRH. Physiologically in

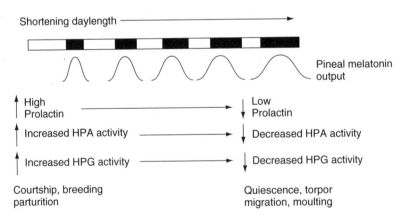

Figure 8.5 *Effect of shortening daylength on neuroendocrine circuits and the associated behaviours.*

the short term, thyroid hormones and glucocorticoids act together to redistribute energy where it is required and to maximize the use of energy production. In the longer term, both hormone classes induce adaptive measures for changes in energy use and production and thermogenesis. Glucocorticoids vary in response to season. For example, in yellow pine chipmunks (*Tamias amoenus*), glucocorticoids are at minimal value at the time of mating. The steroids peak during late lactation with cortisol rising almost twofold and corticosterone increasing more than threefold. These levels then decline until hibernation. However, it is not clear whether the change in glucocorticoids is due to seasonal changes, for example, daylength, *per se*, or rather due indirectly to the behaviours associated with the seasonal event (Chapter 9).

In vertebrates, prolactin appears to play a significant role in regulating the onset of seasonal behaviours. For example, prolactin inhibits torpor in Siberian hamsters. Daily torpor is characterized as a decrease in body temperature, from a euthermic value of 37 °C to about 18–25 °C. Torpor bouts last about four to eight hours starting at dawn and occurring daily at circadian intervals. Prolonged exposure to short days elicits daily torpor, whereas ablation of the SCN terminates torpor expression, producing hyperprolactinemia. On long days, daily torpor can be elicited by restricting hamster food intake, but bouts are shorter and less frequent than on winter short days, when prolactin levels are lower. Elevated levels of prolactin on short winter days therefore cause inhibition of daily torpor. Lactating mammals with high prolactin concentrations generally do not undergo torpor, although bats appear to be a notable exception.

Ground squirrels implanted with oestradiol lose weight and the period of their circannual rhythm can be reduced. In rats, changes in oestrogen concentrations during the oestrous cycle can modify the dendritic spinal density in the ventromedial hypothalamus (VMH) or dorsal hippocampus (Chapter 7). Spinal density is highest during oestrus and pro-oestrus when oestradiol levels are highest and lowest during di-oestrus when oestrogen levels are lowest. Testosterone influences the control of seasonal hibernations and daily torpor in hamsters. Testosterone and prolactin inhibit its expression. In females, oestradiol has the same effect. Elevated testosterone can also reduce the length of hibernation.

Changes in pelage

A number of species show annual changes in pelage depending on the conditions. The coats of minks are thicker as a result of greater number of hair follicles in winter, but thinner with fewer hair follicles in warmer seasons. The prairie vole, *Microtus ochrogaster*, also experiences long cold winters and hot summers. Adjustments that enhance winter survival include a reduction in body weight, metabolic rate and the development of winter pelage. The effect of daylength on pelage is mediated, in part, by changes in prolactin secretion. A number of studies suggest that other mammals also develop winter pelage on short days by inhibiting prolactin secretion in, for example, Siberian hamsters and mink. In these species, the development of a winter coat during short days coincides with a decrease in circulating prolactin, an effect that can be blocked by daily injections of prolactin. The suppression of the seasonal increase in prolactin secretion by the administration of the dopamine agonist, bromocriptine, can delay the onset of the spring moult in the Djungarian hamster and the Red deer. The increasing prolactin concentrations in spring are thus an important component of the endocrine signal that induces moult in Red deer from winter to summer coat. In the Djungarian hamster the concomitant administration of prolactin induces the spring moult.

Clock circuitry in vertebrates

The clock mechanisms of metazoans are composed of several distinct oscillators receiving environmental input. Many cells in the body possess a molecular clock mechanism that becomes entrained by the central clock mechanisms. A number of CNS sites are responsible for the temporal regulation of neuroendocrine rhythms.

Molecular mechanisms of cellular oscillators

The most fundamental oscillator in any species is found in individual cells. As we have previously discussed, there is an intrinsic periodicity in molecular interactions. Direct molecular interactions possess a discrete period for completion. This time interval can be lengthened by increasing the complexity of the reaction. In vertebrates, the cellular oscillator is based around the interplay of a relatively small number of regulatory genes (Fig. 8.6). In this model, the expression of the protein products of *Bmal1* and *clk* act downstream to facilitate the transcription and expression of *Rev-erbα*, *Per* and *Cry* genes. Their protein products then attenuate the expression of the *Bmal1* and *Clk* genes. Once the expression

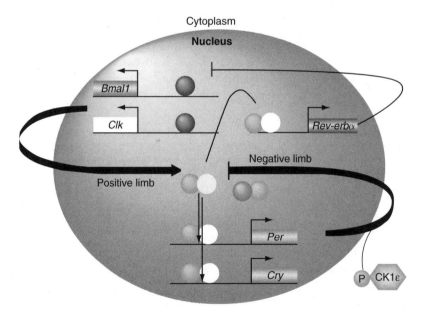

Figure 8.6 *Molecular aspects of clock mechanisms. The expression of* Bmal1 *and* Clk *proteins facilitate the expression of the* Rev-erbα, Per *and* Cry *genes which then inhibit the* Bmal1 *and* Clk *genes. Reprinted from Albrecht and Eichele (2003) with permission from Elsevier Science, Ltd.*

products of these genes fall to a sufficiently low enough level, then the expression of the *Rev-erbα*, *Per* and *Cry* genes fall, thus decreasing the attenuation of the *Bmal1* and *Clk* gene expression. The cycle then begins all over again.

In mammals there are three Per paralogues, of which the proteins show the capability to heterodimerize with each other. There is evidence that the expression of these genes can vary among animal groups. For example, rhythmic Per2 gene expression in the house sparrow hypothalamus is not restricted to the SCN but is also found in an additional nucleus in the lateral hypothalamic nucleus. Per2 expression in the SCN appears to be expressed in the rostral portion of the nucleus before lights on. In the lateral hypothalamus Per2 expression is delayed. The overall circadian Per2 expression pattern is not significantly affected by pinealectomy although it may modulate both the phase and amplitude of rhythmic Per2 expression.

Hypothalamic nuclei

The SCN plays a pivotal role at generating and integrating periodicity in most vertebrates. The rat SCN contains about 8000 cells per side that make extensive connections with each other. If the SCN is isolated from the brain, it will continue to fire in a circadian pattern and can continue for several weeks. Individual cells within the SCN are circadian oscillators. In mammals, the major afferent projections to the SCN come from the retina, raphe nucleus of the midbrain and intergeniculate leaflet in the diencephalon. Although the SCN is the pacemaker fundamental to the regulation of circadian rhythmicity in mammals, it is the pineal gland that serves as the primary circadian clock in birds and reptiles. However, the SCN can disrupt rhythm in some birds. SCN lesions in some species can disrupt circadian rhythms while leaving annual rhythms relatively intact (Fig. 8.7).

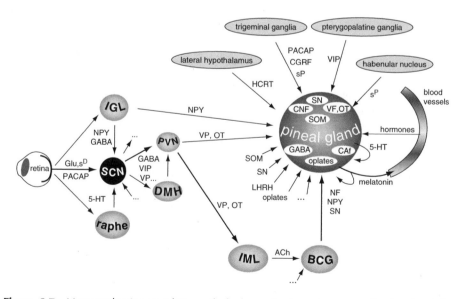

Figure 8.7 *Neuroendocrine regulation of clock mechanisms in mammals. Reprinted from Simonneaux and Ribelayga (2003) with permission from the American Society for Pharmacology and Experimental Therapeutics.*

A number of neurotransmitters have been shown to phase-shift the SCN. NMDA receptor-mediated glutamate transduction can delay the rhythm in neuronal activity during the early subjective night an advances the rhythms during the early subjective day. Several hormones have been implicated in the regulation of SCN function. In mammals, vasoactive intestinal peptide (VIP) increases prolactin secretion and rapid eye movement (REM) sleep whereas VIP inhibitors block these processes. VIP increases hypothalamic prolactin mRNA not associated with pituitary prolactin. NPY concentrations are reported to rise several hours before the onset of the activity period. Oestradiol can alter the daily running activity by female hamsters.

VIP and gastrin-releasing peptide (GRP) are located in the ventrolateral SCN, an area that contains input from the retina via the retinohypothalamic tract (RHT). Microinjections of VIP or GRP into the SCN causes phase delays of the locomotor rhythm when injected during the early subjective night and phase advancement when injected during the late subjective night. The phase-shifting response of VIP or GRP is similar to that of light. GRP levels in the SCN are highest during the day but the phase-shifting effects of GRP occur during the night. The effects of light on the retina may be conveyed to GRP- and VIP-containing neurons in the SCN resulting in a paracrine action on local cells.

Prolactin concentrations are determined by light intensity in a number of species. In rats, there is a distinct expression of prolactin linked to mid-day that can be abolished by SCN lesions. In a greater number of species, however, there is a surge in prolactin secretion near the onset of dark hours. Prolactin is linked to an animal's breeding season where it is associated with the onset of reproductive activity. Prolactin can influence the sleep process, by influencing REM, and prolactin blockers will inhibit the expression of REM sleep.

Pineal complex

The pineal complex plays a major role in the regulation of circadian activity. The structure of the pineal gland was described about 2300 years ago and over that time it has been an object of intense speculation (Chapter 1). Only in the last 50 years its function has become known. The pineal gland is unusual in that it is unpaired. Embryonically, it arises as an evagination of modified ependymal cells from the roof of the caudal aspect of the third ventricle. The blood–brain barrier is absent in the pineal gland. The pineal is highly vascularized and has a remarkably high rate of blood flow. Blood to the pineal comes from vessels that originate in the choroid plexus.

In 1965, Wartman and Axelrod advanced the 'melatonin hypothesis' that suggested that the pineal gland acts as a transducer responding to circambient light by changing the rate of melatonin output. Isolated pineal glands of some birds, lizards and fish can maintain circadian rhythms of melatonin synthesis for many days in constant darkness. There is considerable variation in the structure and size of the pineal gland. For example, it is well developed in animals associated with polar and temperate regions, but small or absent in animals living near the equator.

There has been considerable evolution of function of the pineal complex in the chordates. The pineal complex of vertebrates can influence a number of physiological mechanisms including regulation of circadian rhythms, seasonal reproduction, metamorphosis and body colour change. Hagfish as members of the most phylogenetically oldest group of chordates do not possess a pineal complex. However, locomotor activity rhythm is disrupted in the hagfish *Eptatretus burgeri* in which surgical lesions of the preoptic nucleus were made. The preoptic nucleus (PON) in this species receives input from the retina and appears to act, in part, in a manner analogous to the SCN of phylogenetically more recent chordates. In lamprey, where a pineal body is present (*Lampetra japonica*), pinealectomy abolishes the circadian rhythm of locomotor activity.

In some fish, amphibians and reptiles, the pineal possesses a lens- and retina-like structure that acts as a third photosensory organ analogous to the eyes. The pineal gland may be directly photosynthetic as in fishes, amphibians, reptiles and birds or it may receive photic information via sympathetic neural pathways as which occurs in mammals. Reptiles possess a number of circadian photoreceptors including a photoreceptive pineal gland, an extracranial parapineal organ (parietal eye) and deep brain photoreceptors. A remarkable feature about reptiles is the redundancy of the photoreceptor systems. The retinas of the lateral eyes, pineal and parietal eyes all contain photoreceptors. *Iguana iguana*, when kept in constant ambient temperatures, displays endogenously generated circadian rhythms of body temperature and locomotor activity. Removal of the parietal eye and pineal gland completely abolishes the rhythm of body temperature and abolishes the circadian melatonin rhythms and significantly lowers plasma melatonin concentrations. However, the rhythm of locomotor activity is only slightly affected. In the lizard *Podarcis sicula* melatonin secretion from the pineal varies with high values in spring compared to low values in summer and autumn. *In vitro* the presence of a circadian melatonin rhythm occurs in winter although such a rhythm is absent *in vivo* in winter. The pineal melatonin production may be, therefore, influenced by an extra-pineal oscillator in the intact animal. Pinealectomy can also abolish circadian body temperature and locomotor activity rhythms in the house sparrow (*Passer domesticus*) and can disrupt circadian rhythms in other passerines.

Retina

The retina has been comparatively well studied and pacemakers have been found in the retina of most chordate classes, molluscs and arthropods. Given the ubiquity of this mechanism it is likely that it was comparatively well evolved in the common ancestor to these lineages. Eyes of Xenopus, chicken, quail, fish (e.g. *Esox lucius*) and mammals also contain self-sustained circadian oscillators that regulate melatonin synthesis. In the duck retina, for example, dopamine and its main metabolite 3,4-dihydroxyphenylacetic acid (DOPAC) peak during the light phase. Melatonin and AANAT activity occur maximally at night. Acute exposure to light at night increases dopamine and DOPAC but decreases melatonin and AANAT.

In mammals, the retina also plays a fundamental role at the perception of photoperiodic information and relays it to the integrative centres of the CNS. Light entering the retina can be absorbed by photopigments in the rods and cones or by the retinal ganglion cells. A subset of the retinal ganglion cells express melanopsin and cryptochrome pigments. These cells can therefore relay photic, but non-visual information to the LGN and SCN via PACAP (Chapter 7) and glutamate-mediated systems (Fig. 8.8).

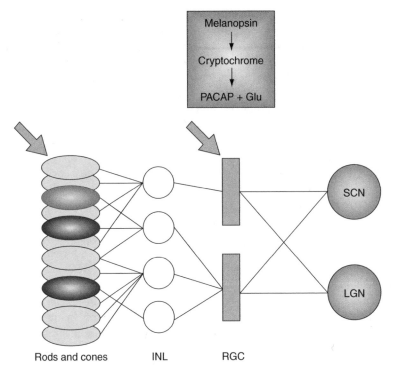

Figure 8.8   *Non-visual pathways from the retina. Light entering the retina can be absorbed by photopigments in the rods and cones or by retinal ganglion cells. A subset of retinal ganglion cells expresses melanopsin and cryptochrome. These cells relay photic but non-visual information to the suprachiasmatic nucleus using PACAP and glutamate. Reprinted from van Gelder (2003) with permission from Elsevier Science Ltd.*

The role of melatonin

Melatonin (*N*-acetyl-5-methoxytryptamine) was named for its ability to induce the aggregation of melanin in the melanophores to induce a pallor of skin in amphibian tadpoles and lampreys during the dark hours. Melatonin and serotonin are indoleamine neurohormones. Melatonin is derived from serotonin by a two-step enzymatic process whereby serotonin is converted to the *N*-acetylserotonin intermediate by the enzyme arylalkylamine *N*-acetyltransferase (AANAT, serotonin *N*-acetyltransferase), then to melatonin by hydroxyindole-*O*-methyltransferase (HIOMT) (Fig. 8.9). Soon after the discovery of the production of melatonin in the bovine pineal gland, the control of melatonin production was shown to be photoperiod dependent. This prediction was made on the basis of a presumed 24-hour rhythm in the HIOMT present in the rat pineal organ. Studies subsequently confirmed that the production of melatonin was higher at night than during the day for most vertebrates. In mammals, the nocturnal rise in blood melatonin is derived primarily from the pineal gland. In non-mammalian vertebrates, other organs may also influence to the 24-hour serum melatonin rhythm (Fig. 8.10).

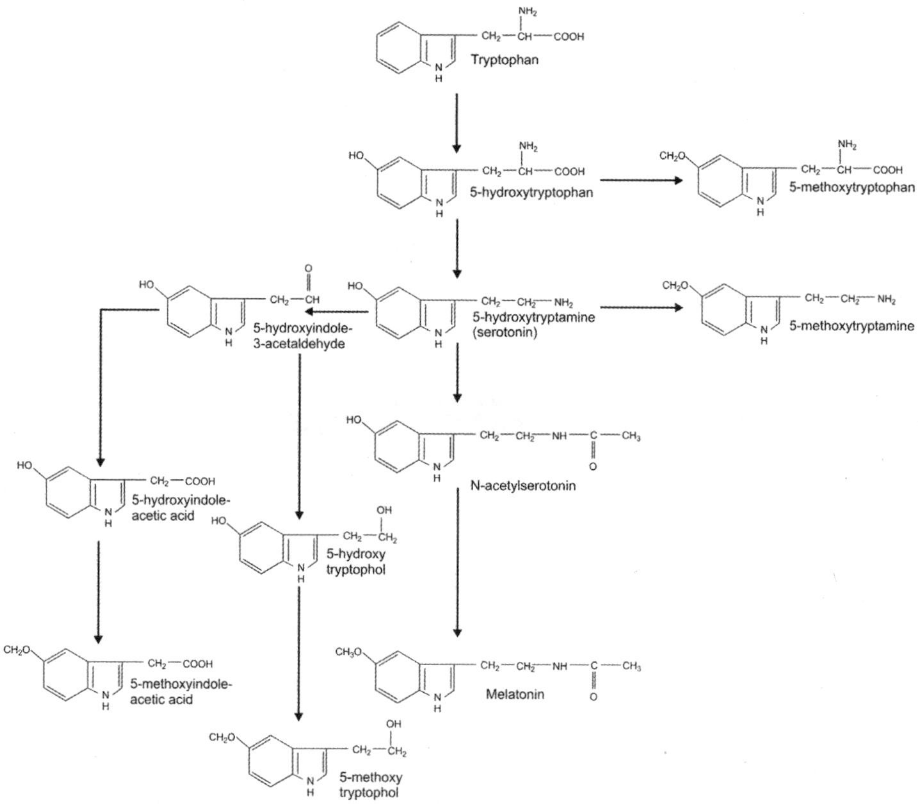

Figure 8.9 *Synthesis of melatonin and metabolites.*

Evolution of melatonin

Melatonin is usually described with its role in biological rhythms in mammals and vertebrates. However, a hormonal role for melatonin is actually phylogenetically relatively recent. Cellular and likely some organismal clock mechanisms evolved well before melatonin became associated with periodicity. Melatonin is an ancient hormone that has multiple functions. The biosynthetic pathway leading to the synthesis of serotonin and melatonin appears to have evolved early in eukaryote history. Melatonin is present in several species of fungi, protistans, algae and throughout the vertebrates. It has also been found in prokaryotes indicating that this pathway was present in an ancestor well before the prokaryote and eukaryotes diverged into separate lineages.

Although it is unlikely that melatonin evolved as part of the rhythm-inducing machinery in primitive organisms, it may have been present around the time, or slightly after the evolution of the first molecular oscillators and organismal clocks. Because melatonin is so ubiquitous, we might expect that the presence of melatonin led to selective survival of the organisms that evolved the ability to synthesize it. As we alluded to earlier in this

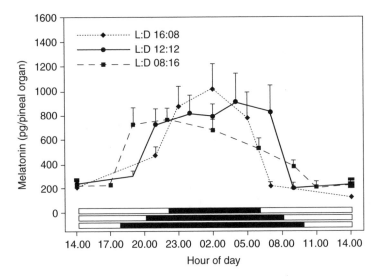

Figure 8.10 *Melatonin synthesis in trout. Melatonin accumulation in the pineal organ varies as a function of the light–dark period. Reprinted with permission from Ceinos* et al. *(2002), Monduzzi Editore.*

chapter, periodicity may have developed in part to allow DNA replication to occur at night when the incidence of mutagenic events is lower. In addition, the evolution of molecular detoxification systems to coincide with DNA replication could enhance the survivability of these organisms. In fact, a number of studies indicate that melatonin can inhibit mutagenesis induced by radiation and by indirect chemical mutagens. Melatonin can also inhibit the development of spontaneous and chemically induced tumours in mice and rats.

Ionizing radiation can induce the formation of a number of highly reactive oxygen radicals (Chapter 7). The formation of these molecular variants has been associated with much of the biological damage induced by radiation. Melatonin has been implicated as an antioxidant in the dinoflagellate *Lingulodinium*, the ciliate *Paramecium*, the rotifer *Philodina* and also in *Drosophila*. Melatonin may have a secondary action on antioxidation by lowering the metabolic rate of cells and hence proliferation rate. For example, melatonin can reduce the proliferation of Chinese hamster ovary (CHO) cells in a dose- and time-dependent manner. The natural antioxidants, resveratrol and vitamin E, which appear in edible plants, can mimic the effect of melatonin. Melatonin treatment can reduce the number of cells in S phase and increase cells both in Go/G1 and G2/M phase. Glutathione, a natural antioxidant, levels are increased after melatonin treatment but do not play a role in the proliferative changes. Melatonin appears to function as a non-receptor mediated free radical scavenging factor. It can also be ingested in foodstuffs such as vegetables, fruits, rice, wheat and herbal medicines. Therefore, as a nutrient, melatonin could also be classified as a vitamin. Melatonin probably evolved first as an antioxidant, then became a vitamin in the food chain and multicellular organisms utilized it as a paracrine factor where it eventually took on hormonal properties. Its complementary role with the night at reducing mutagenic actions on DNA may have been the evolutionary impetus to intertwine the actions of melatonin with photoperiodicity.

The role of melatonin in periodicity

The role melatonin plays in rhythmicity varies among metazoans. It has not been established however how much of a role, if at all, melatonin plays in transducing environmental periodicity into a hormonal signal in invertebrates. Although maximal synthesis at night has been observed in a number of cases, for many other invertebrate species, melatonin secretion is associated with the light hours. In the first stages of melatonin evolution it was likely synthesized constituently or perhaps indirectly in a periodic manner. In vertebrates, it is the enzyme arylalkylamine N-acetyltransferase (AANAT) that converts the perception of day and night into a hormonal signal in the form of melatonin (Fig. 8.11). A putative enzyme in the yeast, *Saccharomyces cerevisiae*, has a similar enzyme activity although the substrate preference pattern is less specific. It has 47% sequence

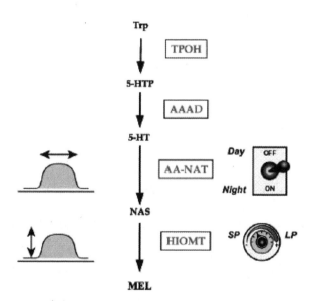

Figure 8.11 *Relationship of melatonin-synthesizing enzymes and the effect on the amplitude and duration of melatonin synthesis and release. The species-specific regulation of these enzymes acts in part to induce the species-dependent effect on melatonin-release profiles. Reprinted from Simonneaux and Ribelayga (2003) with permission from the American Society for Pharmacology and Experimental Therapeutics.*

identity to ovine AANAT. This enzyme appears to be present in a number of fungal species but orthologues have not been identified in the *D. melanogaster* or *C. elegans* genomes. The *S. cerevisiae* enzyme appears to be distinct in that it lacks the specific domains of the vertebrate enzymes that are essential for the regulatory role the enzyme plays in photochemical transduction. Thus, a direct periodic synthesis for melatonin may have evolved in the metazoa after the bifurcation of the animal and fungal kingdoms and possibly during the genome duplications that gave rise to the triploblastic metazoans.

In mammals and many vertebrates, pineal secretion of melatonin is inhibited by light and therefore is elevated at night. Although this is not necessarily the case in all metazoans, a number of marine species in particular show alternative patterns of secretion. For example, in the colonial anthozoan, *Renilla kollikeri*, no daily rhythmic changes of melatonin are found. However, seasonal variations of melatonin are found in both colonial and non-colonial forms. Spring and summer levels are four to five times higher than autumn and winter values. The annual rise coincides with the first stages of sexual maturation. Immunoreactive melatonin occurs exclusively in a neuronal distribution in the endodermal septal filaments present around gametophores, in the endodermal walls of the rachis and in the ectodermal polyps. In the mollusc, *Aplysia californica*, melatonin is high in the eyes during the day but rises in the cerebral ganglia during the night. The photosensory organs from this species, if maintained in culture, will exhibit a diurnal rhythm of melatonin release activity over a three-day period. In the snail, *Helix aspera maxima*, melatonin is low in the cerebroid ganglia, visceral ganglia and ocular tentacles except during the night when there is a small peak of melatonin in the cerebroid ganglia. However, 5-methoxytrypophol (5-ML) is undetectable in cerebroid and the visceral ganglia, but shows a diurnal pattern in the ocular tentacles with low values in the middle of the lighter period and a high value at night. These values are opposite to the known daily variations of 5-ML in vertebrates. 5-ML may be released into the haemolymph, suggesting it could act as a hormone.

Central actions of melatonin in vertebrates

In vertebrates, melatonin is produced locally in the retina, Harderian gland, gut and blood platelets but only the pineal source of melatonin appears to contribute to the systemic circulation of melatonin. Melatonin levels rise with night-time in the pineal in virtually all mammals. Unless there is a genetic absence of enzymes mediating its production, the pattern of nocturnal rise varies among species. Three different patterns of nocturnal melatonin production have been described. Type A is typified by a delay of several hours in the onset of melatonin synthesis following the onset of darkness. Melatonin levels rise to a peak quickly and soon after return to daytime levels at the time of lights on. This type of rhythm occurs in the Syrian hamster and is probably the least common pattern. A Type B pattern is indicated by a gradual rise in pineal production of the indole starting at about the time of lights off. The melatonin peak is reached during the middle of the dark phase, followed by a gradual reduction in production during the second half of the night; examples of this pattern include the domestic rat (*Rattus norvegicus*) and humans.

In Type C, high melatonin synthesis occurs virtually all night. Within 30 minutes of dark onset, the melatonin peak is achieved. Late in the dark-phase levels decline precipitously, as observed in the cotton rat, sheep and wallaby.

Hence in some species melatonin levels are at their highest when the animal is asleep, whereas in others it peaks when the animal is most active. In all mammals so far studied (with the exception of reindeer), the melatonin rhythm is endogenous and persists in the absence of time cues. Although there may be a phylogenetic propensity for some species to be active diurnally, and some species to be active nocturnally, a number of species show both nocturnal and diurnal activity. Humans are a notable example, but so are Green turtles (*Chelonia mydas*). Green turtles can exhibit nocturnal activity in addition to their diurnal activity. In captivity, a nocturnal rise occurs in melatonin and a diurnal rise occurs in cortisol. When induced to perform nocturnal activity, there is a decrease in melatonin compared to the inactive controls. Plasma cortisol also increases with nocturnal activity. The increase correlates with the intensity of nocturnal behaviour that typically includes nesting, mate searching, feeding and swimming behaviours. Generally, plasma melatonin and cortisol show little or no daily fluctuation.

The pattern of melatonin synthesis at night appears to be a major cue in transducing seasonal information into a physiological signal. Regardless of the melatonin secretion pattern, an extension of the dark phase, for example, during the winter nights, prolongs the melatonin peak. The synthesis of melatonin by the pineal is controlled by the circadian system, in that the nocturnal peak of secretion varies in direct proportion to the length of the dark phase, thereby providing an endocrine representation of season. The response to short photoperiods in the Syrian hamster, which is associated with a decline in serum gonadotropins and prolactin, gonadal atrophy, can be blocked by pinealectomy and reproduced by systemic infusions of melatonin, which restore the long-duration melatonin profile characteristic of short daylength.

Melatonin exerts its actions via specific receptors whose subtype and specificity vary considerably among vertebrates. No specific binding of iodinated melatonin has been found in either the hagfish (*Myxine glutinosa*) or amphioxus (*Branchiostoma lanceolatum*), both of which lack a pineal complex. However, in the optic tecta of lamprey, skate and trout, there are specific high-affinity low-capacity binding sites for melatonin. In stark contrast to hagfish, the melatonin binding pattern in the brain shows an elaborate distribution. In lampreys, specific melatonin binding is found in optic tectum and also in the preoptic nucleus, particularly in the parvocellular division. In the larval brain, the binding was less intense and consistent. In the little skate (*Raja erinacea*), intense specific binding is found in the optic tectum, lateral geniculate body, diencephalic, preoptic and supraoptic nucleus, basal hypothalamus and medial pallium. The absence of melatonin receptors in *Amphioxus* and hagfish suggests that the melatonin receptors arose after the divergence of species leading to the Myxini (hagfishes), but before the development of the lampreys. The formation and development of the melatonin receptors may have coincided with a round of genome duplication that is thought to have occurred around this time. Thus the hormonal role of melatonin appears to have developed after the formation of the pineal body, and its ability to synthesize melatonin. If this is in fact the situation, then much of the melatonin role in non-vertebrate metazoans may be primarily involved with anti-oxidation.

Studies in amphibians have indicated that although in a gross sense the neuroanatomical distribution of melatonin binding is similar, there are numerous differences that need to be considered. The crested newt, *Triturus carniflex*, and the green frog, *Rana esculenta*, showed that the highest amount of melatonin-binding occurred in the optic tracts, SCN and optic tectum of both species. Low or no melatonin binding occurred in the POA, tuberal hypothalamus, medulla oblongata, septum or dorsal pallium. In the crested newt, higher melatonin binding occurred in the amygdaloid nucleus pars lateralis and striatum, whereas in green frog, higher levels occurred in the hindbrain. The melatonin receptor distribution then likely reflects the neurological loci required for the transduction of environmental events significant for niche adaptation.

The melatonin receptor is a G-protein-coupled receptor, however in contrast to serotonin, only possesses a few subtypes. Melatonin receptors have been cloned in representative actinopterygian and sarcopterygian species. In the chick brain, for example, a putative melatonin receptor CK-A is 80% identical at the amino acid level to the human Mel1a receptor and CK-B is 80% identical to the *Xenopus* melatonin receptor and may define a new receptor subtype, the Mel1c receptor, which is distinct from the Mel1a and Mel1b subtypes. Polymerase chain-reaction studies suggest that a melatonin receptor family consisting of three subtypes appears to be present among both sarcopterygian and actinopterygian lineages. A potentially novel melatonin receptor subtype, Mel 1d may exist in *Xenopus*. It is only 61% identical with the human Mel 1b receptor.

Physiological actions of melatonin

Melatonin brain circuitry, as we have alluded to previously, varies considerably among species and ultimately reflects their niche adaptation. Mammals are unusual in that the pineal body does not get direct photoperiodic input, in contrast to other amniotes and amphibians. A rather elaborate set of indirect pathways is employed. In mammals, photoperiodic information is perceived by the retina where it is relayed directly to the SCN, intergeniculate leaflet and raphe nucleus. The SCN also receives indirect information from the intergeniculate leaflet via NPY and GABAergic pathways and via a serotonergic pathway from the Raphe nucleus. Photoperiodic information can be relayed indirectly to the pineal body by an NPY dependent circuit from the intergeniculate leaflet (Fig. 8.12). However, the SCN also sends GABA and VIP-mediated efferents that innervate a subpopulation of vasopressin and oxytocin cells of the paraventricular nucleus (PVN). Vasopressin and oxytocin efferents may course directly to the pineal or secondarily via an indirect route that stimulates acetylcholinergic cells of the IML, which subsequently act on a number of neuron types of the BCG. Ultimately NE and NPY efferents issuing from the SCG impinge on the pineal gland. Additional physiological information to the pineal gland is mediated by the efferents from the lateral hypothalamus, habenulae and other loci. Melatonin synthesis and release characteristics are modified by the integrated response of these circuits where it is released into the capillaries surrounding the pineal body.

Given the essential role melatonin plays in transducing both photoperiodic and seasonal information into the appropriate physiological signals, it is not surprising how many

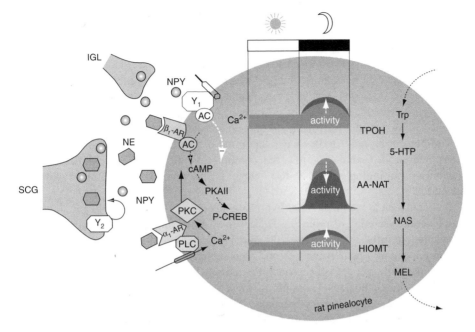

Figure 8.12   *Actions of NPY on melatonin synthesis in rat pinealocytes. Reprinted from Simonneaux and Ribelayga (2003) with permission from the American Society for Pharmacology and Experimental Therapeutics.*

neuroendocrine circuits are modulated by melatonin. The role of melatonin on reproduction and courtship has been particularly well studied. Melatonin appears to have a number of distinct actions on the reproductive system (Chapter 10). Early studies showed that elevated concentrations of melatonin will, for example, decrease testosterone and oestradiol although the mechanism by which this occurred was not understood. As a result many studies focused on the melatonin regulation of the pituitary gonado-trophins LH and FSH (Chapters 5 and 10). For example, studies on sheep have provided evidence that melatonin acts within the mediobasal hypothalamus or in the pars tuberalis of the pituitary gland to regulate the secretion of LH, FSH, prolactin and other hormones from the anterior pituitary gland. In these studies, melatonin was administered chronically into specific sites of the brain and pituitary gland in sheep exposed to long days in a situation where the endogenous pattern of melatonin secretion dictated the endocrine state. The localized administration of melatonin in the mediobasal hypothalamus and pars tuberalis, but not in other areas of the brain (i.e. septum, pre-optic area, anterior and lateral hypothalamus) and the pars distalis of the pituitary gland, induced a full spectrum of endocrine changes as normally observed following a switch from long to short days. In rams, the responses include an increase in the circulating concentrations of FSH and growth of the testis, and a decrease in prolactin and the associated develop-ment of longer winter pelage. The changes reverse following the removal of exogenous melatonin.

However, release of the gonadotrophins are under ultimate control by the hypothalamic-releasing factor, gonadotrophin-releasing hormone (GnRH). Many studies on a variety of vertebrate species have pointed to a circadian modulation of GnRH release. Many of the studies suggested an indirect circadian action on GnRH release. However, it has been unclear whether the circadian rhythm of GnRH release, which peaks in the afternoon, is amplified by the oestrogen surge or if circadian input causes an increase in GnRH sensitivity to the positive feedback effects of oestrogen. Although it is likely that GnRH output is regulated by circadian-influenced input on steroid or peptide (i.e. NPY) actions on the GnRH neuron, new studies have supported a direct melatonin regulation onto the GnRH neuron in mammals. How the combination of indirect and direct circadian information impinging on the GnRH neuron is integrated at the cellular level is not understood.

Melatonin acts in the mediobasal hypothalamus or pars tuberalis of the pituitary gland to regulate the secretion of prolactin. Denervation of the pineal gland disrupts the ability of daylength to influence prolactin secretion. Treatment with the hormone melatonin or a short-day melatonin pattern inhibits prolactin secretion. Anterior deafferentation of the SCN in ewes does not disrupt seasonal prolactin secretion. Although lesions of the SCN and retrochiasmatic nucleus do not block infused effects of melatonin on prolactin secretion, lesions to the anterior hypothalamus prevent the effects of exogenous melatonin on delayed implantation. Lesions of the SCN also disrupt the LH surge thereby causing permanent anoestrus.

Circadian signals, melatonin and hormones associated with the adrenal steroids are intrinsically linked (Fig. 8.13). In rats, photoperiod information via the retina is relayed to the paraventricular nucleus where the release of corticotrophin-releasing factor (CRF) is stimulated from the nerve terminals of the median eminence. This induces the release of ACTH from the corticotrophs of the anterior pituitary into the blood stream, thereby stimulating glucocorticoid synthesis and release from the pituitary. Melatonin as described above is also released in response via oxytocin and vasopressin pathways from the PVN. Melatonin acts directly upon the adrenal gland to suppress secretion of glucocorticoids

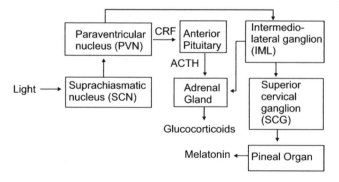

Figure 8.13   *Circadian regulation of the HPA axis. From Larsen et al. (1998).*

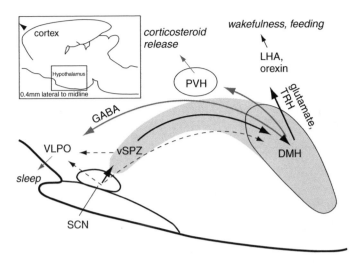

Figure 8.14   *Major Connections between the suprachiasmatic nucleus and dorsal medial hypothalamus regulating circadian control of sleep, wakefulness and hormone section. Reprinted with permission from Chou* et al. *(2003).*

(Chapter 9). Glucocorticoids are regulated by the clock mechanisms and are elevated during the active phase of the light–dark cycle when glucose metabolism and energy utilization are high. Type I but not Type II glucocorticoid receptors appear to be under circadian control. Melatonin will also inhibit the thyroid hormone axis at the neuroendocrine level. This mechanism may be conserved in amniotes. In the soft-shelled turtle, *Lissemys punctata punctata*, for example, melatonin concentrations reduce the thyroid gland weight, plasma thyroxine levels and thyroid peroxidase.

In humans, melatonin synthesis at night is associated with the onset of sleep (Fig. 8.14). Melatonin injections facilitate the onset of sleep in humans. The incidence of jet lag when moving across several time zones over a short period appears to be due to the initial lack of corroboration between the perceived time of day, and the internal representation of the time of day. In other words, the synthesis of melatonin is out of phase with the photoperiod. Overtime last about 3–10 days and the internal clock will eventually become entrained to the cues of the new time zone. A similar situation can occur in shift workers where the adaptation to a particular shift is lost, once the worker tries to adapt to the normal photoperiod during days off, or the beginning of a day shift. Both jet lag and shift work has been associated with decreased cognitive performance, anxiety and depression, and appetite irregularities. Although some studies have indicated that the condition can be alleviated somewhat by oral administration of melatonin, there has been a tendency also to abuse the amount of melatonin ingested which can lead to additional neuroendocrine complications. The neuroendocrine regulation of melatonin is complex, utilizing both photic and non-photic pathways for regulation (Fig. 8.15).

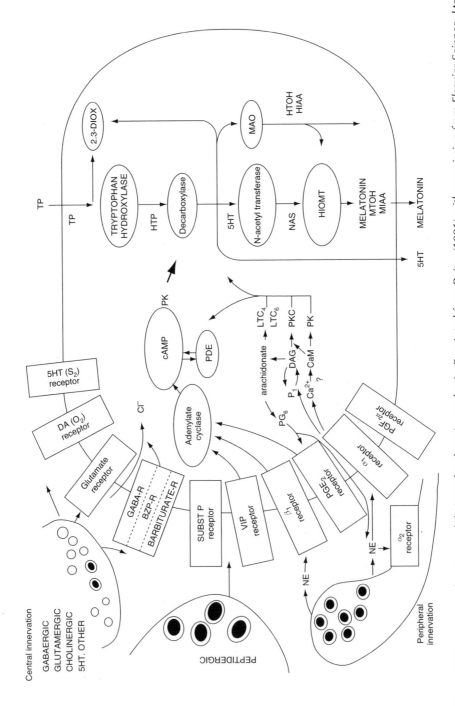

Figure 8.15 Neuroendocrine modulation of melatonin synthesis. Reprinted from Reiter (1991) with permission from Elsevier Science, Ltd.

Chapter summary

All metazoans possess a series of biological oscillators that serve as internal clocks that allow the organism to become temporally adapted to its environment. These biological clocks occur at the molecular, cellular and tissue level to provide time-keeping cues that span the order of minutes to months. Functional biological clocks may have originated in photosensory organs under selection pressure to partition the physiological activity of an organism into active and quiescent periods, where growth and cell division could occur during the quiescent periods, and at night, when the mutagenic potential of ionizing radiation and oxygen radical formation was at a minimum. Melatonin, the fundamental hormone associated with the neuroendocrinology of time-keeping, may have evolved initially as an antioxidant, and only became functional as a hormone after the pineal organ evolved in vertebrates. The pineal organ began initially as a photosensory organ to transduce the day–night period into a neuroendocrine signal. This signal incorporated the serotonin–melatonin biosynthetic pathway, and after the evolution of the melatonin receptors during the genomic expansion events of the basal vertebrates, melatonin superseded serotonin as the fundamental time-keeping signal. Melatonin regulates most of the key neuroendocrine circuits in vertebrates to coordinate organismal physiology with the changing temporal conditions of the environment.

Hamster Tau mutant
Martin Ralph

The circadian period mutation, *tau*, was identified in golden hamsters as an abnormality in the animal's pattern of entrainment. This is a point mutation in the gene, *casein kinase 1ε*, that reduces the function of the protein, resulting in dominant-negative expression. The mutation reduces the period of overt circadian rhythms from the 24-hour wild type to 22 hours in heterozygous and to 20 hours in homozygous carriers. This was the first demonstration of a genetic mutation of a mammalian circadian system. It demonstrated that mammalian clocks were likely to be built with the same molecular structures that were already being elucidated for the systems in insects (*Drosophila*) and fungi (*Neurospora*). Importantly, it prompted researchers to start looking vigorously for the molecular clock in mammals. As a research tool, the mutation was critical for neural transplantation studies that proved the location of the mammalian clock to be the hypothalamic suprachiasmatic nucleus. This work stands as the single definitive demonstration that circadian rhythms of behaviour in the hamster are driven by the SCN clock. The work has been cited extensively and featured in numerous textbooks on Neuroscience and Biology.

More recently, the mutant hamster has led to the finding that chronic disruption of circadian rhythms that is caused by the animals' inability to synchronize with 24-hour light cycles reduced the life expectancy of the animals. At least one potential cause of this is profound cardiovascular deterioration, and we now have verified that poor circadian rhythms can both exacerbate primary heart disease as well as be the primary cause of disease when the disturbance is chronic.

Neuropeptides and Circadian Rhythms
Hugh Piggins

Circadian rhythms in mammalian physiology and behaviour are generated by the dominant circadian pacemaker contained in the suprachiasmatic nuclei of the hypothalamus (SCN) and by the synchronization (entrainment) of this circadian pacemaker by environmental time cues such as variation in daylight levels. The SCN has a distinct distribution of reciprocally connected neuropeptide-synthesizing neurons and a key problem is to determine the role of these intrinsic neurochemicals in biological time-keeping. Neurons of the dorsomedial SCN contain arginine-vasopressin (AVP), whereas cells in the ventral SCN synthesize vasoactive intestinal polypeptide (VIP) and/or gastrin-releasing peptide (GRP). Many GRP and VIP neurons are retinorecipient, while neurons in the dorsomedial and dorsal SCN are sparsely innervated by retinal efferents. All three neuropeptides are present in SCN efferents. These neuroanatomical differences imply interconnected subregions in the SCN.

Functional studies have added further credence to this idea. Exogenous AVP alters SCN neuronal activity but does not alter the phase of the SCN circadian pacemaker. By contrast, GRP excites SCN neurons and resets the phase of the SCN circadian clock in a manner similar to light. GRP neurons are activated by retinal stimulation and exogenous GRP excites SCN neurons and mimics the phase-shifting effects of light on the SCN circadian pacemaker. These effects of GRP are mediated via the BB_2 receptor as antagonists to this receptor block these actions of GRP while transgenic mice lacking BB_2 receptors do not respond to GRP and are less sensitive to the retinal illumination. These studies firmly establish that AVP is an output signal of the SCN, while GRP-BB_2 signalling is important for conveying photic information through the SCN.

The most striking findings on the role of neuropeptides in biological timing have come from investigations of VIP, a peptide present in SCN neurons in most mammalian species. VIP can signal via three subtypes of receptor, PAC_1, $VPAC_1$, and $VPAC_2$. Of these, PAC_1 and $VPAC_2$ are expressed in the rodent SCN. Earlier studies implicated VIP in photic entrainment of the SCN since exposure to short-duration light pulses activates VIP-containing SCN neurons and VIP applied directly to the SCN resets hamster behavioural rhythms in a pattern resembling the phase-shifting actions of light on wheel-running rhythms.

More recent investigations using transgenic mice with impaired VIP-$VPAC_2$ signalling have revealed more fundamental roles for VIP in circadian rhythm processes. Mice deficient in VIP have an accelerated SCN pacemaker and increased probability of becoming behaviourally arrhythmic in constant conditions. Mice lacking $VPAC_2$ receptors also have abnormal circadian rhythms; these mice show diminished profiles of core clock gene expression in the SCN and lack clear rhythms in wheel-running activity. Suprachiasmatic neurons from these mice have unusually low levels of spontaneous activity when recorded *in vitro* and the SCN of these mice respond at inappropriate phases to pulses of light. By contrast, circadian function is largely intact in mice lacking the PAC_1 receptor. Taken in sum, these studies reveal that contrary to conventional belief, intercellular communication via neuropeptide signalling appears crucial to normal SCN circadian function at behavioural, cellular, and molecular levels. Determining the signal transduction events linking activation of VIP and GRP receptors to the core molecular clock works is a key goal for future research in circadian neurobiology.

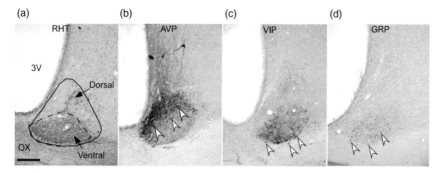

Figure 1

Photomicrographs of coronal sections through the suprachiasmatic nuclei (SCN) region of the rat. (A) The retinal innervation of the SCN (delineated by the solid line). The retinohypothalamic tract (RHT) conveys environmental lighting information to the SCN. This project is shown by dark immunostaining for the tracer choleratoxin subunit B in the SCN (injected into the retina seven days earlier). Note the dense innervation of the ventral SCN (outlined by the broken line oval), whereas the RHT is sparse in the dorsal SCN. The SCN lie dorsal to the optic chiasma (OX) and lateral to the third ventricle (3V). (B) Immunostaining for arginine-vasopressin (AVP). Note the numerous AVP-immunopositive cell bodies (highlighted by the white arrowheads) in the dorsomedial SCN. (C) Immunostaining for vasoactive intestinal polypeptide (VIP). Note the many VIP-containing neurons in the ventral (highlighted by the white arrowheads) SCN. (D) Immunostaining for gastrin-releasing peptide (GRP). GRP is found in cells of ventral SCN (indicated by white arrowheads). Calibration bar in A = 100 μm.

References

Piggins, H.D., Antle, M.C. and Rusak, B. (1995) Neuropeptides phase shift the mammalian circadian pacemaker. *J. Neurosci.* 15, 5612–5622.

Piggins, H.D. and Cutler, D.J. (2003) The roles of vasoactive intestinal polypeptide in the mammalian circadian clock. *J. Endocrinol.* 177, 7–15.

Colwell, C.S., Michel, S., Itri, J., Rodriguez, W., Tam, J., Lelievre, V., Hu, Z., Liu, X. and Waschek, J.A. (2003) Disrupted circadian rhythms in VIP- and PHI-deficient mice. *Am. J. Physiol.* 285, R939-R949.

Hughes, A.T., Fahey, B., Cutler, D.J., Coogan, A.N. and Piggins, H.D. (2004) Aberrant gating photic input to the suprachiasmatic circadian pacemaker of mice lacking the VPAC$_2$ receptor. *J. Neurosci.* 24, 3522–3526.

9

Stress, arousal and homeostatic challenge

Introduction

To us, as humans, the stress response manifests as a variety of perceptions such as anxiety, irritability and the inability to concentrate on tasks that are frequently required of us. We think of stress as an inherently bad thing. However, all organisms, from a single cell to the most complex metazoans, such as humans, show a stress response. The more complex the animal, and in particular, the central nervous system, then the more complex the stress response becomes. Evolutionarily, the goal of the stress response is to protect the organism from danger and to shunt the energy reserves where it is needed the most. Arousal and motivation are also elements of the stress response. It is this aspect of stress physiology that allows us to mount the behavioural and physiological responses that allow us to deal with crisis situations such as natural disasters, engage in high performance sports or even studying and completing our final exams, or writing this book for example, within a given time frame. In a homogenous environment, where there are no predators, no competition for resources, favourable climate and sufficient shelter, we might not need the elaborate stress response we possess. Of course, such a utopian existence does not exist. Our stress response facilitates adaptation to novel situations and hence the evolution of a species.

The neural and endocrine component of the stress response can affect virtually every signalling system in the organism either directly or indirectly. A stress response in an organism may be defined as any event, whether real or perceived, that acts to disturb the

Neuroendocrinology: An Integrated Approach   David A. Lovejoy
© 2005 John Wiley & Sons, Ltd

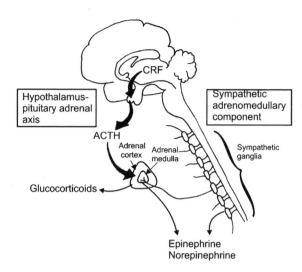

Figure 9.1   *Sympathetic adrenomedullary and hypothalamus–pituitary–adrenal axis components of the homeostatic stress response.*

homeostatic balance. Two main fundamental endocrine responses are elicited when a stressor is encountered. These may be loosely grouped into homeostatic and generalized responses. Homeostatic responses, mediated by the autonomic nervous system, are specific to a stimulus and are, therefore, predictable. In contrast, severe or persistent disturbances that are not corrected by homeostatic responses will evoke generalized responses that include sympathetic-adrenomedullary and adrenocortical activation (Fig. 9.1). The physiological goal of the stress response in animals is to divert energy to those tissues and organs that are required to resolve the homeostatic challenge event.

Physiology and behaviour associated with stress

Historically, the identification of the stress response came from medical studies (Chapter 1). As a young medical student, Hans Selye noticed that a common set of symptoms were associated with patients regardless of the type of illness. He referred this as 'the syndrome of being sick'. According to Selye, many stereotypes and behavioural adaptations displayed by severely ill patients arose from particular combinations of distressful events that exceeded the organism's ability to cope. Furthermore, pathologies associated with a breakdown in homeostatic tolerance could be attributed to both psychological and physiological events that interacted to typically externalize the locus of control. In other words, if the patient felt powerless to resolve a particular set of situations then the negative aspects of stress, such as anxiety and depression, became exacerbated. However, within this paradigm, an additional definition was required to differentiate stressors beneficial to the gross welfare of the individual from those of an obvious deleterious nature. Selye coined the term 'biological stress', borrowing the word 'stress' from physics, although many years afterwards he admitted that his lack of understanding of English led to selecting the incorrect word. 'Strain' and the 'strain syndrome' was a better choice, he argued. However, by that time, the notion of biological stress was already ensconced in the scientific literature. Advantageous perceptual cues, such as aversive stimuli provoking flight reactions from predators, Selye termed instances of 'eustress', whereas manifestations of events typically detrimental in nature, for example, the circumstances associated with protracted bereavement-induced depression, were classified as 'distress'. More specifically, Selye proposed that the attenuation of reproductive activity, often observed during stressful incidents, was indicative of activation of the sympathetic nervous system. With the sympathetic nervous system activated during exposure to stressful experiences, salivation, digestion and sexual arousal are quickly inhibited, the pupil dilates, heart-rate accelerates and the adrenal gland is stimulated to secrete epinephrine. Stored proteins are reintroduced back into the blood stream as amino acids, glycogen becomes re-mobilized as glucose, and triglycerides, derived from the consumption of fats, provide the fatty acids, glycerol and ketone bodies essential for instigating the 'fight or flight' response. The physiological responses to stressors involve all levels of animal organization. The integrated stress response has been classically described as having a catecholamine component or 'flight or fight response' and a glucocorticoid component or 'general adaptation' response.

The stress response in vertebrates may be described as having three discrete components (Fig. 9.2). The initial phase following the perception of a stressor is characterized by the rapid release of catecholamines via the autonomic nervous system and a few minutes later the release of the glucocorticoids into circulation. Subsequent to this is the response of organs to the catecholamines and glucocorticoids. This involves changes in cardiac output, oxygen uptake, energy mobilization and hydromineral balance (Chapters 6 and 7). The final stage involves long-term effects such as inhibition of growth, reproduction and immune activity and tolerance to additional stressors.

Prolonged stress can manifest in a number of different ways. Predators can have indirect effects on a prey population by affecting the behaviours, reproduction and foraging patterns of the prey. Chronic activation of stress, particularly by psychological factors, can affect the long-term survival and fitness of species in the wild. Continuous exposure to glucocorticoids has been associated with a number of metabolic and neurological disorders and may manifest as infertility, growth inhibition and impaired resistance to

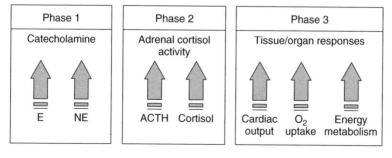

Figure 9.2   *Three basic phases of a stress response.*

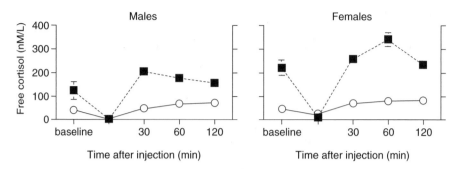

Figure 9.3   *Response in plasma cortisol by ACTH injection in ground squirrels living in open alpine regions compared to those living in the boreal forest. Modified after Hik et al. (2001).*

disease. For example, snowshoe hares typically show a ten-year population cycle in the Canadian Yukon Territory. During the decline, virtually every hare that dies is killed by a predator. During these declines, the animals show higher levels of plasma cortisol, reduced testosterone response and increased glucose mobilization (Fig. 9.3). Similarly, mature male arctic ground squirrels and some birds will show an increased stress response during breeding season that can act to compromise their survival. A stress response in fish can be stimulated by a variety of physical characteristics such as salinity, temperature turbidity, chemical and heavy metal pollution, and pH, as well as biological components such as competition for food and space, the presence of predators and parasites.

In humans, mental illness associated with stress and anxiety is increasing at an alarming rate in western industrialized nations. Women are twice as sensitive to stress and anxiety than men. Psychosocial stress due to family, work and health concerns and physical stress can induce a variety of anxiety-related illnesses. Moreover, women have long episodes of stress and anxiety, and have a lower rate of spontaneous remission. The World Health Organization reported in 1990 that major depression is the single largest cause of morbidity for women and the leading cause of disability worldwide. Depression and other anxiolytic disorders afflict women predominantly in their child-bearing and child-rearing years and may be the result of several cultural and economic factors. Women are more likely than men to be covered as dependants, to work part time, or to provide work for small businesses that do not provide health insurance. Thus, women are more susceptible to disruption of coverage through divorce, death and job loss. Such psychological stressors act to chronically stimulate the stress-response system.

Components of the stress-response system

Depending upon the metazoan, the stress response may involve a number of different nervous and endocrine components. Much of what we know of the integrated mechanisms of the stress response has been derived from studies involving chordates, and, therefore, the emphasis has been placed on the vertebrate stress response. However, many of the molecular components that are part of this system have also been found throughout invertebrate species.

Hypothalamus–pituitary–adrenal/interrenal axis

As we discussed in Chapter 5, the modern development of neuroendocrinology as a separate discipline was motivated, in part, by our desire to understand the mechanisms of the pituitary–adrenal axis. Much of the integration of the organismal stress response occurs via the hypothalamus–pituitary–adrenal/interrenal (HPA/I) axis (Fig. 9.4). After the appropriate stimulus, the hypothalamic peptide, corticotrophin-releasing factor (CRF), is secreted into the vascular system of the median eminence in most vertebrates, or by direct neurosecretory interaction in most teleosts. This subsequently induces the pituitary corticotroph cells to release adrenocorticotropic hormone (ACTH) into the systemic blood. In most vertebrates, the vasopressin and oxytocin-like peptides also stimulate ACTH release. In some mammals, depending upon the

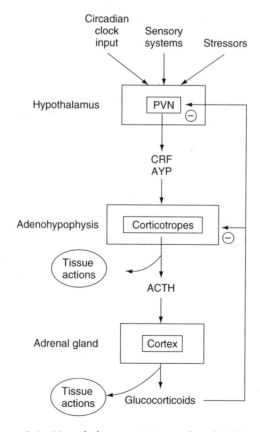

Figure 9.4   *Hypothalamus–pituitary–adrenal (HPA) axis.*

type and duration of the stressor, and the species, vasopressin may act as the primary ACTH-releasing hypothalamic peptide. In the rainbow trout, *Oncorhynchus mykiss*, CRF and arginine vasotocin will synergize to release ACTH, a situation similar to that seen in mammals.

The release of ACTH into the systemic circulation stimulates the synthesis and release of the glucocorticoids from the adrenal/interrenal gland. This mechanism is well conserved in amongst chordates, with the basic mechanism similar in both actinopterygian and sarcopterygian/tetrapod lineages. Little is known about the HPA/I axis in the cartilaginous fish, but it is likely more or less intact because the essential components are present in lampreys. The situation is not clear in hagfishes. However, some of the neuroendocrine stress axis elements are present in tunicates, thus one assumes that hagfish have at least some rudimentary system.

The metabolic actions of the glucocorticoids are to provide the animal with enough energy to survive a stressful situation. Glucocorticoids possess a number of actions associated with the utilization and flow of energy (Fig. 9.5). The *de novo* synthesis of glucose, gluconeogenesis, is increased in the liver following mobilization of proteins from skeletal muscle and consequent deamination of amino acids that are released from protein breakdown. However, glycogen can be also deposited in the liver because of an increase in glycogen synthetase reaction. In tandem with this, glycogenolysis is inhibited. The actions of the glucocorticoids are based on a short-term need for energy (Fig. 9.6). During a stress reaction, energy is obtained via protein breakdown. Glucose stores in the form of glycogen in the liver are, therefore, protected. In birds, increased adrenocortical secretion in response to stress can redirect activity by facilitating an increase in food searching and food intake needed to meet periods of increased energy demand. In the rainbow trout, apoptosis and cell proliferation are influenced by glucocorticoids. Low levels stimulate apoptosis whereas high levels stimulate proliferation.

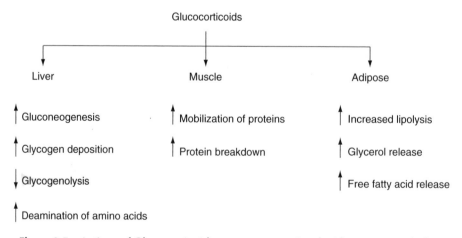

Figure 9.5 *Actions of Glucocorticoids on organs associated with energy metabolism.*

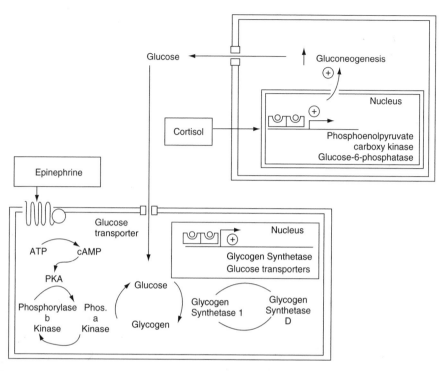

Figure 9.6 *Actions of epinephrine and cortisol on glucose metabolism in the liver. Cortisol will tend to antagonize the actions of epinephrine on glucose usage diverting the energy usage away from stored glucose.*

Sympathetic nervous system

As we have discussed in Chapter 4, the sympathetic nervous system is the branch of the autonomic nervous system that is essentially responsible for arousal in vertebrates. Many of its effects are mediated by the catecholamine hormones. The synthesis of epinephrine (adrenaline) begins with tyrosine. Tyrosine is taken up by chromaffin cells and converted to dihydroxyphenylalanine (DOPA), which is subsequently decarboxylized to dopamine. The rate-limiting step in the synthesis of catecholamines is the conversion of tyrosine to DOPA catalysed by tyrosine hydroxylase. Through the enzymatic action of dopamine β-dehydroxylase, it is then converted to norepinephrine (noradrenaline) and is then converted to epinephrine. Secretion of epinephrine from the chromaffin cells is stimulated directly by acetylcholine release from preganglionic sympathetic fibres innervating the adrenal medulla.

The actions of the sympathetic nervous system and the parasympathetic nervous system are functionally antagonistic to each other. The sympathetic nervous system acts to increase the mobilization of energy and redistribution of the blood supply that are essential for response. The parasympathetic nervous system promotes the digestion of food and storage of energy (Fig. 9.7). The sympathetic nervous system may be considered to possess

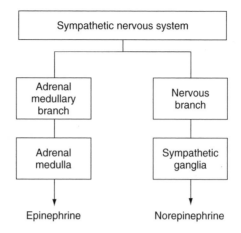

Figure 9.7   *Branches of the sympathetic nervous system.*

two distinct branches. The sympathetic adrenal medullary branch is associated with the synthesis and release of catecholamines from the chromaffin cells of the adrenal medulla in vertebrates, or the head kidney of fishes. Epinephrine is the primary catecholamine that is released. The neural branch consists of the sympathetic nerve terminals impinging primarily upon the cardiovascular system. Norepinephrine is mostly released from these nerve terminals. Upon stress, the sympathetic nervous system and adrenocortical response are activated simultaneously. Their time-course of actions follows different routes. The catecholamines released from the adrenal medulla and sympathetic nerves act immediately, whereas the adrenal glucocorticoids take effect about 20–30 minutes later in humans, for example.

The teleost homologue of the adrenal gland is located in the head kidney and consists of the catecholamine-synthesizing chromaffin cells and the glucocorticoid-synthesizing interrenal cells. Both cell groups are intermingled. The autonomic nervous system regulation is similar to that in mammals. The primary effects of the catecholamines are on respiration, branchial blood flow, heart rate and oxygen transport capacity, as well as metabolic actions on free fatty acid and blood glucose levels via glycogenolysis in the liver mediated by β-adrenergic receptors although several teleost species may also utilize α-adrenergic receptors.

Some evidence suggests that emotional stress is more related to the activation of the adrenal medullary branch of the sympathetic nervous system and a physical workload more to the activation of the neural branch of the sympathetic nervous system (Fig. 9.8). For example, administration of 5-HT agonists into the PVN of resting rats increases both the activity of the HPA axis and the adrenal medullary branch of the sympathetic nervous system. Administration of 5-HT agonists into the PVN of exercising rats, on the other hand, leads to a reduction of the activity of the neural branch of the sympathetic nervous system. Emotional stress is accompanied by increased 5-HT activity in the hypothalamus. If a workload is of moderate intensity, then about 70% of the total energy expenditure is a result of free fatty acid breakdown. Lipolysis and free fatty acid production are

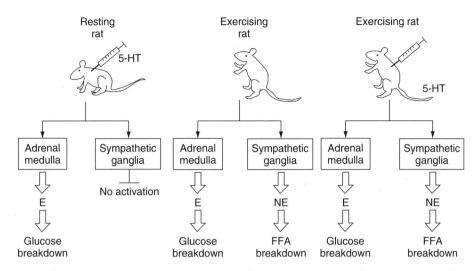

Figure 9.8 *Emotional stress utilizes glucose for energy, whereas physical stress tends to utilize fatty acids for energy.*

maintained during long periods by continued activation of the nervous branch. But for emotional stress, the increased CNS activity is entirely glucose-dependent, thus the adrenal branch is preferably activated.

However, the organization and function of these systems in mammals may differ considerably from other vertebrates. For example, norepinephrine injection into a carp under normal conditions can lead to a suppression of plasma free fatty acid levels. A number of animals can survive under hypoxic and anoxic conditions, such as in cyprinid fishes. Carbohydrates become the major substrate for all energy expenditure and this leads to depletion of glycogen states. During hypoxia, free fatty acid levels decline in spite of a large increase in plasma norepinephrine.

Caudal neurosecretory system (CNSS)

The caudal neurosecretory system or urophysis in teleosts has been implicated in the regulation of glucocorticoids. Urophysectomy of the goldfish can induce an increase in plasma cortisol. This may be due to enhanced secretion of urotensin-I from the goldfish hypothalamus. Indeed, after urophysectomy of *Catostomus commersoni*, urotensin-I mRNA levels are elevated in the lateral tuberal nucleus (LTN) whereas CRF mRNA in the preoptic nucleus and LTN remained more or less constant. These observations are consistent with an earlier report of a four-fold increase in the number of parvocellular urotensin-I neurons in the LTN after urophysectomy.

However, urotensin-I may also stimulate the HPI axis directly at the level of the inter-renal tissue. Urotensin-I appears to stimulate cortisol secretion directly and interact synergistically with ACTH to promote cortisol secretion in saltwater-adapted trout isolated interrenal preparations. In both trout and flounder, urotensin-I injection *in vivo* leads to a dose-dependent increase in plasma cortisol secretion, suggesting that such

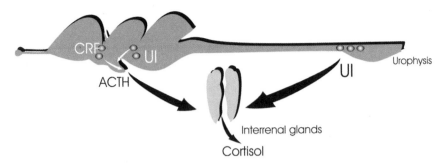

Figure 9.9 *Combined actions of CRF and Urotensin-I on interrenal regulation in fishes. Reprinted from Lovejoy and Balment (1999) by the permission of Elsevier Science (USA).*

responses are of physiological relevance. Thus, the CNSS may provide a pituitary-independent route to regulate cortisol secretion, affording alternate, perhaps, stimulant-specific mechanisms to modulate plasma cortisol. This may be particularly important in fish groups which lack the hypothalamus–pituitary portal blood link and thus lack the complex regulatory input of a cocktail of hypothalamic factors delivered to ACTH cells in tetrapods. The fixed and direct innervation of ACTH cells of the fish pars distalis inevitably restricts the variety of stimulants or moderating factors that can affect ACTH, and thus interrenal secretion. The CNSS provides an additional mechanism to allow other stimulant-specific inputs to modulate cortisol secretion (Fig. 9.9).

Hypothalamo intermediate lobe regulation

Melanocyte-stimulating hormone (MSH) is the principal hormone secreted from the intermediate lobe of the pituitary. In many non-avian and non-mammalian vertebrates, MSH is responsible for the colour change associated with background colour adaptation and camouflage. This colour-change mechanism is associated with elements of the stress response. The melanotropes are under regulatory control by a host of stimulatory and inhibitory factors from the hypothalamus (Fig. 9.10). The regulation of MSH from the pars intermedia has been particularly well studied in anuran species. In frogs and toads, a subset of NPY cells of the suprachiasmatic nucleus (SCN) directly innervates the pars intermedia. In these cells, NPY is co-localized with the dopamine and GABA. In both *Rana ridibunda* and *X. laevis*, NPY acts as an α-MSH release inhibiting factor. The term 'melanostatin' has been used to describe NPY in amphibians. In Xenopus, the melanotrope-inhibitory neurons of the SCN appear to receive direct photic input from the retina. Thus, this pathway appears to be associated with the perception of background colour although it is not clear if is regulated, in part, by clock systems residing in the SCN.

A number of physiological systems in vertebrates appear to employ CRF and NPY in opposition to each other. In Chapter 6 we examined this relationship in relationship to appetite in feeding. A similar situation appears to occur with respect to MSH-release regulation in the pars intermedia. Thus, in addition to CRF- and urotensin-I-like peptides

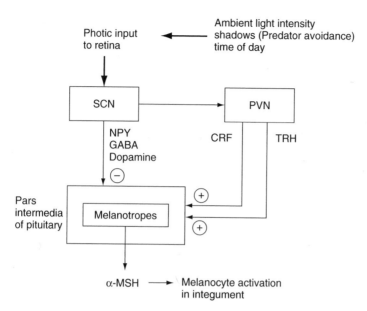

Figure 9.10 *Regulation of α-MSH release from pars intermedia.*

stimulating of HPI axis, these peptides also stimulate teleost pituitary melanotropes that release numerous peptides including ACTH, MSH, LPH, CLIP and endorphins (Chapter 5). In superfused columns of dispersed goldfish neurointermediate lobe cells, pulses of urotensin-I can cause concomitant release of MSH and ACTH. Superfusion of the neurointermediate lobe tissue of the pituitary gland of *X. laevis* with CRF and urotensin-I can produce similar, rapid and dose-dependent stimulation of MSH and endorphin secretion. Animals adapted to a white background show much greater sensitivity to CRF and sauvagine than those adapted to the black background.

Corticotrophin-releasing factor and TRH have a number of overlapping functions. In amphibians and fish, TRH, like CRF, is a potent stimulator of α-MSH. In pituitary cells, TRH can stimulate a number of secondary messenger pathways, including adenylyl cyclase Ca^{2+}/calmodulin-dependent protein kinase II, phospholipase A_2 and protein tyrosine kinase. It stimulates a phospholipase C and induces a biphasic increase in cytosolic Ca^{2+} resulting from both Ca^{2+} influx and mobilization of intracellular sources. However, there are a number of important species differences. For example, cAMP-mediated pathways appear not to play a role in the frog *R. ridibunda*.

Although not part of the pars intermedia, the melanin-concentrating hormone (MCH) plays a complementary role to MSH with respect to pigmentation. MCH plays a significant role in the regulation of teleost pigmentation in the integument but also appears to play a separate role in the regulation of the stress response. In both rats and trout, exogenous MCH decreases the ACTH release as well as inhibits melanin dispersion in the melanophores of the integument. This effect appears to be mediated at the hypothalamus level.

Corticotrophin-releasing factor superfamily of peptides

The structure of ovine CRF was reported in 1981 after numerous attempts were made to purify it during the preceding 30 years. However, two years earlier, the structure of sauvagine, a CRF-like peptide from frog skin, was reported, and shortly after the CRF report came a report on the structure of urotensin-I from the urophysis. Suddenly then, within a three-year period, CRF-like peptides were known to be found in the brain, the urophysis and the skin of different species.

Corticotrophin-releasing factor

Corticotrophin-releasing factor is acknowledged as the primary hypothalamic factor mediating stress-induced adrenocorticotropin (ACTH) secretion from the anterior pituitary in vertebrates. The majority of these investigations have utilized mammals. The situation in non-mammals is less well understood. CRF is present in all actinopterygian and sarcopterygian/tetrapod species investigated to date. CRF orthologues have not been found in the cartilaginous fish; however, the elaborate CRF networks present in the brains of basal actinopterygians and sarcopterygians, and investigations of CRF immunoreactivity in the forebrain of the elasmobranch, *Scyliorhinus canicula*, indicate that CRF is likely to be present in the cartilaginous fish and plays a similar functional role.

The CRF neurons that regulate ACTH release are found in the parvocellular cells of the paraventricular nucleus (PVN; Chapter 8) of the hypothalamus (Fig. 9.11). These cells are sensitive to glucocorticoid feedback from the adrenal cortex and, therefore, form the neuroendocrine negative feedback loop resulting from high plasma concentrations of the

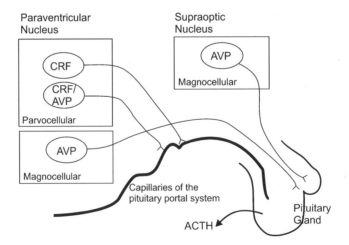

Figure 9.11 *ACTH release by CRF and vasopressin.*

glucocorticoids in response to ACTH stimulation. CRF is also present in a number of locations in the brain including the bed nucleus of the stria terminalis, central nucleus of the amygdala and in a number of other hypothalamic and brainstem regions (Fig. 9.12; Chapter 11).

Corticotrophin-releasing factor is well conserved for a 41-reside peptide. The primary structure is identical in primates, carnivores, rodents and perissodactyl ungulates (i.e. horse). However, the primary structure apparently underwent several residue changes within the artiodactyl ruminant (sheep, cattle) lineage, similar to the situation that occurred in the evolution of growth hormone. Presently, the structures of CRF in birds and reptiles have not been reported. CRF in amphibians is known only by two sequences obtained from *Xenopus* where the two sequences appear to be a result of the tetraploid genome in this species. Two forms of CRF from the white sucker,

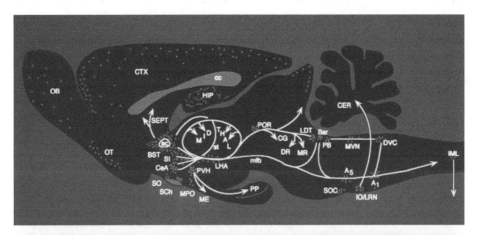

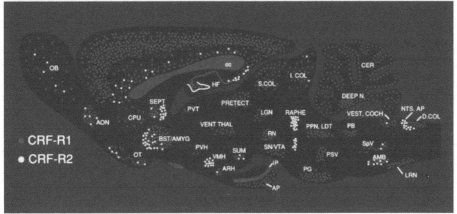

Figure 9.12 *Expression of CRF (top panel) and CRF receptors (bottom panel). Modified after Sawchenko and Swanson (1989) and Bittencourt et al. (2001).*

Catostomus commersoni, and sockeye salmon, *Oncorhynchus nerka*, also appear to be the result of tetraploidization. In teleosts, there is considerably less conservation of the CRF sequence.

CRF paralogues

Urotensin-I is a CRF-like peptide originally isolated from the urophysis of fish, and since then, an orthologue termed 'urocortin' has been cloned from mammal brain. Urotensin-I/urocortin peptides are a direct paralogue of CRF as the result of gene duplication. Although in fishes most of the urotensin-I in the nervous system is present in the urophysis, the majority of cells expressing the hormone in the midbrain occur within the nucleus of the medial longitudinal fasciculus (nMLF). In mammals, urocortin is found in the Edinger-Westphal (EW) nucleus (Fig. 9.13). The actual boundary of this nucleus has not been resolved and may include parts of what is termed the nMLF. The functional role of the midbrain urocortin/urotensin-I is not clear, but does play a role in a number of stress- and anxiety-related functions including suppression of appetite. Urophyseal urotensin-I in fishes is implicated with interrenal physiology at a peripheral level. Peripheral urotensin-I and urocortin have both been implicated in cardiovascular responses.

The CRF/urotensin-I lineage is paralogous to a second lineage of CRF-like peptides. This lineage includes urocortin-II and urocortin-III and probably occurred during the same duplication event that led to CRF and urotensin-I/urocortin. Insects possess apparent orthologues of both the CRF/urotensin-I lineage and the urocortin-II/urocortin-III lineage suggesting that two separate CRF-like genes were present well before the metazoa split into distinct paths leading to the deuterostomes and to the ecdysozoans. Thus, the CRF peptide lineage represents another ancient hormone that evolved before the Precambrian explosion. It is really not clear how much the urocortins II and III play in the stress response. At this point their putative role is based primarily on the structural similarity these peptides have with CRF and the experiments that have been performed to show similar modes of action to CRF.

There is some evidence that the CRF lineage may form a sister lineage to the calcitonin group of peptides. CRF and calcitonin receptors bear the closest structural similarity to each other. In Chapter 6 we discussed the structural similarity of one lineage of insect diuretic peptides that bear structural similarity to both urocortin II/III lineage and to calcitonin. Moreover, recently a new group of neuropeptide-like sequences have been identified in the Metazoa. A single copy appears to be present in *Drosophila*, but four conserved copies are present in the vertebrates. This peptide sequence, termed 'teneurin C-terminal associated peptide' (TCAP), is present on the extracellular tip of the teneurin transmembrane proteins (Fig. 9.14). This peptide may be cleaved from its proprotein by a membrane-bound enzyme, in the same manner as described for some cytokines, such as tumour necrosis factor a and fractalkine. TCAP possesses clear structural similarity for both the CRF and calcitonin group of peptides. Physiologically, however, its actions in the brain are quite distinct from CRF and may act in part as an antagonist to CRF-mediated systems.

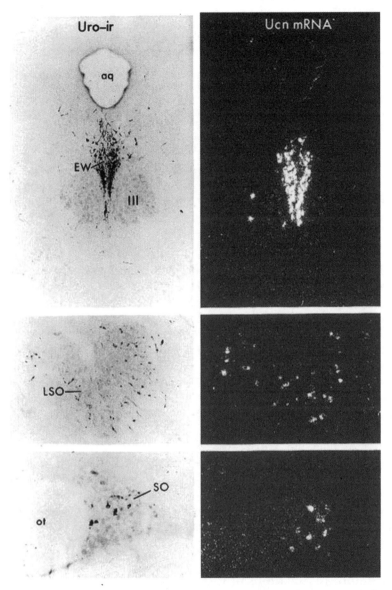

Figure 9.13 *Expression of urocortin in the brain. Top panel: Edinger Westphal Nucleus, Middle panel: Bottom panel: Superior olivary complex. Reprinted from Vaughan et al. (1995) by the permission of Nature Publishing Group.*

Arginine vasopressin as a ACTH-releasing factor

In most mammals there is a subpopulation of parvocellular cells in the PVN that secretes both CRF and vasopressin into the median eminence. CRF actions may be potentiated by the presence of vasopressin. Vasopressin can also be released, in response to the

```
human TCAP 1      QQLLSTGRVQGYDGYFVLSVEQYLELS DSANNIHFMRQSEI-NH₂
human TCAP 2      QQLLSTGRVQGYEGYYVLPVEQYPELA DSSSNIQFLRQNEM-NH₂
human TCAP 3       QLLSAGKVQGYDGYYVLSVEQYPELA DSANNIQFLRQSEI-NH₂
human TCAP 4      QQVLSTGRVQGYDGFFVISVEQYPELS DSANNIHFMRQSEM-NH₂

mouse TCAP-1      QQLLGTGRVQGYDGYFVLSVEQYLELS DSANNIHFMRQSEI-NH₂
mouse TCAP-2      QQLLSTGRVQGYEGYYVLPVEQYPELA DSSSNIQFLRQNEM-NH₂
mouse TCAP-3       QLLSAGKVQGYDGYYVLSVEQYPELA DSANNIQFLRQSEI-NH₂
mouse TCAP-4      QQVLNTGRVQGYDGFFVTSVEQYPELS DSANNIHFMRQSEM-NH₂

human CRF         SEEPPIS LDLTFHLLREVLEMARAEQLAQQAHSNRKLM EII-NH₂
human urocortin   DNPSLS IDLTFHLLRTLLELARTQSQRERAEQNRIIF DSV-NH₂
human urocortin 2    IVLS LDVPIGLLQILLEQARARAAREQATTNARIL ARV-NH₂
human urocortin 3    FTLS LDVPTNIMNLLFNIAKAKNLRAQAAANAHLM AQI-NH₂
```

Figure 9.14   *Comparison of the human and mouse TCAP sequences with the human CRF peptide family.*

appropriate stressor, from the magnocellular cells of the paraventricular nucleus, and also from magnocellular cells of the supraoptic nucleus. Thus, there are distinct subpopulations of vasopressin-secreting cells that are secreted into the portal system of the median eminence, and also directly to the neurohypophysis and stored in the neurosecretory terminals there. As discussed in Chapter 6, neurohypophysial arginine vasopressin is secreted directly into the systemic blood and plays a role in osmoregulation. In fishes, CRF appears to act as the primary releasing factor, but like mammals, the vasopressin (vasotocin)-related peptides also act as ACTH-releasing factors under some conditions. Arginine vasotocin and isotocin can produce additive actions but do not appear to potentiate the ACTH response to urotensin-I or CRF in goldfish. In teleost fish, the release of ACTH in perfused columns of goldfish (*Carassius auratus*) pituitary cells is sensitive to CRF and also urotensin-I. CRF, rather than urotensin-I, is also apparently the major stimulant for ACTH secretion in perfused frog pituitary cells. Leaf- and monkey-frogs in the Phyllomedusinae subfamily of tree frogs (Hylidae) possess a CRF-like peptide (sauvagine) in skin glands. However, it has not been determined if this peptide is present in the brain and acts as an ACTH-releasing factor. Currently, all attempts to clone the gene or cDNA for this peptide have not been successful.

Neuroanatomical locations of CRF-like peptides

A comparative neuroanatomical analysis suggests a relationship between the nMLF and the EW nucleus in vertebrates. There is considerable confusion in the literature as to what constitutes the EW nucleus, which is generally used to describe a cell group within the oculomotor complex. The nMLF is recognized in hagfish, lampreys, cartilaginous fish, actinopterygians and sarcoptyerygians. EW-homologous regions as defined by pupillary input are recognized in elasmobranchs and actinopterygians suggesting that, in mammals, the EW nucleus may include aspects of the nMLF. Studies on bullfrog (*R. catesbeiana*) and white sucker (*C. commersoni*) suggest that the major descending autonomic pathway by urotensin-I peptides appears to be the urotensin-I-expressing system of the nMLF. Therefore, the expression of urocortin in the EW nucleus and urotensin-I in the nMLF suggests these loci may be, in part, homologous. In phylogenetically older vertebrates and actinopterygians in general, urotensin-I expression is predominant in the spinal cord and brainstem sites where CRF appears to be not present. In amniotes, however, CRF expression is associated with nuclei that contribute descending autonomic fibres. Many of these fibres eventually terminate upon cell groups that innervate smooth and cardiac muscle, various glands and body viscera. The main nuclei that produce these descending autonomic fibres include the paraventricular and posterior hypothalamic regions of the diencephalon, visceral nuclei of the ocular motor complex (EW nucleus), the locus coeruleus (LC) and parts of the nuclei of the solitary tract. Fibres from the PVN and posterior hypothalamus project to visceral nuclei in the medulla as well as to the spinal cord levels. Descending fibres from the EW nucleus send fibres that descend to the lumbar regions. CRF expression in the PVN, LC and in the caudal nucleus of the solitary tract has been well characterized in rats and mammals in general. Similarly in the pigeon, *Columbus livia*, and in domestic fowl, *Gallus domesticus*, the homologous regions display CRF immunoreactivity.

In contrast, in fishes, CRFergic descending fibres from the neuroanatomically equivalent regions appear not to be widespread. In elvers, *Anguilla*, CRF-immunoreactive fibres were noted in brainstem and spinal cord but this network appeared vastly reduced in adults and few CRF-immunoreactive fibres were noted in caudal regions of the green molly (*Latipinna poecilia*) brain. In the brown ghost, *Apteronotus leptorhynchus*, CRF immunoreactivity was not observed in any regions caudal to the posterior diencephalon. Mesencephalic CRF is, however, expressed in tectal regions of the tiger frog (*Rana tigrina*), cerebellum and nucleus interpeduncularis in *Ambystoma mexicanum*, *Pleurodeles waltii*, *X. laevis* and *R. ridibunda*. Thus, though the Amphibia show evidence of CRF extending to caudal regions of the brain, there is a paucity of studies in reptiles to corroborate these findings. Amphibians may represent a transitional state with respect to descending CRFergic systems.

CRF receptors

The two primary subtypes of CRF receptor (R1, R2) show the greatest sequence similarity to the class II group of G-protein–coupled receptors (GPCR) (Fig. 9.15). At least four isoforms of the CRF-R1 receptor have been identified. The three primary variants α, β

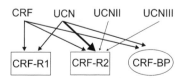

Figure 9.15 *Affinity relationship among CRF-like ligands and their receptors.*

and γ all vary with respect to each other in the amino acid sequence of the first 50–60 residues. The R1δ form possesses a shorter deletion between residues 81 and 99 at the N-terminus, but retains low affinity for several of the CRF-related ligands. At least four subtypes of the CRF-R2 receptor have also been identified. But unlike the R1 receptor, the R2 subtypes show considerable selectivity among the CRF-related ligands. The R1 receptors have been implicated in the onset of anxiogenic-type behaviours, whereas the R2 receptors have been associated with a number of peripheral events. For example, the inhibition of epidermal oedema by urotensin-I-CRF peptides, which appears to be mediated by R2 receptors, is consistent with the much higher potency of urotensin-I than CRF in this action. The greater potency of urotensin-I in stimulating cAMP production in neonatal cardial myocytes is similarly associated with the presence of R2 receptors in this tissue. The presence of R2 receptors in the peripheral vasculature is also considered responsible for the vasodilatory actions ascribed to urotensin-I-CRF peptides.

Much of what is known about CRF receptors has been based upon a corticotrope cell model where our understanding of the CRF-receptor physiology has been constrained by the predominance of the R1 receptor in corticotrope membranes and by the unusual embryonic development of the corticotrope cells (Chapter 4). These aspects, with numerous studies now supporting a universal ability of G-protein-coupled receptor to heterodimerize (p. 137), suggest that the corticotrope model may not be appropriate to understand the molecular mechanisms of the CRF receptor in a neuronal membrane. However, even given the differences between corticotrope and neuronal CRF-receptor function, some pituitary functions are left unanswered by our current model of CRF function in corticotropes. For example, many studies indicate a lack of correlation between pituitary responsiveness and the number of CRF receptors in the anterior pituitary. Discrepancies between changes in CRF receptors and pituitary responsiveness have been shown during chronic osmotic stimulation, ACTH response to novel stressors and CRF injections. Thus, CRF-receptor number appears not to be an essential factor influencing corticotrope responsiveness, and other molecular mechanisms, such as dimerization, may be involved. For example, the somatostatin sst 3 receptor can be inactivated by heterodimerization with the sst 2a receptor (Fig. 9.16).

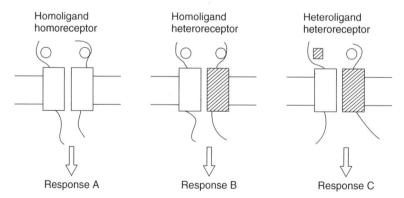

Figure 9.16 *Signal transduction responses may vary depending upon the heterodimerization or homodimerization of both the ligands and receptors.*

Proopiomelanocortin and adrenocorticotrophic hormone

Proopiomelanocortin (POMC) is the precursor for adrenocorticotrophic hormone (ACTH), β-lipotropin, melanin-stimulating hormone (MSH; melanotropin) and β-lipotropin. There are several variants of these peptides among the different vertebrate species. Tetrapod POMC possesses pro-γ-MSH, ACTH and lipotropin. γ-MSH is present in pro-γ-MSH, α-MSH is part of ACTH and β-MSH is cleaved from the β-lipotropin precursor. However in actinopterygians, the POMC precursor may contain one to four different variants of MSH including a unique form, δ-MSH. Elasmobranchs also appear to possess all four variants of MSH. In lampreys, two POMC-related precursors are expressed, proopiocortin (POC) and proopiomelanotropin (POM). POC is expressed in the pars distalis whereas POM is found in the pars intermedia. In gnathostomes, the pars distalis and pars intermedia express the same precursor; however, tissue-specific processing yields different peptide products. The POMC gene appears to have evolved early in metazoan evolution as two lophotrochozoan species, leech and mussel, both possess POMC peptides that have the same basic peptide sequences found in the same order on the precursor.

Five subtypes of receptors have been isolated that bind MSH- and ACTH-related peptides. The MC1 receptor has been implicated in pigmentation and may also mediate the anti-inflammatory actions of the melanocortins. The MC2 receptor is found exclusively in the adrenal glands and mediates the glucocorticoid synthesizing and releasing effects of ACTH. The MC3, 4 and 5 receptors are found in the brain although MC5 is found in a number of tissues as well. MC5 may also mediate some exocrine functions in the mouse (Chapter 13). The MC3 and MC4 receptors have been implicated in the regulation of feeding, appetite and metabolic rate. The melanocortin receptors possess natural agonists in the form of the agouti peptide, and the agouti-related peptide (Chapter 7).

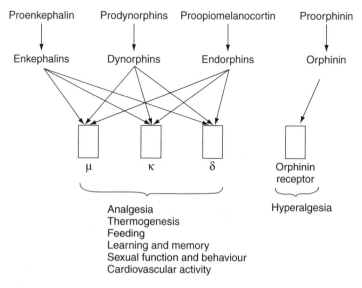

Figure 9.17 *Relationship of opioid prohormones, their receptors and their physiological functions.*

POMC belongs to a family of four related prohormones. Proenkephalin is the precursor for the opioids leu-enkephalin and met-enkephalin; prodynorphin is cleaved to yield a number of dynorphin-related peptides; and pro-orphinin is the prohormone for orphinin LQ. All peptides act upon the opioid receptors μ, κ and δ, with the exception of orphinin LQ that acts on its own specific receptor to mediate hyperalgesia (Fig. 9.17). These hormones have been implicated in a variety of functions including algesia, thermogenesis, feeding, learning and memory, sexual function and behaviour, cardiovascular and respiratory actions. There are also a number of other peptides with opioid functions that are processed from proteins that are unrelated to the POMC-family of peptides. Notable examples are the casomorphins, endomorphins and the amphibian dermophins and deltorphins. Non-peptide opioids appear to be present throughout the Metazoa. Morphine and morphine-6-glucuronide, a morphine metabolite, are present in the blue mussel, *Mytilus edulis*, pedal ganglion. This species also appears to possess a variant of the μ-opioid receptor.

Integration of HPA/I components with other systems

The onset of a stress response is highly integrated with other physiological systems. In general, such a response acts to inhibit parasympathetic-related functions and stimulate parasympathetic-related functions.

Osmoregulation

In fish, altered external salinity often leads to changes in urophyseal stored urotensin-I content. By comparison with saltwater-maintained *Gillichthys mirabilis*, fish transferred to freshwater exhibits increased urophyseal urotensin-I content after 24 hours. This apparent osmotic sensitivity of urotensin-I secretion and/or synthesis is associated with a direct action on transporting epithelia. Urotensin-I causes significant reduction in water and NaCl absorption in isolated anterior intestinal segments of freshwater-adapted but not saltwater-adapted tilapia. Active chloride transport by the opercular skin of *G. mirabilis* is stimulated by urotensin-I, an important component of ion balance in marine fish. In mammals, extravasation and oedema following injurious stimuli can be inhibited by urotensin-I and CRF through an unusual action of apparently reducing the permeability of small blood vessels during inflammation. Perhaps more dramatic are the vasodilatory effects of urotensin-I in mammals, reported in a series of pharmacological studies. In anaesthetized dogs, urotensin-I induces a specific dilatation of the mesenteric vascular bed. Urotensin-I is also effective in lowering systemic blood pressure in spontaneously hypertensive rats. Although urotensin-I was used in these studies, recent studies have indicated that it is urocortin that carries out these actions. In the spotted dogfish, *S. canicula*, bolus injections of a synthetic version of the endogenous urotensin-I produces a transient decrease in arterial pressure followed by a sustained rise in pressure, although no changes in heart rate appear to occur. Such actions on the renal vascular system are likely to be responsible for the observed urotensin-I-induced decreases in urine production and glomerular filtration rate and renal plasma flow, which are independent of vasopressin. Vasorelaxation induced by urotensin-I has also been reported in isolated strips of bird dorsal aorta.

Glucocorticoids, by themselves, do not induce sodium uptake in rats, but can do so when they are administered to rabbits or sheep. Rats subjected to immobilization stress will ingest more sodium than would be expected from compensating for their sodium loss, when released. Whereas CRF decreases food appetite, it does not for Na^+ ingestions. Infusions of CRF can elicit sodium ingestions that are independent of sodium loss. Hypertonic saline infusion will decrease CRF in the central nucleus of the amygdala and in the PVN. The central nucleus of the amygdala plays a role in the integration of signals from both angiotensin-II and CRF in generating a sodium need.

Together, subthreshold doses of angiotensin-II and a mineralocorticoid (deoxycorticosterone) can elicit Na^+ ingestion, indicating that the two systems may be synergistic. Glucocorticoids and mineralocorticoids are synergistic in rabbits at stimulating sodium ingestion. However, the combination of angiotensin and aldosterone peripherally does not produce synergistic effects on Na^+ ingestion. One mechanism for this synergism may occur at the receptor level. For example, mineralocorticoids increase the number of angiotensin receptors in the brain. This is mediated by the Type I receptor. Cortisol potentiates angiotensin-II-induced water intake as well as mineralocorticoid-induced Na^+ intake. Cortisol can potentiate angiotensin-II-mediated water intake that occurs via the AT2 receptors. Cortisol may increase the amount of angiotensinogen synthesis (found in glial cells) by binding to the Type II glucocorticoid receptors. Cortisol binding to the Type II receptors can also increase Type I glucocorticoid receptor expression.

Feeding and appetite

Food deprivation will activate the HPA axis and activation of the HPA axis attenuates feeding behaviour. Low concentrations of corticosterone will stimulate food intake, high concentrations will inhibit food intake. Lesions to the ventromedial hypothalamus produce hyperphagic and overweight animals. Adrenalectomy abolishes the hyperphagia whereas cortisol replacement reinstates it. The glucocorticoid-mediated actions on feeding appear to be mediated primarily via the Type II glucocorticoid receptor. The rise in plasma glucocorticoids appears to impart preferences in the diet. For example, protein intake is unaffected by corticosterone treatment although fat intake is. Short-term intake is associated with the Type II cortisol receptors linked to carbohydrate intake. Type I receptors may also play a role for fat ingestion and long-term regulation of energy balance.

The actions of CRF and NPY are antagonistic in appetite regulation (Chapter 6). CRF will inhibit appetite and feeding, whereas NPY will tend to promote feeding. Adrenalectomy can abolish NPY-induced feeding and cortisol replacement reinstates it. Stimulation of the Type II glucocorticoid receptors using specific agonists increases NPY gene expression in the basomedial hypothalamic region or arcuate nucleus. Both regions send projections to the PVN. NPY is regulated under conditions in which food access is compromised and rats are hungry. Elevated NPY may be associated with the enjoyment of rewards such as food intake.

Insulin and leptin are both part of a feedback loop linking feeding and the HPA axis. Adrenalectomy will reduce insulin secretion but cortisol will restore or increase it. Insulin receptors are present in PVN and arcuate nucleus, where they appear to modulate the sensitivity of leptin and other factors on CRF and NPY respectively (Fig. 9.18). Leptin has modulatory actions on the HPA axis. It alters the expression of CRF in the hypothalamus, interacts with

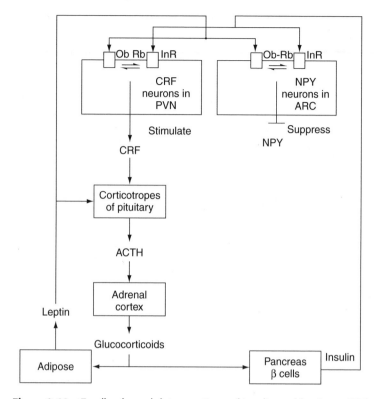

Figure 9.18   *Feedback modulatory actions of insulin and leptin on CRF.*

ACTH at the adrenal level and is regulated by glucocorticoids. Plasma leptin and cortisol concentrations show inverse circadian rhythms to each other and may receive photoperiodic input independently from each other. For example, glucocorticoids play a modulatory but not essential role in generating the leptin diurnal rhythm. Glucocorticoids can act directly on adipose tissue and increase leptin synthesis and secretion in humans. Glucocorticoids appears to act as one of the key modulator of body weight and food intake promoting leptin secretion by adipocytes, limiting central leptin-induced effects and favouring those of the NPY system.

Actions of the HPA axis on other systems

The neuroanatomical arrangement of the urotensin-I/urocortin cells in the midbrain suggests an association with locomotor activity. CRF can stimulate locomotor activity in urodeles. For example, in the roughskin newt, discharges of neurons in the raphe nuclei, associated with walking and swimming behaviours, can be modified by injections of CRF into the lateral ventricles. Although the midbrain population of urocortin neurons appears to be associated with the neural stress response, as evidenced by its interactions with nucleus of the solitary tract, and with the CRF neurons of the PVN, its primary role appears to be associated with motor control and sensorimotor integration.

A number of recent studies have implicated the activation of the HPA axis as a significant factor in the epigenetic development of some behaviours. During breast-feeding, women are less responsive to activation of the HPA axis. During lactation, cortisol concentrations are largely independent of the hypothalamic pituitary activations. In rodents, cortisol can enhance the responsiveness to infant cues. Corticosterone has been implicated in the facilitation of attachment behaviours in the male prairie vole. Infants separated from their mothers exhibit decreased secretions of growth hormone and prolactin as well as elevated cortisol concentrations. They will also lose weight. Stress in mothers can be passed to offspring. These behaviours may include decreased motor performance and lower body weight. Other effects can include a lower production of growth hormone and greater fear-related responses to unfamiliar events. The central nucleus of the amygdala, bed nucleus of the stria terminalis and paraventricular nucleus have higher concentrations of CRF in pups of mother who have experienced stress during pregnancy. Neonatal rats that are separated from their mothers will synthesize greater amounts of CRF as adults than pups who have not been separated. Macaques exposed to unpredictable foraging outcomes as youngsters also tend to have higher concentrations of CRF in the cerebrospinal fluid. ACTH and cortisol concentrations are lower in adult rats that have been handled as pups compared to those animals that have not been handled. In rabbits, the stress of high predation pressure experienced by the mothers appears to be passed to the next generation who show more sensitive HPA axes and reduced fertility. There are evolutionary reasons for such a relationship. Enhanced sensitivity of HPA axis in the offspring will manifest as increased wariness of novel situations, or of strangers. There is, therefore, a trade-off between survival and fertility.

In addition to the systemic actions of urotensin-I and CRF-like peptides on cardiovascular activity, a rapidly expanding array of central effects is reported. The intracerebroventricular (ICV) administration of urotensin-I and sauvagine but not CRF in conscious dogs produces long-term increases in mesenteric blood flow and slightly elevated mean arterial pressure, underscoring separable central and peripherally mediated effects of urotensin-I and sauvagine on mesenteric blood flow. Some of this effect may be mediated by the central nucleus of the amygdala which is also important for the cardiovascular regulation.

Centrally administered CRF-related peptides elicit thermogenic responses in the rat. Centrally and peripherally injected CRF induces a dose-dependent hypothermia in rats. The dopamine receptor agonists, haloperidol and spiperone block this action suggesting that a D2 dopamine receptor-mediated mechanism is activated by the CRF peptides. The adrenergic receptor blocker, phentolamine, and adrenergic antagonist, yohimbine, enhance the actions of sauvagine on thermogenesis, indicating the existence of a synergistic catecholaminergic pathway regulating thermogenesis. The effects of CRF peptides on thermogenesis may be related, in part, to their interaction with TRH. In mammals, CRF and TRH are closely situated within the PVN and appear to regulate each other's release of reciprocal connections; thus some of these thermogenic responses may be mediated by TRH and the thyroid axis.

Complementary neuroendocrine circuits associated with stress

Although we have focused almost entirely upon the role of the CRF-like peptides at regulating the stress response, there are numerous other neuropeptide and neurohormone systems that act in a parallel and complementary fashion to potentiate the stress response. Other peptides, such as NPY and the recently discovered TCAP peptides, appear to act in an antagonistic manner and act to inhibit the stress response. Others such as cholecystokinin and the calcitonin-related peptides are complementary and, in some cases, synergistic with CRF-mediated systems.

Thyroid axis

We have discussed the close relationship of CRF and TRH with respect to the induction of metamorphosis, regulation of feeding and appetite and control of MSH in the pars intermedia. Thus, during periods of HPA activation the HPT axis is frequently activated. Typically, circulating T3 levels are highly regulated by peripheral tissues, however stresses such as trauma, burns, infections, diseases, myocardial infarction, chronic diseases or metabolic disorders will elicit thyroid hormone response resulting in low serum T3 levels. This is due to the decreased conversion of T4 into T3. T4 is instead directed towards alternative metabolic pathways. The resulting lowered T3 levels allow for conservation of protein and also the initiation of gluconeogenesis. If the illness progresses, levels of both T3 and T4 will occur as T4 clearance levels will increase. An inverse relationship exists between serum T4 levels and mortality rate. There are three main potential mediators of low T3/T4 levels. Infection or trauma leads to increased cytokines that induce low levels of thyroid hormones. Secondly, surgery or burns promote an increase in serum cortisol concentrations that produce low T3 levels. Nutritional status is another factor capable of inducing serum thyroid hormone changes. Fasting initiates a fall in serum T3 levels. In this case, uncontrolled diabetes mellitus, which has the same effect as fasting, will also cause a decrease in serum T3 levels.

The mechanism by which CRF interacts with TRH in mammals appears to have been derived from regulatory mechanisms already in place in non-mammalian vertebrates. The CRF-mediated induction of TSH secretion in amphibians, reptiles, birds and actinopterygians suggests that this is a fundamental mechanism in vertebrates. In coho salmon (*Oncorhynchus kisutch*), ovineCRF, sauvagine, and urotensin-I increase TSH *in vivo*, where urotensin-I appears to be the most potent. The release of TSH from salmon pituitary cell cultures is antagonized by the α-helical CRF antagonist, suggesting that this action is mediated by a CRF receptor. In birds, injections of oCRF to chick embryos on day E19 leads immediately to increased pituitary glycoprotein and TSH concentrations, although LH and FSH levels remain unchanged, *in vivo*. The thyroid hormones T3, T4 and rT3 are subsequently increased one-hour post injections. Similar increases in glycoprotein induced by oCRF occur *in vitro* with cultured chick pituitary cells.

Prolactin and HPA

Prolactin appears to play an intrinsic role in the activation of the HPA axis. Restraint stress can decrease levels of plasma prolactin in rats and sheep. However, although, in rats, injections of CRF stimulate the release of both ACTH and prolactin from the anterior pituitary, its presence may not regulate pituitary prolactin mRNA synthesis. Furthermore, in humans and sheep, CRF does not have a direct effect on pituitary prolactin, but prolactin may instead regulate the release of CRF via a centrally located mechanism. This possibility is supported by studies that show that prolactin stimulates CRF from rat hypothalami *in vitro*, which suggests that a reciprocal interaction occurs between CRF- and PRL-mediated systems within brain regions innervating the hypothalamus.

Prolactin has a number of modulatory actions on the immune system (Fig. 9.19). Exposure to short days reduces blood prolactin levels in mammals and has a pronounced effect upon immune function in a variety of species. Generally, it enhances normal immunological activities, but can also compromise immune function, particularly at high or low circulating levels. As exposure to short days suppresses prolactin levels it could be the source of some of the seasonal changes that occur in immune function. Hypophysectomy of rats results in compromised humoral and cell-mediated immunity, which was restored by prolactin-replacement therapy. Prolactin receptors are present on lymphocytes, and prolactin-like substances have been identified in mouse splenocytes and human lymphoblastoid cell lines. Prolactin elevates the respiratory burst and phagocytosis of peritoneal macrophages for young and old mice. Suppression of prolactin with bromocriptine in rodents causes a decrease in immunological responses manifested as delayed type hypersensitivity, primarily antibody responses, T-cell dependent macrophage activation and *ex-vivo* T-lymphocyte and B-lymphocyte proliferation. Cyclosporin A and glucocorticoids have the same immunocompromising effects. But these can be reversed by treatment with factors that stimulate endogenous prolactin release or exogenous ovine prolactin. The immunological effects of prolactin might interact with the immunological effects of steroid hormones to mediate seasonal fluctuations in immune function.

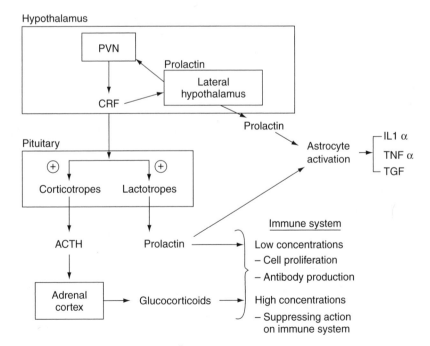

Figure 9.19 *Relationship between CRF, prolactin and immunocompetent cell systems.*

Astrocytes are the most common cell type in the mammalian brain. They increase in number and size in response to infection or trauma. Astrocytes act as immunocompetent cells in the CNS and secrete cytokines. Hypoprolactinemia induced by hypophysectomy, or by administration of bromocriptine, impairs humoral, cell-mediated and auto-immune responses, for example, producing decreases in antibody production in rats and thymus weight. In experimental allergic encephalomyelitis (EAE), which causes autoimmune demyelination, prolactin acts as an immunoregulatory hormone. Serum prolactin concentrations are five times higher prior to the onset of the neurological disease. Administration of bromocriptine reduced the incidence and acuteness of EAE and its re-occurrence in rats. Prolactin can act as a mutagen in cultured astrocytes. It induces the expression of interleukin 1α (IL-1α), tumour necrosis factor-α (TNF-α) and transforming growth factor-α (TGF-α) in cultured astrocytes. Administration of prolactin into a CNS wound increases the expression of astrocyte specific protein GFAP, as well as TNF-α. Further infliction of the wound results in increases in prolactin content and prolactin mRNA in the surrounding tissue.

In lymphocytes, prolactin increases hormonal and cellular immunity, reversing the anaemia, leukopenia and thrombocytopenia caused by hypophysectomy. Prolactin also increases antibody formation. In addition to stimulating cell proliferation, prolactin will inhibit apoptosis of lymphocytes. In the mammary gland, prolactin enhances IgA-secreting plasma cell activity.

Seasonal fluctuations in immune function has been well documented, for example, the number of circulating leukocytes in mice, rats, voles and humans are thought to be elevated during autumn and winter. Also spleen and thymus masses have been observed in deer mice (*Peromyscus maniculatus*) and prairie voles (*Microtus ochrogaster*) during autumn and winter. These changes appear to be mediated by daylength. Short day exposure increases splenic masses in deer mice and the Syrian hamster (*Mesocricetus auratus*), as well as elevating total lymphocyte and macrophage counts.

Galanin

Galanin coexists with CRF in the hypothalamic paraventricular nucleus. These findings support the hypothesis that galanin and CRF are simultaneously involved in regulation of ACTH secretion from the anterior pituitary. Galanin administration to normal rats results in a marked rise in the blood levels of ACTH. In human anterior pituitaries, galanin is present in corticotrophs scattered throughout the gland, but not in lactotrophs, somatotrophs, thyrotrophs or gonadotrophs. Galanin can inhibit ACTH release in cultured rat anterior pituitary cells, whereas the immunoneutralization with galanin antiserum will remove this effect. Furthermore, low plasma concentrations of ACTH can increase galanin release from the anterior pituitary of male adult rat, but the high concentrations of ACTH will suppress galanin release. At the adrenal gland level, galanin stimulates adrenal glucocorticoid secretion in rats directly. Thus galanin may be acting, in part, as an autocrine modulatory factor at the hypothalamic and pituitary level.

Galanin has been implicated in the response to stress in several studies. Limbic forebrain structures important for the expression of fear and anxiety, such as the central nucleus of the amygdala (CeA) and the bed nucleus of the stria terminalis (BNST), show a rich expression of galanin and galanin receptors. Furthermore, galanin coexists in 80–90% of the norepinephrine-containing neurons in the locus coeruleus (LC). Moreover, galanin mRNA signal is also evident in some stress associated hypothalamic nuclei such as the paraventricular nucleus, supraoptic, dorsomedial, arcuate nuclei and the lateral hypothalamus. By observing the effects of acute and chronic restraint stress on preprogalanin mRNA expression in the CNS of normotensive (Wistar Kyoto; WKY) and spontaneously hypertensive rats (SHR), it was found that, following acute restraint, preprogalanin mRNA expression was significantly increased by approximately 135% in CeA of WKY rats. In SHR, significant increases of up to 300% were observed in the CeA and supraoptic nucleus following chronic restraint. In addition, expression of preprogalanin mRNA was significantly decreased in the LC of SHR following acute restraint. These results provide the evidence that both acute (LC) and chronic (CeA, SON) restraint stress is associated with alterations in preprogalanin mRNA expression. On the other hand, in some other experiment models, the galanin expression increased in the rat LC during chronic stress, in the medial subdivision of CeA following formalin-evoked pain and in rat LC after treadmill exercise training. Furthermore, some behaviour studies have added to our understanding of the effects of galanin on stress response. For example, administration of galanin antagonists into the lateral bed nucleus of the stria terminalis, or central nucleus of the amygdala before stress attenuates the anxiogenic-like effects of immobilization stress, or the anxiolytic influence of the adrenergic autoreceptor antagonist yohimbine pre-treatment. Immobilization stress, that typically increases plasma ACTH, is also attenuated by the administration galanin antagonists into the BNST prior to stress.

Galanin is present in a small population of dorsal root ganglion (DRG) neurons. Galanin levels in DRGs are high prenatally and are down-regulated postnatally. In adult rats, galanin expression increases dramatically in the lumbar 4 and 5 DRGs after transection of the sciatic nerve. And also, there is a moderate increase in the number of galanin-positive primary afferent terminals in laminae I and II, with a limited expansion of galanin-like immunoreactivity into lamina III of the spinal cord. In normal animals in which the sciatic nerve is intact, exogenous galanin exerts both facilitatory and inhibitory effects. Inhibitory effects have been recorded from dorsal horn neurons. Intrathecal injection of a high dose of galanin increased the pain threshold in mice. By contrast, painful reaction to light touch and a decreased mechanical nociceptive threshold with no effect on thermal nociception have been found following intrathecal injection of galanin; the latter effect is, at least in part, mediated via galanin-induced release of substance P. In addition, chronic intrathecal delivery of a low dose of exogenous galanin to nerve-intact adult rats induces persistent mechanical and/or thermal hypersensitivity. On the other hand, in animals with peripheral nerve injury, the inhibitory component of exogenous galanin is enhanced significantly, suggesting increased importance of galanin-receptive mechanisms mediating antinociception. Animals with peripheral inflammation are less well studied. Exogenous galanin at a high dose reduces inflammation-induced hyperexcitability. The galanin-induced inhibition of reflex facilitation following conditioning stimuli is much less potent after inflammation than in normal rats. Recently, studies have indicated that the sensitivity to noxious stimuli is significantly higher in galanin knockout mice than in wild-type mice.

Studies also suggested that galanin may interact with other neurotransmitters in the transmission of presumed nociceptive information in the spinal cord. The opioid receptor antagonist, naloxone, and the μ-opioid receptor antagonist, β-funaltrexamine, can block the increased hind-paw response latencies induced by galanin. Taken together, these findings suggest a possible role for galanin in processes that are important during development and for the survival and regeneration of damaged neurons.

Cholecystokinin-gastrin family

The cholecystokinin-gastrin family of peptides has been implicated in a number of stress-inducing and anxiety-associated mechanisms. Cholecystokinin (CCK) was originally discovered in the I or CCK cells of the duodenum, but has since been found in the CNS of all vertebrates. CCK homologues are also present in the CNS of a number of invertebrate species. Gastrin was found initially in the G-cells of the gastric antrum. It is found in all main regions of the pituitary gland. In the intermediate and anterior lobe it is co-localized with POMC neurons and is regulated by gastrin-releasing peptide (GRP). The human CCK gene is found on chromosome 3 whereas the human gastrin gene is present on chromosome 17. Gastrin is 17 residues long whereas CCK is 8 amino acids in length. Both possess the common sequence GWMDP-NH2 at the carboxy terminus (Chapter 7). This sequence is necessary for the basic biological activity of both hormones, whereas the potency is determined by N-terminal sequences. Two variants of gastrin have been isolated. Gastrin II that has the identical amino acid sequence to gastrin I but has instead a sulphated tyrosine residue. The preprohormone of both neuropeptides possess the same basic organization of three exons and two introns. Both peptides are present as different length chains that appear to be due to post-translational cleavage of the prohormone at monobasic (i.e. lysine or arginine) residues.

Thus, both neuropeptides appear to be the result of a gene duplication in vertebrates that occurred before the emergence of the cartilaginous fishes. Separate genes encoding gastrin and CCK have been identified in the bullfrog. The spiny dogfish (*Squalus acanthias*) and porbeagle shark (*Lamna cornubica*) also possess separate genes for gastrin and CCK. Thus, the common ancestor for this gene appears to have evolved over 400 million years ago possibly before the emergence of jawed vertebrates. The spiny dogfish version of CCK-8 is identical to the mammalian form of the peptide. Three separate cDNAs encoding CCK have been identified in the rainbow trout, *Oncorynchus mykiss*. The skin of the tree frog, *Hyla caerulea*, contains CCK-like decapeptide called caerulein. The gene is not known but appears to be more related to CCK than gastrin. Many of the anurans show varying degrees of polyploidy relative to other jawed vertebrates, and possess unusual variants of neuropeptides in their skin, as defence mechanisms. This is discussed in greater detail in Chapter 13.

Currently, only a single form of a gastrin/CCK-like peptide has been isolated from invertebrate species. A single CCK/gastrin like octapeptide has been isolated from the neural ganglion of the protochordate *Ciona intestinalis*. This peptide is unusual in that it possesses sulphated tyrosine residues in both positions 6 and 7, relative to the C-terminus. It, therefore, possesses both CCK- and gastrin-like attributes. A common ancestor to this gene, however, appears to have evolved sometime before protostomes and deuterostomes diverged as CCK/gastrin-like peptides have been isolated from the Madeira cockroach, *Leucophora maderae*, and fruitfly, *Drosophila melanogaster*.

Two CCK/gastrin receptors have been identified in vertebrates (Fig. 9.20). CCK-A receptor was originally found in the alimentary tract and the CCK-B receptor in the brain. Since then, the CCK-A receptor has also been found in the brain. CCK-A receptors have

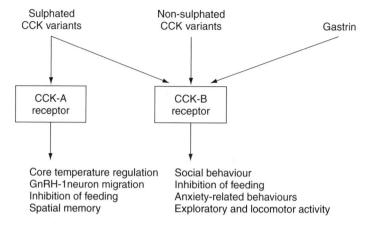

Figure 9.20 *Actions of Cholecystokinin-related peptides.*

high affinity for the sulphated variants of CCK, but not gastrin. CCK-B receptors are less discerning and bind both sulphated and non-sulphated forms of CCK and gastrin. Both receptors possessed belong to the G-protein-coupled receptor family and are transcribed from genes consisting of five exons and four introns. The two receptors were presumably the result of a duplication of a receptor gene with less specificity for its ligand. CCK/gastrin receptors in mako shark and rainbow trout, *O. mykiss*, have been identified with these characteristics but currently little is known about the receptor genes in non-mammalian species.

Other systems

The endozepines are a family of peptides that are derived from the diazepam-binding inhibitor and its proteolytic fragments such as triakontatetraneuropeptide (TTN) and octadecaneuropeptide (ODN). They are present in the brain and most endocrine glands and are found in all terrestrial vertebrates. They appear to act as local regulators of hormone secretin. They were originally identified by their ability to displace benzodiazepines from their binding sites. In the mammalian adrenal gland, the endozepines act as intracrine factors that promote cholesterol transport via stimulation of benzodiazepine receptors located on the outer mitochondrial membrane. Endozepine receptors have also been found in the plasma membrane indicating that they also act as autocrine and paracrine agents. In the frog adrenal gland they bind to a non-benzodiazepine receptor to induce Ca^{2+} influx leading to an increase in corticosteroid secretion.

The calcitonin gene-related peptide (CGRP) has been implicated, like calcitonin in aspects of the stress response. Two forms of CGRP have been characterized in mammals. A single variant has been isolated from the brain of the frog, *R. ridibunda*. Frog CGRP is a potent stimulator of corticosteroid and aldosterone secretion from frog adrenal slices. In frogs, the tachykinin, ranakinin and neurokinin A also stimulate cortisol and aldosterone from adrenal tissue. The tachykinins are a family of regulatory peptides related to substance P. They are present throughout vertebrate and invertebrate species.

Chapter summary

The stress response evolved early in metazoan ancestry as a means to regulate energy production and transport to physiological systems that require it. The stress response allows animals to mount a defensive response to events in the environment that act to challenge homeostatic balance and survival. The elements of the organismal stress response have been the most comprehensively studied in vertebrates. The central neuroendocrine circuit of the stress response is the hypothalamus–pituitary–adrenal (interrenal) axis. Hypothalamic corticotrophin-releasing factor (CRF) stimulates the synthesis and release of POMC-associated peptides from the corticotrophs and melanotrophs from the pars distalis and pars intermedia respectively. ACTH release into the systemic blood supply mediates the synthesis and release of glucocorticoids from the adrenal gland of tetrapods or the interrenal tissues of fishes. CRF is part of a large gene family that includes urotensin-I, urocortin-II and urocortin-III. POMC is also part of a gene family that include proenkephalin, prodynorphin and proorphinin. CRF and POMC-like peptides have been found in invertebrates although it is not known if they form similar interregulatory relationships as is found in the vertebrates. In vertebrates, activation of the sympathetic nervous system branch of the autonomic nervous system is responsible for the 'flight or fight' response. A number of other hormonal systems such as galanin, thyrotrophin-releasing hormone, prolactin, cholecystokinin and calcitonin gene-related peptide play complementary roles to the HPA and sympathetic nervous system activation during homeostatic challenge.

Proopiomelanocortin
Robert M. Dores

Proopiomelanocortin (POMC), the common precursor for the opioid, β-endorphin, and the melanocortins, has been one of the most thoroughly investigated neuroendocrine precursor proteins, yet the origin of this ligand-coding gene remains unresolved. POMC is placed in the opioid/orphanin gene family, which includes the proenkephalin gene, the prodynorphin gene, and the proorphanin gene. Like other members of this gene family, the POMC gene encodes at least one opioid core sequence (YGGF) that is present in the N-terminal of the β-endorphin sequence. However, unlike other members of the gene family, POMC also encodes multiple melanocortin-related sequences (i.e., α-MSH/ACTH, β-MSH, γ-MSH, δ-MSH) that all have the core sequence HFRW. POMC cDNAs have been cloned from representatives of every major class of the gnathostome vertebrates, and it is well established that this gene is expressed in the corticotropic cells of the anterior pituitary, the melanotropic cells of the intermediate pituitary, and subsets of neurons in the central nervous system. The orthodox view on the spatial expression pattern for the POMC gene has been that: the primary function of the corticotropic cells is to produce ACTH (adrenocorticotropin) for the purpose of regulating the production of glucocorticoids from adrenalcortical cells; the primary function of the melanotropic cells is to produce α-MSH (α-melanocyte stimulating hormone) for the purpose of regulating physiological colour change in amphibians and some reptiles; and the primary purpose of the POMC neurons in the CNS is to produce β-endorphin, an inhibitory neurotransmitter, that influences analgesia. The realization that POMC neurons in the CNS also project to appetite centres in the hypothalamus, and that the melanocortins can influence feeding behaviour, lipid metabolism, and glucose homeostasis underscores the multi-functional properties of the POMC gene, and provides additional opportunities for comparative analyses on the metabolic actions of end-products derived from this precursor.

Although there is agreement that the POMC gene was derived from some ancestral opioid gene (Fig. B9.1), the origin of the melanocortin sequences has not been resolved. One thing is clear, however. There are no melanocortin-like sequences in any of the other members of the opioid/orphanin gene family (i.e. proenkephalin, prodynorphin, or proorphanin). In the scenario presented in Fig. B9.1, it is assumed that the ACTH/a-MSH sequence was the original opioid sequence, and that as a result of a series of unequal crossing over events, the α-MSH sequence was duplicated. The presence of α-MSH-like and β-MSH-like sequences in the POM (proopiomelanocortin) form of the POMC gene in the lamprey, *Petromyzon marinus*, coupled with the absence of a γ-MSH-like sequence suggests that the α-MSH/β-MSH duplication event happened during the radiation of the ancestral agnathan vertebrates and that the γ-MSH duplication event happened during the early radiation of the ancestral gnathostomes (Fig. B9.1). The presence of ACTH/α-MSH, β-MSH, and γ-MSH (the ancestral gnathostome condition) has been found in the Sarcopterygii (lobe-finned fish and tetrapods), and secondarily modified in two lineage specific ways in the cartilaginous fish (class Chondrichthyes) and the ray-finned fish (class Actinopterygii).

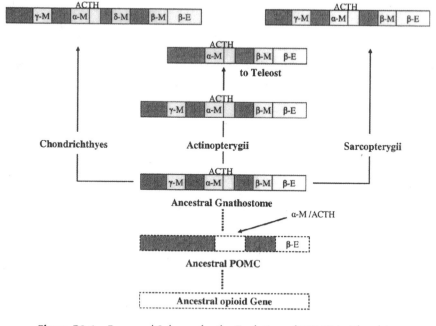

Figure B9.1 *Proposed Scheme for the Evolution of POMC in Chordates.*

(Continued)

In the cartilaginous fish there has been an additional melanocortin duplication event that gave rise to the δ-MSH sequence early in the radiation of the cartilaginous fish. By contrast, in the ray-finned fish, there has been a progressive degeneration of the γ-MSH sequence that has resulted in the complete loss of this melanocortin in teleosts. The selective pressures that have influenced these modifications in the organization of POMC have not been established. However, correlating the co-evolution of the melanocortin receptors and the opioid receptors may explain the lineage specific features of the POMC gene.

In this cartoon of radiation of the Proopiomelanocortin (POMC) precursor protein in phylum Chordata, the relative positions of the melanocortin sequences (ACTH; γ-MSH: γ-M; α-MSH: α-M; β-MSH: β-M; and δ-MSH: δ-M) and the opioid β-endorphin (β-end) are shown. The cartilaginous fish (Chondrichthyes), ray-finned fish (Actinopterygii) and lobe-finned/tetrapod (Sarcopterygii) precursors are framed with a solid line because these representations are based on actual amino acids sequences. The cartoon for the predicted ancestral gnathostome POMC is also framed with a solid line because this representation is the most parsimonious interpretation of the current data. The hypothetical representations for the ancestral POMC and the ancestral opioid precursor are framed with a dashed line.

References

Dores, R.M., McDonald, L., Steveson, T.C. and Sei, C.A. (1990) The molecular evolution of neuropeptides: Prospects for the '90s. *Brain Behav. Evol.* 36, 80–99.

Danielson, P.B. and Dores, R.M. (1999) The evolution of the opioid/orphanin gene family. *Gen. Comp. Endocrinol.* 113, 169–186.

Dores, R.M., Lecaude, S., Bauer, D. and Danielson, P.B. (2002) Analyzing the evolution of the opioid/orphanin gene family. *Mass. Spec. Rev.* 21, 220–243.

10

Reproduction

Introduction

Once the basic survival needs of an individual are met, then reproductive needs become
the primary motivator for behaviour for many metazoans. In the last four chapters,
we discussed the neuroendocrine mechanisms that were essential for the survival of
the organism under differing environmental situations. In this chapter, we discuss the
neuroendocrine system that is responsible for the perpetuation of the individual,
and ultimately the population and its species. At some point or another, every signalling system associated with sensory systems impinges on and acts to modulate the
reproductive neuroendocrine system. Events that act to favour the health and well-
being of the individual tend to facilitate aspects of reproductive physiology and
behaviour, whereas situations compromising the health of the individual have the
opposite effect.

Reproduction is probably the most studied of all the physiological systems; despite this
there are still vast areas of neuroendocrine regulation of reproduction that is not understood. Clearly, all the intricacies of the regulation of reproduction cannot be covered in a
short chapter in a small book; however, many of the core essentials can be discussed.
Many of the basal metazoans employ non-sexual reproduction, for example, the budding
process in hydra; however, only the neuroendocrine elements of sexual reproduction will
be discussed in this chapter.

Neuroendocrinology: An Integrated Approach   David A. Lovejoy
© 2005 John Wiley & Sons, Ltd

Selection of sexual reproduction

Sexual reproduction mixes genes. Different combinations of genes from the parents lead to numerous variations inherited by the progeny. The widespread occurrence of organisms' sexual reproduction, relative to the few species that do not, indicates that the genes regulating sexual reproduction were more successful than those regulating other strategies. Parthenogenetic or asexual species have a much smaller gene pool compared to sexual species, because they are essentially clones of their parent and possess the same complement of genes. As a result they would be expected to have limited niche adaptation abilities relative to sexual species. Asexual reproduction also reduces sibling competition since they are genetically similar and will tend to respond to a given stimulus in a similar manner. Thus, early in the origin of a species, genomic variability is selected for. For sexual species, the chances for survival increase as the population in general has less susceptibility to disease or predation due to the genetic and, hence, phenotypic variability of the population.

Sexual reproduction is also a way to remove harmful mutations. In asexual species, the number of mutations can only increase. In sexual species, however, the offspring may have lower mutations than parents due to the genetic recombination. In the event where genetic recombination will statistically produce a number of individuals with higher than normal mutations, many of these individuals may have a compromised reproductive ability and will eventually be removed from the population along with their genes. This will reduce the overall mutation load in the population and increase the overall fitness of the population relative to asexual reproduction.

One of the requirements of sexual reproduction is the production of haploid gametes from both of the sexes. However, the production of haploid sex cells was only possible once meiosis evolved. The sexes were basically similar but each had two types of cells: diploid somatic cells and haploid sex cells. Fusion of the sex cells produced a diploid cell. In the most ancestral sexual organisms the structure of gametes were likely similar in shape and size. However, over time, two size morphs would have been selected for. Gametes on the larger size would have the advantage of survivability in that they would possess a larger store of nutrients. Thus, these genes would be selected for. At the other extreme, smaller sizes could be produced more quickly with fewer nutrients. Their long-term survivability would not be that important as they could fuse with the larger gametes. Intermediate-sized gametes would have no selective advantage and would eventually be eliminated. Large gametes would become the female form whereas small gametes would become the male form. Thus, females become selected for the ability to produce larger but fewer gametes. Physiologically, systems aimed at increasing nutrients of eggs, their protection and hence survivability are selected for. On the other hand, males become selected for a system that produces larger numbers of small gametes.

Regulation of reproduction

There are two or three main components to the regulation of reproductive cycles, depending upon the complexity of the organism. Initially, a neuroendocrine factor is secreted from the brain in response to the appropriate environmental stimuli to initiate the reproductive

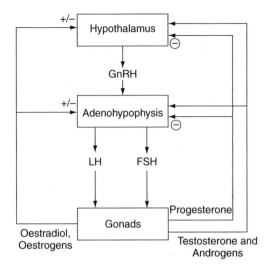

Figure 10.1   *Basic arrangement of the hypothalamus–pituitary–gonadal (HPG) axis.*

cycle. This factor then may stimulate the gonads directly, or act via a secondary endocrine organ to regulate the gonads. The neuroendocrine factors are typically neuropeptides. The gonads act to regulate the synthesis and release of the neuropeptides by a steroid feedback mechanism (Fig. 10.1). In vertebrates, there is a three-tiered system consisting of a gonadotrophin-releasing factor in the brain that stimulates the gonadotrophins from the pituitary gland, which subsequently stimulate the gonads to synthesize and release steroid hormones.

Reproduction in invertebrates

The regulation of reproduction in insects appears to utilize a number of similar molecular components analogous to what has been found in vertebrates. However, it is not clear where these hormones are orthologous to their vertebrate counterparts. Despite the presence of gonadotrophin-releasing hormone (GnRH) peptides in protochordates and molluscs, GnRH-like peptides in yeast, and GnRH immunoreactivity in other invertebrates, GnRH-like peptides have not been found in arthropods. GnRH immunoreactivity has been found in some parts of the *Drosophila* brain (Fig. 10.2), although the epitope has not been identified. There is evidence, however, for gonadotrophins in insects. A peptide, 65 amino acids in length, was originally discovered in *Locusta migratoria* pars intercerebralis and is called ovary-maturing peptide (OMP). This peptide appears to act like a gonadotrophin and can regulate the synthesis and release of the ecdysteroids. Although the role of ecdysteroids in metamorphosis and moulting is well established, these steroids can also stimulate vitellogenin synthesis. Juvenile hormone can also stimulate vitellogenin synthesis (Fig. 10.3).

There are two principal steroids that have been identified in insects that play a role in sexual differentiation and reproduction. Ecdysone is the predominant ecdysteroid in males whereas 20-OH ecdysone has been implicated with vitellogenin synthesis (Fig. 10.4). Thus, these steroids may be the arthropod equivalent of androgens and oestrogens, respectively.

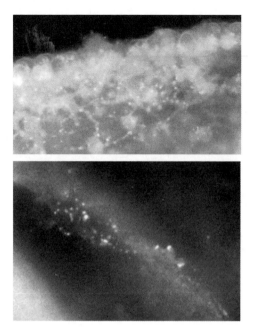

Figure 10.2 *GnRH immunoreactivity in the nervous system of a cnidarian,* Aurelia *(top) and an arthropod,* Drosophila *(bottom). Images courtesy of Dr. Roswitha Marx, University of Victoria (top) and Dr. Wendi Neckameyer, St Louis University (bottom).*

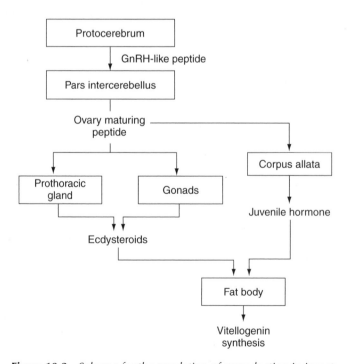

Figure 10.3 *Scheme for the regulation of reproduction in insects.*

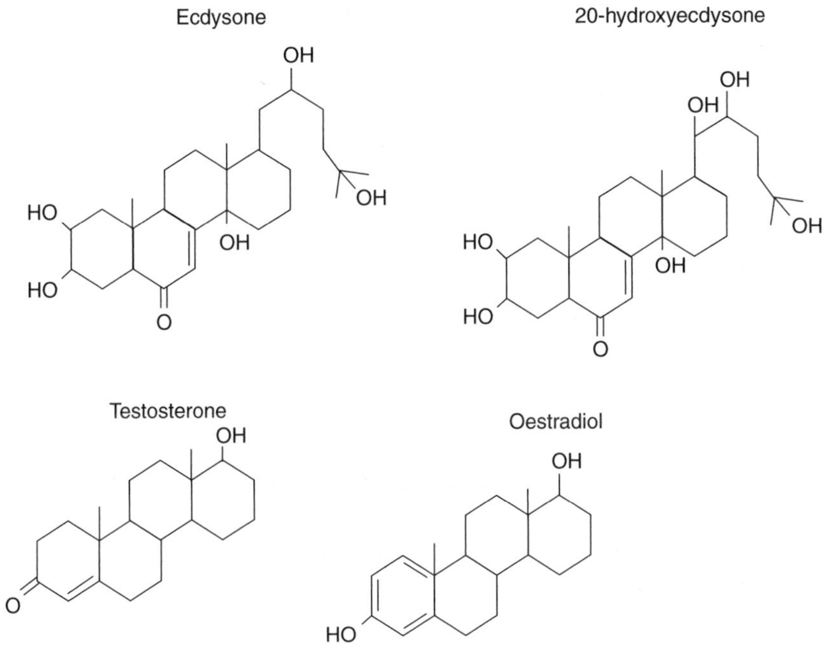

Figure 10.4   *Comparison with the principle sex steroids in insects and mammals.*

Ecdysone is the precursor for 20-OH ecdysone. This biosynthetic arrangement is similar to oestrogen being biosynthetically downstream from testosterone. In the moth, *Oryzia postica*, the ecdysone/20-OH ecdysone ratio increases in males as the sexual differentiation process progresses. The twin actions of these hormones on reproduction and moulting likely reflect the physiological need to coordinate these two mechanisms. Moulting continues throughout adulthood in arthropods, and therefore reproduction and moulting need to be closely integrated.

Mushroom bodies are paired structures found in the dorsoposterior part of the insect brain. These structures are thought to play a role in learning and memory. In the dorsal part of the mushroom bodied in the cricket, *Acheta domesticus*, there are a cluster of undifferentiated cells primarily in the form of neuroblasts and ganglion mother cells that continue to undergo mitosis throughout adult life. In this species both JH (III) and ecdysone regulate the rate of mitogenesis in the adult mushroom bodies. Oviposition behaviour in crickets is independent of the presence of ovaries. Removal of the corpora allata prevents egg-laying behaviour but it can be restored by injection of JH. The onset of these behaviours may be due to neurogenesis in the mushroom bodies and the formation of novel synaptic circuits.

Regulation of reproductive cycles in vertebrates

The basic scheme for the regulation of reproductive cycles in vertebrates is largely conserved, although the details of the interaction and the subsequent timing between events can vary enormously. In mammals, reproductive cycles are initiated by the pulsatile release of GnRH from hypothalamic and forebrain regions into the portal vasculature of the median eminence. In males, this induces the release of follicle-stimulating hormone (FSH) and luteinizing hormone (LH) from the gonadotrophs of the pituitary gland into the systemic circulation. In males, FSH acts to stimulate the activity of Sertoli cells in the seminiferous tubules of the testes to aid in spermatogenesis. The Sertoli cells, in response to FSH, secrete a peptide hormone, inhibin, and a small amount of oestradiol into the blood stream (Fig. 10.5). Inhibin acts to selectively attenuate the release of FSH from the pituitary gonadotrophs. LH, on the other hand, stimulates the production of testosterone from the Leydig cells of the interstitial region of the testes. Most testosterone secreted from Leydig cells passes into the blood stream. However, a small amount passes into the seminiferous tubules. Testosterone, being a steroid and highly lipophilic, passes freely across the blood–testes barrier. Sertoli cells secrete androgen-binding protein to maintain local high concentrations of testosterone. Testosterone circulates in plasma bound to sex steroid binding proteins or other plasma proteins. In tissues, testosterone can be converted to dihydroxytestosterone (DHA), 5α-androstenedione or oestradiol. The major targets of testosterone include the accessory organs of the male reproductive tract such as the prostate, seminal vesicles and epididymis. Testosterone also has an effect on a number of non-reproductive tissues such as the liver, heart, skin, skeletal, muscle, bone and brain (Fig. 10.6). If plasma testosterone levels rise too high, then they inhibit the release of the pituitary

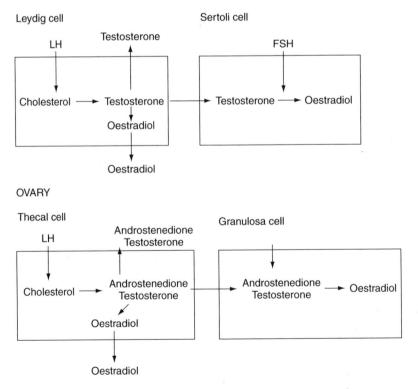

Figure 10.5 *Comparison of sex steroid synthesis in testes and ovary.*

Testosterone
    Foetus   Epididymus growth and development
              Vas deferens growth and development
              Seminal vesicle growth and development
    Puberty   Larynx development
              Penis enlargement
              Skeletal and musculature development

Dihydroxytestosterone
    Foetus   External genitalia
    Puberty   Secondary sex characteristics
              Further development of scrotum and prostate

Androstenedione
    Puberty   Hair and skin changes

Oestradiol
    Foetus   Masculinization of brain

Figure 10.6   *Actions of testosterone and its metabolites on tissues in mammals.*

gonadotrophins, and also the release of GnRH from the hypothalamus. This feedback mechanism is ongoing, such that testosterone production and spermatogenesis remain more or less consistent during the lifetime of a non-seasonal breeding mammal.

In females, the reproductive cycle is somewhat more complex. GnRH initiates the reproductive cycle as in males; however, its pulsatile characteristics are modulated to focus the stimulation on FSH or LH release (p. 290).

During foetal life, the primordial germ cells of the ovary form and continue mitotic proliferation. By the time of birth the total number of primordial germ cells is complete. In the foetus, primordial germ cells are known as oogonia. The oogonia enter the first meiotic division and become oocytes. Oocytes become surrounded by mesenchyme cells, and a basement membrane (basal lamina) is formed. This is then called a primordial follicle. Oocytes in the primordial follicle remain arrested at the first meiotic phase until reproductive maturity (puberty). Towards the end of the preantral stage, the granulosa cells develop receptors for oestrogens and FSH. The thecal cells, on the other hand, develop receptors for LH. Both gonadotrophins are required for the preantral follicle to develop into an antral follicle. In response to the gonadotrophins, the thecal and granulosa layers proliferate and begin to differentiate. Granulosa cells secrete fluid around the oocyte. In antral follicles where the thecal cells are under control of LH, the internal thecal layer (theca interna) begins to secrete testosterone, androstenedione and small amounts of oestrogens. In some non-mammalian species (e.g. elasmobranchs), the granulosa cells may also synthesize a small amount of androgens. The androgens from thecal cells diffuse to granulosa cells that convert these hormones into oestrogens. Much of the oestrogens diffuse into the blood stream and act to further stimulate the production and release of GnRH and gonadotrophins. Granulosa cells are under the control of FSH. Thus, the granulosa cells are analogous to the Sertoli cells in the male, and the thecal cells are analogous to the Leydig cells. In the preovulatory follicle, LH receptors appear in granulosa cells in preparation for ovulation. Several follicles develop to this stage but only one is selected to enter the preovulatory stage. The remainder atrophy and die. The preovulatory stage lasts 36 hours in humans. The oocyte finally completes the first meiotic division and now becomes a secondary oocyte. The secondary oocyte is ovulated. In preovulatory stage, the granulosa cells begin synthesizing progesterone. The follicle subsequently forms the

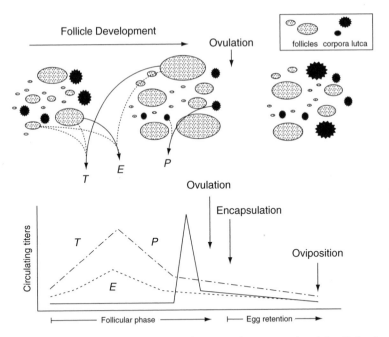

Figure 10.7   *Plasma steroid levels during the reproductive cycle of the little skate,* Raja erinacea. *Reprinted with permission from Koob and Callard (1999), Wiley Liss Inc.*

corpus luteum and this becomes the primary progesterone-synthesizing tissue in the body. Progesterone inhibits both GnRH and gonadotrophins. Then, once primed by progesterone, the GnRH neurons and gonadotrophs are inhibited by the oestrogens as well. This then acts to turn off the cycle until the corpus luteum atrophies, and the progesterone inhibition is removed.

Although we might consider this to be a model of a generalized endocrine response of a reproductive cycle, the timing and the amount of steroid secretion varies considerably among vertebrate classes and even between families with classes. For example, in the little skate (*Raja erinacea*), testosterone is also produced in significant quantities by the ovaries and appears to play a role in the regulation of the reproductive cycle in females. In addition in this species, the progesterone and testosterone concentrations show a peak plasma level well before the preovulatory oestradiol surge (Fig. 10.7).

Gonadotrophin-releasing hormone

Gonadotrophin-releasing hormone (GnRH) is the hypothalamic-releasing factor that is responsible for the initiation and functional maintenance of the reproductive system in virtually all vertebrates. However, evidence is accumulating that it also plays a significant role in the regulation of reproduction for a number of invertebrate species.

Evolution of GnRH

Gonadotrophin-releasing hormone is found in multiple forms all through chordates and protochordates. Recently, a GnRH variant was isolated and structurally characterized in the octopus. GnRH immunoreactivity has also been observed in the molluscs, arthropods and cnidarians. The structure of yeast α mating factor shows a significant structural similarity to GnRH and is active at releasing gonadotrophins from rat anterior pituitary cells. However, not all mating factor peptide orthologues found in fungal species show the same level of identity to the GnRH family of peptides, and the evolutionary relationship of the yeast mating factors to GnRH remains tenuous. If additional evidence appears where the orthology of the yeast peptides can be established with confidence, then we might postulate that GnRH-like peptides were present before the bifurcation of the fungi and animals.

Gonadotrophin-releasing hormone is unusual among neuropeptides in that it does not appear to be paralogous to any other known peptides outside of its immediate peptide family. Genetically, it did not appear to be subjected to the other genomic or chromosomal duplications in the chordates that led to the expansion of so many other neuropeptide families. One possibility is that the gene did duplicate and that the paralogous genes have been silenced via an accrual of mutations. If this were the case, then it may be an example of a situation where the formation of paralogues reduces the reproductive fitness of a population or species. There is, however, some evidence that initially GnRH underwent a paralogous expansion in some chordate lineages. In elasmobranchs, although two forms of GnRH have been characterized, a number of other studies indicate that five to seven different forms of GnRH may be present. However, the level of polyploidization in sharks is not known, and therefore it is not clear whether the apparent high numbers of GnRH variants in sharks represent derived traits of sharks. Ray-finned fishes appear to generally possess three forms of GnRH but this too may also reflect tetraploidization or partial tetraploidization that has occurred in many actinopterygian lineages.

The terrestrial vertebrates appear only to have two forms of GnRH that have been highly conserved. Because GnRH consists of only ten amino acids and has been highly conserved, for many years it was difficult to determine which variants were orthologous or paralogous. Since the cloning of the genes, paralogy can be determined. However, the classification of GnRH is confusing and there is little consensus in the literature (Table 10.1).

Ontogeny and neurological distribution of GnRH peptides

Gonadotrophin-releasing hormone is also unique in that it appears to be the only releasing factor that migrates into the forebrain from outside the brain. The migration of GnRH from the olfactory system to the brain is conserved in all vertebrates and may reflect an evolutionary connection between olfaction and reproduction. There are two distinct GnRH populations that migrate from this region. Although the migration was discovered first in mammals, it is easier to understand the pattern of migration using a fish brain example. In the sea bream, for example, the salmon (s)GnRH (Table 10.1) expressing subpopulation is detected first, about seven days after hatching, then begins a migration along the terminal nerve towards the telencephalon and eventually to the preoptic area (Fig. 10.8). Fibres extend throughout the brain and towards the brainstem and a few are present in the pituitary. About 18–20 days after the first appearance of the sGnRH subpopulation,

Table 10.1   *Gonadotropin-releasing hormone nomenclature*

Structure	Structural name	Trivial name	Other names
pEHWSYGLRPG	[Arg^8]-GnRH	Mammal GnRH	GnRH-1 Luteinizing hormone- releasing hormone (LHRH) luliberin-releasing factor (LRF)
pEHWSYGLQPG	[Gln^8]-GnRH	Chicken GnRH-I	
pEHWSYGLSPG	[Ser^8]-GnRH	Sea bream GnRH	teleost GnRH-I
pEHWSHGWYPG	[His^5,Trp^{7}Tyr^8]-GnRH	Chicken GnRH-II	GnRH-II
pEHWSYGWLPG	[Trp^7,Leu^8]-GnRH	Salmon GnRH	

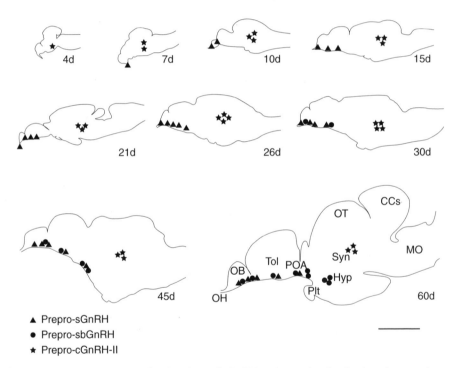

▲ Prepro-sGnRH
● Prepro-sbGnRH
★ Prepro-cGnRH-II

Figure 10.8 *Expression and migration of GnRH neurons in the brain of a sea bream. Reprinted from Gonzalez Martinez (2002) by the permission of Elsevier Science.*

the sbGnRH immunoreactive cells appear in the olfactory bulb and migrate along a similar path as sGnRH. The fibres issuing from the cells are much more restricted to the forebrain, and have extensive innervation of the pituitary.

Mammals also have two distinct subpopulations of GnRH immunoreactive neurons originating in the olfactory placode. The first population to migrate has a distinctly different immunoreactive profile from the second subpopulation that expresses mGnRH. However, only two GnRH genes are found in the mammalian genome and so the early migrating population appears to be expressing a GnRH fragment. The early migrating cells in mammals appear to be homologous to the sGnRH migrating cells of sea bream and other teleosts although a sGnRH form has not been found in the human or mouse genomes. Sea bream GnRH is the sea bream orthologue of mammal GnRH. Thus, the evolutionary relationship between the early migrating cells of fishes and those of mammals are not clear. In both fish and mammals, the same orthologue is present in the later migrating cells. From a comparative evolution point of view, a sGnRH-like form would be expected in the early migrating cells of mammals although there is no concrete evidence to support this. In the dogfish, *Squalus acanthias*, at least four GnRH forms can be identified in the terminal nerve, including GnRH-II and salmon GnRH-like forms. The potential for additional GnRH migrating cells to be discovered, therefore, remains. A comparison of GnRH neuron origins in mouse and lamprey B shown in Fig. 10.9.

Although the GnRH neurons arise in the primordial olfactory epithelium, evidence suggests that this region was initially derived from the neural ectoderm (Chapter 4). The primordial cells of the primary olfactory neurons originate in the inner layer of the anterolateral part of the neural ridge situated on either side of the anterior part of the neural ridge. These cells also give rise to both the nasal epithelium and neurons of the olfactory bulb. Once the neural tube closes, the primordial olfactory tissue extends to form the nasal epithelium and olfactory bulbs. This is followed by the differentiation into primary and secondary olfactory neurons and terminal neurons. Sometime later, a subpopulation differentiates into GnRH neurons. Some of the preoptic cells that originate in the anterior part of the neural ridge undergo an extracerebral migration to the hypothalamus.

In mammals, the migration of the GnRH-I cells from the nasal placode to the rostral forebrain is a journey involving many cues and signals ensuring that the cells reach their

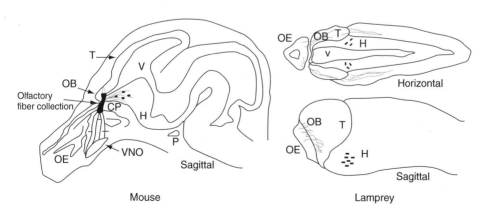

Figure 10.9 *Comparison of GnRH neuron origins in mouse and lamprey. Reprinted from Tobet et al. (1997) by the permission of Elsevier Science (USA).*

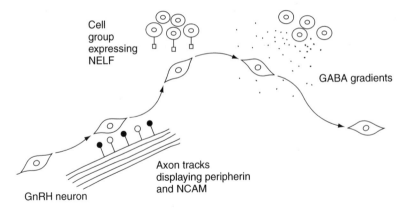

Cell group expressing NELF

GABA gradients

Axon tracks displaying peripherin and NCAM

GnRH neuron

Figure 10.10   *Some of the guidance cues used by the GnRH neurons during the migration from the olfactory placode to the caudal telencephalon.*

final destination (Fig. 10.10). The development of the olfactory system and the GnRH neuroendocrine system is intimately entwined. GnRH-I cells migrate across the nasal region on axons originating from cells in the olfactory pit/vomeronasal organ (Chapter 13). The axon-rich track-like structures act as guidance cues through the expression of the intermediate filament, peripherin, that is characteristic of all olfactory/vomeronasal axons. The association of GnRH-I cells with peripherin-positive nasal axons led to the hypothesis that a cell-adhesion molecule may be involved in the movement of GnRH-1 cells within the nasal region. Olfactory/vomeronasal axons express N-CAM, a cell-adhesion molecule that changes expression during development and cell movement. GnRH-1 cells are associated with N-CAM peripherin-positive olfactory/vomeronasal axons; however, N-CAM involvement in cell movement does not seem to be a pertinent guidance cue. A novel protein, termed 'nasal embryonic LHRH factor' (NELF), has been identified as a guidance cue for the neurophilic migration of GnRH-1 cells through the nasal regions. The expression pattern and extracellular location of NELF suggest a role as an axon outgrowth/migration factor, specifically while the GnRH neurons are migrating across the nasal septum into the developing CNS. Developmentally, many of the regions that express NELF exhibit active neuron migration.

A population of GABAergic neurons terminate at the cribriform plate where GnRH-1 neurons migrate from the nasal region into the forebrain. The expression of this GABAergic population correlates with GnRH-1 neuron migration out of the nasal region. Thus, GABA may act as a migratory stop signal that delays the neuron entrance into the CNS. The reason for this pause may ensure the maturation of GnRH-1 neurons, the establishment or targeting of the migratory pathway to the appropriate brain regions and/or changes in the extracellular milieu composition. In opposition to the effect of GABA, glutamatergic regulation through AMPA receptor activation is also involved. AMPA receptor stimulation enhances the migration of GnRH-1 neurons at the nasal/forebrain junction.

The cues and mechanisms guiding the final establishment of the GnRH system are ambiguous; however, a pathway has been delineated. A peripherin-positive axonal pathway extends from the nasal regions to the ventral surface of the brain, appearing to end at the caudal hypothalamus/median eminence region. The dispersed distribution of the GnRH-1 neurons in the forebrain postnatally corresponds with the peripherin-positive pathway prenatally, therefore, forming a bilateral continuum. The primary targeting of the median eminence by the terminal projections of the neuroendocrine GnRH cells postnatally may involve a number of other chemoattractant factors.

A second form of GnRH ([His^{5}Trp^{7}Tyr^8]-GnRH; GnRH-II; chicken GnRH-II), ubiquitous in vertebrates, has been cloned and characterized in the tree shrew (*Tupaia glis belangeri*), macaque and humans as well as several fish species. Although GnRH-II is the most structurally conserved of all GnRH paralogues, establishing a function for this peptide has proved problematic. Previous studies have suggested it could act as a neuromodulator or neurohormone, regulating reproduction and associated behaviours. Recent studies have implicated GnRH-II as a factor to integrate mating behaviours and energy intake. For example, in female musk shrews, GnRH-II but not GnRH-I can enhance mating behaviour in animals that are food-restricted. Moreover, this effect appears to be mediated by the Type II GnRH receptor.

In the masu salmon, GnRH-II positive cells appear to be present in the nMLF. Studies on the dwarf gourami, on the other hand, suggest that the GnRH-II-expressing cells form a distinct nucleus situated in a more dorsocaudal direction from that of the nMLF. Retrograde tracing of descending neurons established by biocytin injections into the spinal cord labelled cells in the nMLF of which all were negative for GnRH. Most studies, however, report that immunoreactive GnRH cells occur along the medial border of the MLF of various vertebrates (Fig. 10.11).

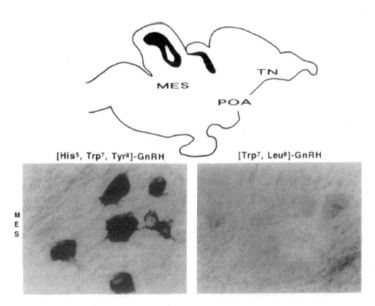

Figure 10.11 *Expression of GnRH-II but not GnRH-III in the midbrain of the cichlid,* Haplochromis burtonii. *Reprinted from White et al. (1994) by the permission of National Academy of Sciences.*

Gonadotrophin-releasing hormone-II has an order of magnitude greater affinity for the Type II receptor than the Type I receptor. It is expressed more widely throughout the brain than the Type I receptor being found preferentially in the amygdala, although expression also occurs in the hippocampus, substantia nigra, subthalamic nuclei and spinal cord. About 69% of LH-expressing cells of the sheep anterior pituitary express the Type II receptor. In monkeys, GnRH-II has been found in supraoptic, paraventricular arcuate nucleusuate and pituitary stalk regions suggesting a potential role in the regulation of the pituitary gonadotrophins. In rams, GnRH-II releases a greater FSH to LH ratio than GnRH-I. Thus GnRH-II may act in part as an FSH-releasing factor. Such a function in mammals is consistent with observations that GnRH-II is the predominant GnRH that circulates peripherally to regulate gonadotrophins in shark species.

Unlike the GnRH-1 system, the GnRH neurons appear to arise locally around the third ventricle during embryonic development. From there, they undergo a short migration to the regions around the nMLF. In the sea bass, the GnRH-II precursor is present in the synencephalon, close to the third ventricle by about four days after hatching. GnRH-II neurons increase in number and size between 10 and 30 days after hatching and reach their final position near the medial longitudinal fascicle. The neurons extend fibres to most areas of the brain and particularly to the brainstem but are not found in the pituitary.

Despite the conservation of the GnRH-II structure throughout metazoan and particularly vertebrate phylogeny, its function as a separate and distinct signalling system is being lost in some lineages. In Chapter 5 we discussed the possibility that after an initial gene duplication, ligands and their receptors will undergo rapid changes, before they begin to co-evolve. This appears to be the situation with GnRH-II. The GnRH-II gene appears to have been silenced in mice, whereas in humans, chimpanzees, cattle, sheep and rat, the GnRH-II receptor has been silenced or disrupted. However, a number of other primates such as marmosets, African green monkeys and rhesus monkeys do possess functional GnRH-II receptors, suggesting that the silencing does not occur along phylogenetic lines. It will be interesting to determine how widespread the silencing of the receptor and ligand is, as all species noted so far are highly social species.

Gonadotrophins and their regulation

The gonadotrophins, synthesized and released from the anterior lobe of the pituitary gland, are the peptides responsible for carrying out the systemic and gonadal actions associated with the reproductive cycles.

Gonadotrophin structure and location

In terrestrial vertebrates, the two principle pituitary gonadotrophins are follicle-stimulating hormone (FSH) and luteinizing hormone (LH). In ray-finned fishes, gonadotrophin-I is orthologous to FSH, whereas gonadotrophin-II is orthologous to LH. Although the piscine gonadotrophins have structural similarity to the corresponding tetrapod gonadotrophins, there appear to be significant functional differences among fishes. For a number of species, it is unclear how much gonadotrophin II participates in the regulation of the reproductive cycles. Little is known about the gonadotrophins in the cartilaginous fish, so it is not clear what the ancestral condition was. Although immunoreactive gonadotrophins have been detected in the ventral lobe of the pituitary in elasmobranchs and in the buccal lobe of holocephalans, attempts to extract and purify the hormones or to clone the genes have not been successful. Thus, there is a considerable gap in our knowledge of understanding how evolution of the HPG axis in vertebrates came about.

Luteinizing hormone and FSH are members of the glycoprotein peptide family. This group also includes TSH and the placental chorionic gonadotrophin (CG) (Fig. 10.12). Chorionic gonadotrophin only appears to be present in primates and equine species. Each member of the glycoprotein family is a heterodimer formed by the non-covalent association of α and β subunits, of which each are encoded by separate genes. The α subunit is common to all members of the glycoprotein family, except for certain fish species. The β subunits confer hormone specificity and identity. These peptides are relatively rare among peptide signalling molecules in that they are glycosylated. The glycosylation on both subunits is essential for receptor recognition and activation.

The gonadotroph cells of the pituitary express both gonadotrophins. Some of the secretory granules contain both gonadotrophins, whereas other secretory granules may contain either one gonadotrophin or the other. In mammals, the gonadotrophs are found scattered throughout the pars distalis, although a significant amount are also found in the pars tuberalis. In teleost fishes, the gonadotrophins are generally clustered together in the pars distalis. The cartilaginous fishes show an anatomical separation of the pituitary lobe that contains the gonadotrophins. In elasmobranchs, the gonadotrophins are present in a separate and ventrally located lobe of the pituitary. It does not possess a vascular or neural connection to the rest of the brain. There is a similar situation in holocephalans, where the gonadotrophins are present in the buccal lobe. The buccal lobe is entirely separated from the rest of the pituitary by a layer of cartilage and has no direct vascular connection to the hypothalamus. Coelacanths, a sarcopterygian, appear to have a pituitary lobe similar to that as found in some holocephalans (Chapter 4). In all cases, the gonadotrophins are regulated by GnRH that is secreted into systemic circulation. In these species, the concentration of

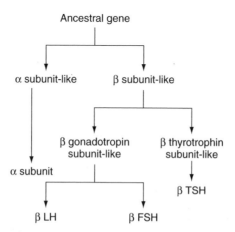

Figure 10.12 *Evolutionary relationship among the glycoprotein hormone genes.*

GnRH in the systemic circulation is similar to the GnRH concentration of the mammalian portal system.

GnRH regulation of gonadotrophins

After GnRH was first discovered and the peptide synthesized, it was noticed that GnRH had a preferential LH-releasing ability. Hence, the peptide was originally named luteinizing hormone-releasing hormone or LHRH. However, this suggested to many of the researchers that there may also be a follicle-stimulating hormone-releasing hormone (FSHRH). This search continued for at least 20 years after the reporting of the first GnRH, although no strong evidence was found for a separate FSHRH that acted alongside GnRH to release the gonadotrophins. Instead, some rather interesting properties of the GnRH neuron were discovered.

Gonadotrophin-releasing hormone is released into the portal system in a pulsatile manner. Low frequency pulses favour the release of FSH, whereas high-frequency pulses promote LH release (Fig. 10.13). There are a number of neuroendocrine factors that act to modulate GnRH pulse frequency to ultimately affect gonadotrophin secretion. The pulsatile nature of GnRH release appears to be an intrinsic property of GnRH neurons. Investigations with the GT1-7 GnRH-secreting cell line indicate that it will release GnRH in a pulsatile manner in the absence of other cell types. Coordination of secretion between GnRH neurons may be achieved by reciprocal axo-dendritic connections. Some modelling studies have suggested that coordination of release could be achieved with as few as 3% of cells

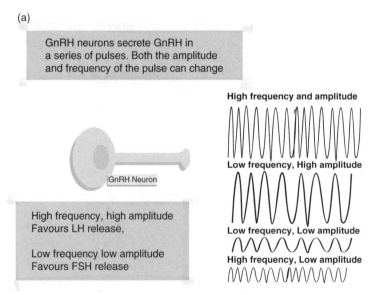

Figure 10.13   (a) Frequency and amplitude modulation of gonadotrophins by GnRH neurons; (b) Neuroendocrine modulation of the pulsatile release of GnRH. Reprinted from Terasawa (1998) with permission from Elsevier Science Ltd; (c) Changes in plasma steroid and gonadotrophin concentrations in humans during developmental states. Reprinted from Huhtaniemi and Warren (1990) with permission from Elsevier Science, Ltd.

(b)

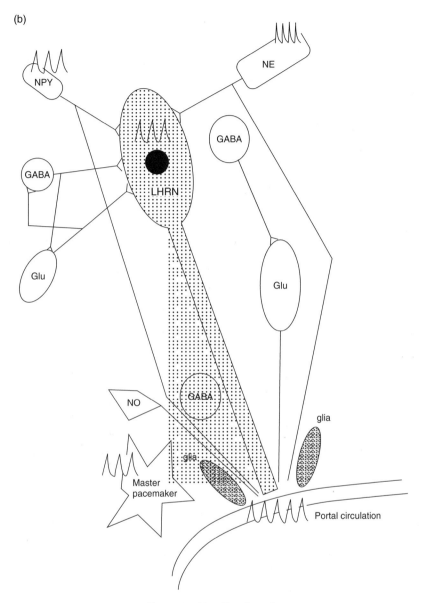

Figure 10.13 *(Continued).*

making connections with one another. GnRH neurosecretory terminals converge at both the median eminence and organum vasculosum of the lateral terminalis (OVLT) (Chapter 4) and it is likely the regulation of coordination occurs in these regions. The pulse characteristics of GnRH are modified considerably by a number of other factors, particularly the gonadal steroids. However, a number of other neurohormones including NPY, norepinephrine,

(c)

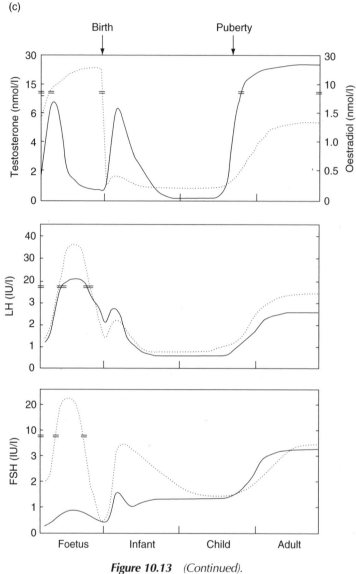

Figure 10.13   *(Continued).*

GABA, glutamate and nitric oxide have all been implicated in the regulation of GnRH pulsatility.

In rats, GnRH can increase the α subunit, LH β and FSH β subunit mRNA. However, the model for GnRH-mediated gonadotrophin release has been based on a single molecular variant of GnRH. In fishes, two and sometimes three variants of GnRH appear to play a role in gonadotrophin release. Different GnRH variants can trigger alternative signal transduction pathways to regulate gonadotrophin synthesis and secretion. For example, in tilapia, GnRH stimulates the transcription of GTH II β using both PKA- and PKC-mediated pathways. sGnRH increases the steady-state levels of the α-glycoprotein subunit via PKA- and PKC-dependent mechanism. In the African catfish, cfGnRH inhibits and cGnRH II has little effect on alpha subunit and LH β transcripts.

When gonadotrophin release is modulated by more that one form of GnRH, then the expression and release of the GnRH isoform that is used may be regulated in a seasonal manner, or by the stage in the reproductive cycle. In the frog, *Rana esculenta*, there are two molecular forms of GnRH: mGnRH and GnRH-II. The annual reproduction period in this species is characterized by long periods of GnRH accumulation followed by long periods of GnRH release. GnRH-II immunoreactivity in the medial septum is high but low in the rostral region of the anterior POA. On the other hand, mGnRH is reversed in these regions. Amphibians generally show a similar pattern in the relative expression of GnRH expression.

GnRH regulation and onset of puberty

During reproductive maturation (puberty), the GnRH neurons typically are activated from a quiescent state to initiate the onset of the reproductive cycles. In mammals, GnRH neurons are active during the latter stages of foetal development. They are turned on near parturition, activating the testes to produce the perinatal concentrations of testosterone required for the masculinization of the brain. In females, the GnRH neurons remain much more quiet than in males during foetal stage, infancy and childhood. After birth, the GnRH neurons become inhibited by neural factors and remain more or less quiescent until puberty when they lose the inhibition and become active again. During the quiescent phase, GnRH suppression appears to be achieved in part by a direct inhibitory action of both NPYergic and GABAergic neurons on the GnRH neuron. In addition, NPY may also inhibit the stimulatory actions of glutamatergic interneurons on the GnRH neurons. Puberty becomes initiated by the removal of these inhibitory mechanisms by both neural and endocrine factors. Increasing plasma leptin concentrations act to inhibit the direct NPY inhibition on the GnRH neuron and the indirect action via the glutamate-secreting interneurons. Additional neural factors appear to be responsible for inhibiting the GABAergic neurons and stimulating the glutamatergic interneurons. There is also evidence to suggest that TNFα from astrocytes plays a facilitatory role in the activation of GnRH neurons (Fig. 10.14).

The African catfish has been particularly well studied in regards to the initiation of reproductive maturity. In this species the developing gonad (anlage) differentiates into the testes at about six weeks of age. They contain spermatogonia stem cells and spermatogonium. By about 12 weeks, spermatocytes are detected indicating the beginning of meiosis. Spermatids are presented by 16 weeks and spermatozoa follow by 22–24 weeks of age. High levels of testicular androgens are present during the initial differentiation stage followed by a gradual decline through stages marked by spermatocytes and spermatid differentiation then a rapid decrease during the final stage of spermatozoa differentiation. In the earliest stages, the Leydig cells are arranged in clusters in the interstitial regions but eventually become dispersed during testes development.

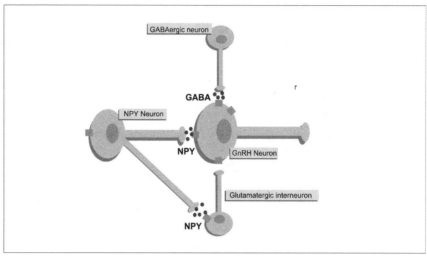

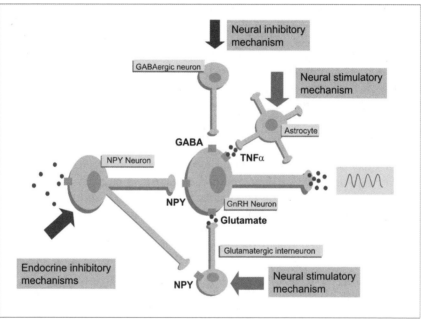

Figure 10.14   *A model for the regulation of the GnRH neuron before and during puberty. Top panel: the GnRH neuron is quiescent during the prepubescent period then becomes activated (lower panel) to initiate reproductive maturity.*

In the immature African catfish testes, the Leydig cells synthesize high local concentrations of mainly 11-β-hydroxyandrostenedione (OHA) (Fig. 10.15). In these species OHA is subsequently converted to 11-ketotestosterone in the liver. As the animal grows and matures, the testes grow disproportionately to the animal's body mass. This leads to an increase in OHA and 11-ketotestosterone concentrations as more Leydig cells become active. The increasing steroids lead to the activation of GnRH and the gonadotrophs

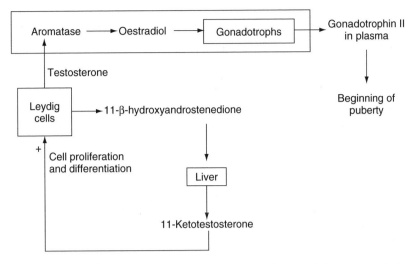

Figure 10.15 *Basic endocrine and neuroendocrine mechanism regulating the onset of puberty in a male African catfish.*

subsequently initiating testicular development. 11-Ketotestosterone appears to act primarily at the testicular level where it stimulates cell proliferation and differentiation. Testosterone, on the other hand, is aromatized to oestradiol in the pituitary where it accelerates the maturation of the gonadotrophins.

In this species, the initiation of puberty is associated with an increase in the expression of the gonadotrophin-II gene and protein as well as the number of immunoreactive gonadotrophin cells in the pituitary. There is a subsequent increase of gonadotrophin-II into the blood. This increase appears to be due to the increase of oestradiol produced in the pituitary by aromatization from circulating testosterone. The circulating sex steroids may act to stimulate the activity and development of the hypothalamic GnRH neurons. At the initial stages of puberty, only gonadotrophin-II is produced and secreted into the blood stream. During puberty, there is a continued activation and recruitment of gonado-trophs as the GnRH neurons become activated.

Neuroendocrine regulation of the HPG axis

Numerous neuroendocrine factors regulate the HPG axis at all levels of organization. In fact, it is likely that virtually all signalling systems in the brain affect the regulation of reproduction at some point or another.

Prolactin

Prolactin exerts a marked effect on the gonads, perhaps by modulating the effects of gonadotrophins (Fig. 10.16). In the rat ovary, prolactin promotes the formation and maintenance of functional corpora lutea acting in conjunction with the gonadotrophins.

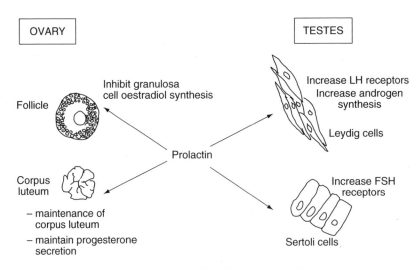

Figure 10.16   *Actions of prolactin on gonadal tissue.*

Progesterone production by the ovaries is obligatory for implantation and fertilization of the ovum, for the maintenance of pregnancy and the inhibition of ovulation. Thus, regulation of prolactin production by the corpus luteum is necessary. Prolactin acts in a luteotropic manner by stimulating progesterone production in luteal cells. Because the maintenance of production of ovarian progesterone involves a luteotropic complex rather than a single gonadotrophin, prolactin acts in conjunction with LH, and probably other factors. Prolactin can inhibit oestrogen production and induce α-macroglobulin via activation of STAT 5 in rat ovarian granulosa cells. As a factor regulating the formation and destruction of the corpus luteum, prolactin plays a major role in modulating the physiological states of oestrus, pregnancy and lactation.

Prolactin possibly acts during ovulation on the competence and maturation of oocytes and also increases the development of organized embryos. It acts also to directly inhibit decomposition and degeneration of surface epithelial cells and the disruption of connective tissue at the apex of the follicle wall. In the uterus, prolactin increases the level of progesterone receptors so enhancing the latter hormone's actions and increases uteroglobin production.

In the rat testis, prolactin modulates Leydig cell function by potentiation of LH-stimulated responses. This is done partly through control of LH receptor expression. Prolactin apparently stimulates steroidogenesis by maintaining or inducing LH receptors in Leydig cells and/or by influencing the activity of specific enzymes involved in androgen biosynthesis. It has been proposed that under natural conditions the high concentrations of prolactin induced by long days in summer has a 'priming' role in the testes and permits the rapid reactivation of testicular function in response to the increase of gonadotrophins in the autumn .

Prolactin has also thought to be involved in sperm capacitation. In Sertoli cells, prolactin increases the number of FSH receptors. Prolactin maintains the mobility and attachment of spermatozoa to the oocyte and reduces the time required to achieve capacitation. The localization of prolactin receptors in rodents occurs in the Leydig cells and interstitial tissues, and is expressed in germ cells in the seminiferous tubules. Prolactin stimulates testicular growth and testosterone secretion in hypogonadal states induced by photoperiod in the Syrian hamster.

The long form of the prolactin receptor is expressed preferentially in the testis, epididymis, prostate, seminal vesicle and mammary glands from lactating animals. Equivalent expression of both forms of the receptor was observed in the ovary, uterus, and the mammary gland of pregnant animals. The high circulating levels of progesterone that occur during pregnancy are probably responsible for limiting the numbers of receptors in the mammary gland.

Galanin

Galanin appears to have an important role in regulating reproductive function (Fig. 10.17). Although several studies showed galanin may have the inhibitory effect on sexual behaviour, its main effect on the GnRH system appears to be stimulatory. The GnRH neurons express galanin mRNA and immunoreactivity or receive galanin input in various species, including rat and mouse. The level of galanin expression is sexually dimorphic in these species with more galanin-immunoreactive GnRH cells in intact, mature female than male animals. Furthermore, studies indicated that the galanin may regulate the reproductive function at three levels. First, galanin can stimulate LH secretion and potentiate the GnRH-induced LH secretion from pituitary gonadotrophs in culture, suggesting a

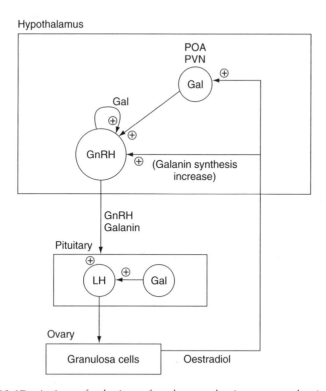

Figure 10.17 *Actions of galanin on female reproductive neuroendocrine circuit.*

stimulatory role for galanin on LH release at the pituitary level. Secondly, exogenous galanin stimulates the release of GnRH into the medium, an effect that can be blocked by galanin antagonist galantide, suggesting that galanin may act at GnRH terminals to further enhance the release of GnRH. Finally, galanin appears to have direct synaptic input to activated GnRH cells in normal female mice, suggesting a somatic level of galanin action on GnRH neuron. The action of galanin on GnRH release may be regulated by the gonadal hormone, oestrogen. 17β-Oestradiol induced a two- to three-fold increase in galanin mRNA in both the paraventricular and medial preoptic area. Studies across oestrus cycle and following various hormone manipulations also found that oestrogen increases the expression of galanin in GnRH neurons.

Pregnancy, parturition and lactation

Lactotrophs are the last anterior pituitary cells to differentiate and are preceded by growth hormone and dual growth hormone/prolactin producing cells. A functional POU, homeo-domain transcription factor Pit-1, is required for development of somatotrophs, lactotrophs and thyrotrophs and its inactivation results in virtual absence of these cell types. Lactotrophs comprise 20–50% of total anterior pituitary cells. Morphologically they are made up of two types: densely granulated cells that function as storage or resting cells, and sparsely granulated secretory cells that are abundant in prolactinaemias. Lactotrophs are located in central or lateral areas of the pituitary and have different responsiveness to releasing and inhibiting factors, indicating regional differences in exposure to hypothalamic or posterior pituitary factors.

In mammals, prolactin is primarily responsible for the development of the mammary gland and lactogenesis (Fig. 10.18). Prolactin induces growth and differentiation of the ductal and lobuloalveolar epithelium, acting in conjunction with oestrogen, progesterone, growth hormone and several growth factors during pregnancy. The terminal stage of mammary gland development, lobuloalveolar growth, is directly regulated by prolactin. Prolactin also maintains lactation during the postpartum period and is the hormone primarily responsible for the synthesis of milk proteins, lactose and lipids, and in association with insulin and glucocorticoids it stimulates milk protein gene expression at both transcriptional and post-transcriptional levels. Circulating prolactin levels are elevated during pregnancy, but lactation is not initiated until after delivery, owing to the effects of high levels of oestrogen and progesterone on lactogenesis. Prolactin levels show a further increase immediately postpartum, followed by episodic increases during each period of suckling. The prolactin secretory pool is made up mainly of the bioactive form of the hormone (MW 23 000 kD) and its release maintains lactogenesis and ensures an adequate milk supply for the next feed. In the mouse mammary gland, the long form of the prolactin receptor mRNA changes cyclically, being highest at oestrus and lowest at dioestrus. As expected the levels of mammary gland prolactin receptor mRNA are low in virgin and pregnant rats but significantly increase on day 21 of pregnancy. This increase continues throughout lactation.

Hypothalamic regulation of prolactin in the pituitary is primary under inhibitory control. In mammals, the main inhibiting factor is dopamine that is produced in the basal

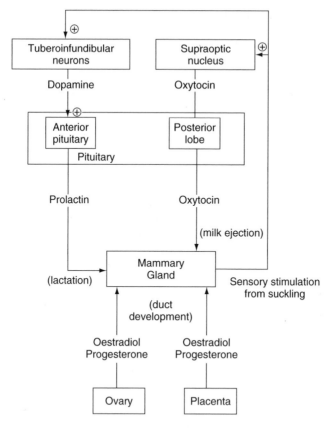

Figure 10.18   *Neuroendocrine regulation of mammary gland function.*

hypothalamic tubero-infundibular group of dopaminergic neurons with terminals in the median eminence. Birds do not contain a tubero-infundibular group of dopaminergic neurons although dopamine-positive neurons are present in the median eminence. Dopamine, norepinephrine and 5-HT have no direct effects on prolactin secretion from the avian pituitary gland whereas TRH, arginine vasotocin and VIP stimulate prolactin release from avian pituitary glands *in vitro*. VIP releases prolactin from the avian pituitary but has no effect on GH or LH release. VIP content in the basal hypothalamus is associated with prolactin secretion in laying and incubating hens. Oestrogen, but not testosterone or progesterone, enhances the stimulatory effect of VIP on prolactin release. In turkeys, intracerebroventricular injection of 5-HT or low concentrations of dopamine can stimulate prolactin secretion from the pituitary. However, dopamine can inhibit the stimulatory effect of VIP in the pituitary gland. This effect appears to be mediated by D2 dopamine receptors.

Galanin is principally synthesized, stored and released by a subpopulation of prolactin producing cells, the lactotrophs, in the rodent pituitary and is extremely sensitive to the oestrogen status of the animal. In contrast to the apparently hypothalamic site of galanin action on GH, galanin acts directly on the pituitary lactotrophs, mediating cell proliferation and prolactin expression as a autocrine/paracrine regulator. Oestrogen upregulates galanin gene expression by increasing both the number of galanin-positive cells and the levels of gene expression. Prolactin secretion from galanin-positive lactotrophs is significantly greater than that from galanin-negative lactotrophs. Moreover, treatment with galanin antiserum significantly attenuates prolactin secretion from galanin-positive cells, and treatment with galanin significantly enhances prolactin secretion from galanin-negative lactotrophs. Also, overexpression of galanin in the anterior pituitary stimulates prolactin synthesis and secretion, but prolactin expression is reduced in the mice carrying a loss-of-function mutation of the endogenous galanin gene.

Galanin may act as a growth factor to trigger and promote the proliferation of lactotrophs in the presence of oestrogen. For example, galanin acts as a mitogen to a lactotroph cell line acting through GALR1 receptor. Targeted overexpression of galanin to the lactotrophs and somatotrophs of transgenic mice induces pituitary hyperplasia and adenoma formation. But the proliferative response of the lactotroph to high doses of oestrogen is almost completely abrogated in the mice carrying a loss-of-function mutation of the endogenous galanin gene. These data support the notion that the galanin may serve a role in regulating the proliferation of lactotrophs.

Seasonal reproduction

Specific environmental cues, such as light, temperature and habitat, underline the phenomenon of seasonal breeding. The use of daylight to regulate reproduction seasonally cues animals in environments where climatic and dietary conditions vary. Regardless of how often an animal reproduces in a year, its reproductive cycle is driven by an endogenous circannual rhythm, which is synchronized by photoperiod (Chapter 8). Biological rhythms of various periodicities occur in all eukaryote organisms. Annual changes in daylength are known to control the timing of breeding of animals living in higher latitudes and temperate regions. This is to ensure that their offspring are born at the most optimum time of year for survival when climate and food availability are at their most favourable levels. For example, deer are seasonal breeders who mate in the autumn when food availability is declining and the weather conditions are deteriorating; thus, giving birth in spring, which is the optimal time of year. Syrian hamsters have a relatively restricted geographic range, and in their natural habitat breed in the spring and autumn and hibernate during the winter. Under laboratory conditions hamsters can remain sexually active throughout the year as long as they are exposed to photoperiods of over 12.5 hours of light a day. However, transferring animals from long photoperiods to short photoperiods induces reproductive quiescence, resulting in decreased levels of plasma concentrations of gonadotrophins and prolactin and gonadal atrophy. The amplitude to these changes is considerable, with reduction of testicular weight by about 80%, cessation of spermatogenesis, reduction in testosterone and loss of libido.

Melatonin and seasonality

Growing evidence shows that melatonin has an effect on the release of GnRH. For example, pinealectomies in goldfish abolishes the daily cycle of plasma gonadotrophin fluctuations.

The basal secretion of GnRH from the hypothalamus decreased during daylight house when melatonin levels are low and increased during the dark period when melatonin levels are highest. Similar rhythmic results were found in the Atlantic croaker. Melatonin influences plasma gonadotrophin-II levels that varied diurnally in the teleosts.

In humans, melatonin can regulate GnRH and GnRH receptor gene expression in human granulosa luteal cells mediated by a MAPK signal transduction mechanism. For example, a 17-year-old girl possessing an absence of secondary sexual characteristics was found to have a cystic lesion in her pineal gland that produced decreased levels of melatonin. As a result she was unable to respond to the external or internal cues to develop properly and did not go through puberty. Young ewes given timed oral administrations of melatonin had increased concentrations of LH in response to GnRH pulses. Melatonin may modify the pituitary responsiveness to GnRH pulses, which may be a possible mechanism by which melatonin influences the onset of puberty in sheep.

Prolactin and seasonality

Most seasonally reproductive breeding mammals show a pattern of prolactin secretion which peaks on long days and falls on short days. Photoperiod influences the secretion of prolactin via the effects of melatonin secretion from the pineal. Although all seasonal breeds show a seasonal change in prolactin secretion, it is unclear whether continuously breeding species do so also, under photoperiodic control. Depending on the species this sensitivity to changes in daylength may lead to a biological endpoint such as seasonal reproduction or pelage growth. In species with obligate seasonal embryonic diapause, the seasonal increase in prolactin acts as a luteotrophin (e.g. mink) or luteostatin (e.g. wallabies). In the Syrian hamster, increases in prolactin in spring may augment the effect of increasing gonadotrophin concentrations in facilitating gonadal growth. Seasonal changes in pelage growth vary with prolactin secretion. The onset of spring and autumn months correlated with increases and decreases in circulating prolactin respectively. On long summer days, prolactin is high, but on short winter days prolactin is low. This is seen in seasonally breeding eutherian species such as Red deer, wallaby and golden hamster. The exception to this generalization is the macropodial marsupials, for example, the Tammar and Bennett's wallabies, in which seasonality is due to an obligatory period of ovarian quiescence resulting in embryonic diapause.

Since the pattern of reproduction varies between species – some breeding in summer when prolactin levels are high, others in winter when they are low – no clear role has been identified for prolactin in seasonal reproduction. There is no single trophic or inhibitory effect of prolactin on the hypothalamus–pituitary–gonadal axis for seasonal species; thus, the seasonal increase in prolactin levels could be a cue for summer.

Reproduction and stress

The modulation of reproductive activity by stress is not a new concept. In fact, the onset of severe stress in mammals and humans has been thought to induce a temporal decrease in reproductive physiology since Selye proposed in 1939 that an activated stress axis was

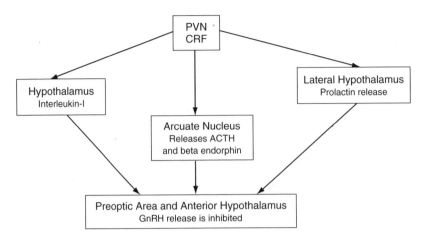

Figure 10.19 *Inhibitory mechanisms on GnRH release associated with stress.*

capable of inhibiting the reproductive axis (Chapter 9). This classical interpretation maintains that the excessive increase of adrenal activity associated with hypothalamic CRF upregulation augments cortisol precursor output and subsequently elevates levels of circulating glucocorticoids. The resulting suppression of LH and GnRH secretion from the pituitary and hypothalamus, respectively, interferes with normal gonadal functions, disrupting menstrual cycles and manifesting as the erratic or abnormal sex drives.

But, although corticosteroid upregulation during stress clearly inhibits GnRH production and subsequently reduces the release of LH at the level of the pituitary, adrenalectomized rats also exhibit decreased plasma LH levels during stressful situations. Furthermore, the failure of peripherally administered CRF to disrupt LH and GnRH release, whereas injections of CRF into the brain, or median eminence (ME), inhibits pituitary LH secretion, also implies that circumventricular organs do not participate in the regulation of certain systemic signals. Moreover, in sheep, ICV injection of CRF can increase the pulse amplitude of plasma LH and decrease the median eminence stores of GnRH. Considering then that the secretion of LH from the pituitary is only inhibited when CRF is released centrally, and that systemic administration of CRF does not affect pituitary LH release, CRF-associated peptides may act directly on GnRH-expressing neurons within the brain (Fig. 10.19).

Sex differences in stress and reproduction

In women, normal menses are required for normal growth, fat deposition, fertility, ageing and general well-being. Physiologically, the regulation of reproductive cycles occurs with the pulsatile release of GnRH from the hypothalamus. Changes in the amplitude or frequency of the GnRH pulse induce variations in pituitary LH or FSH release into the systemic circulation thereby affecting ovarian function. The subsequent steroidal release into circulation modulates both the actions of the HPA axis as well as GnRH-pituitary function. Disruption of normal cycles occurs during periods of increased HPA axis activity associated with, for example, depression, anorexia nervosa and intense exercise. CRF, ACTH and cortisol have all been implicated as causative factors. The cessation of menstrual cycles in women is associated with a decrease in circulating sex steroids, notably oestradiol and progesterone. Sudden changes in the plasma concentration of these steroids are related to an exacerbation of mood disorders and depression, complicating the situation for a patient already at risk for major depression. Numerous studies indicate that the increased stress-response in women appears to be mediated, in part, by the enhanced activation of the HPA axis by oestrogens. In men, an attenuation of the HPA axis may be due to a suppressive effect by androgens. The human oestrogen receptor protein binds to an oestrogenic response element-like sequence in the 5′ flanking region of the human CRF gene, suggesting that there is a direct effect of oestrogens on HPA activation. Studies of gender differences of HPA activity in sleep regulation have also indicated greater CRF neuronal activity in women compared to men. Animal model studies support these observations. In female rats, stress-induced ovarian CRF is present in its highest concentrations, and the CRF-R1 receptor transcription activity in the paraventricular nucleus peaks during pro-oestrous when plasma oestrogens are elevated.

CRF-mediated actions on the reproductive axis

There have been numerous studies over the last 20 years that indicated a direct effect of CRF on GnRH systems. CRF can act directly on GnRH neurons in the arcuate nucleus-ventromedial area of the female rat hypothalamus to inhibit GnRH release. Intracerebroventricular injection of CRF decreased immunoreactive GnRH release into the hypophysial-portal circulation and lowered plasma LH levels in intact female rats on the afternoon of pro-oestrous and in ovariectomized (OVX) rats. In contrast, peripheral injections of CRF have no effect on plasma LH levels in OVX female rats. CRF can induce a dose-related suppression of GnRH release from the rat hypothalamus, *in vitro*, that can be blocked by treatment with the CRF receptor antagonist α-helical CRF_{9-41}. Injection of CRF bilaterally into the hypothalamic medial preoptic area (mPOA) suppresses GnRH release into the median eminence during the pro-oestrous afternoon in female rats whereas administration of CRF into the paraventricular or arcuate nuclei does not. Numerous other studies have shown a significant suppression of LH activity as CRF is increased and have demonstrated a reinstatement of the LH pulse after the subsequent administration of CRF antagonists.

Several sites within the brain may contribute CRF-ergic projections to GnRH-secreting neurons of the forebrain. It was initially thought that because the majority of CRF perikarya of the paraventricular nucleus impinge upon the median eminence and project to the portal hypophyseal vasculature, it would be these neurons which could explain the *in vitro* suppression of GnRH by direct CRF action on neurosecretory terminals within the median eminence. However, complete destruction of the paraventricular nucleus has failed to prevent the inhibition of LH secretion during stress, and moreover, upregulation of CRF in the paraventricular nucleus does not lead to inhibition of LH in the rhesus monkey.

The mPOA of the rat contains the highest density of GnRH neurons making this the most likely site of action of CRF to influence the endogenous activity of GnRH neurons and the hypothalamus–pituitary–gonadal (HPG) axis. The central nucleus of amygdala (CeA), the bed nucleus of the stria terminalis (BNST) and the mPOA itself contain a large number of CRF-expressing cells, which may project to the mPOA. Thus, the CRF-GnRH synapses previously identified in mammals and birds could represent either local connections from CRF- and GnRH-expressing cells located within the mPOA, or CRF projections from other areas, such as CeA and the BNST. Stimulation of the CeA by stress appears to affect the amygdaloid CRF neurons innervating the lateral BNST, and lateral hypothalamic area and possibly the CRF-expressing cells located in the mPOA. Bilateral lesioning of the mPOA and the CeA induces a reduction in plasma corticosterone and a decrease in CRF in the ME, respectively, suggesting that the CRF perikarya of the mPOA and CeA are an integral part of the stress cascade. Given that the mPOA is capable of signalling other hypothalamic regions in the activation of adrenocortical secretion, it is possible that the CeA modulates GnRH activity during severe stress by activating CRF neurons in the mPOA. Such regulation of GnRH may occur with CRF acting as a neuromodulator to influence the efficiency of synaptic transmission, and/or by it impinging directly upon GnRH neurons within the hypothalamus.

Corticotrophin-releasing factor is part of a larger family of structurally similar and functionally related peptides that includes urotensin-I (urocortin). Although urocortin is synthesized primarily in the midbrain, immunoreactive urocortin fibres impinge near GnRH-secreting cells of the septal nuclei, diagonal band, mPOA and ventromedial nucleus. Urocortin has 10- to 20-fold greater affinity than CRF on the R2 receptor and is generally more potent than CRF both *in vivo* and *in vitro* on the R1 receptor. At present, little is known about the role urocortin plays in the regulation of GnRH. It appears to be co-expressed in the same region of the midbrain as a GnRH variant, GnRH-II. Urotensin-I, an orthologue of urocortin, has a potent stimulatory effect on GnRH transcription, in contrast to CRF, on both mouse and chicken GnRH-luciferase reporter genes.

Although CRF-mediated mechanisms appear to regulate GnRH-based reproductive physiology, establishing the appropriate controlled procedures to provide a definitive mechanism for this relationship has proved problematical. This is particularly evident, given that under certain conditions CRF or stress can either increase, decrease or have no effect on LH release. One principal factor in this is that the numerous populations of CRF-expressing neurons dispersed throughout the brain are, collectively, so diverse in their physiological function thereby capable of simultaneously modulating cardiovascular, metabolic, endocrine and behavioural responsiveness to both internally and externally represented stimuli. This difficulty is compounded by the wide range of substances variously regulating GnRH within the brain, interfering with LH-induced LH-release from the pituitary, and/or reducing the production of sex steroids within the gonads.

Other neuroendocrine mechanisms

A number of other neuroendocrine systems have been shown to attenuate reproductive function at the hypothalamic level (Fig. 10.20). Opioid peptides may inhibit the HPG-axis by a direct receptor-specific mechanism on GnRH neurons. Moreover, opiate receptor antagonists, such as naloxone, can block the inhibition of CRF on GnRH release. Treatment of rat hypothalamic slices, *in vitro*, with α-helical CRF$_{9-41}$, resulted in a significant suppression of the release of α-endorphin and Met-enkephalin and a coincident significant increase in the release of GnRH suggesting a reciprocal relationship. However, β-endorphin is less effective than CRF at inhibiting gonadotrophin release. Administration of opiate receptor antagonists bilaterally into mPOA failed to completely reverse the inhibitory influence of CRF on GnRH neuronal activity. Furthermore, in OVX

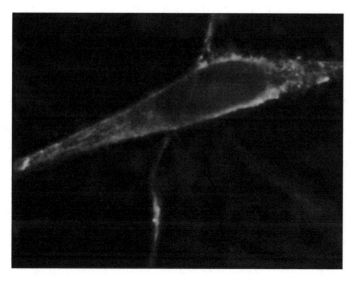

Figure 10.20 *GnRH-expressing neuron showing CRF-receptor Type I immunoreactivity around the periphery.*

oestrogen–progesterone-treated female rats, whereas naloxone pretreatment of the mPOA site prevented the inhibitory effects of β-endorphin, neither the opiate receptor antagonist nor anti-β-endorphin-γ-globulin infused into the mPOA was effective in completely preventing the inhibition of lordosis produced by CRF.

A number of other neurohormonal systems also act to regulate GnRH. For example, norepinephrine can inhibit the HPG axis through a CRF-dependent mechanism. Norepinephrine administered within the paraventricular nucleus suppressed the pulsatile release of LH in female rats via α-adrenergic receptors. Prolactin can also inhibit HPG axis by stimulating CRF secretion possibly via an adrenergic mechanism. Interleukin-I (IL-1) is a major inhibitor of the HPG axis, particularly during periods of inflammation, and may act directly upon GnRH perikarya of the hypothalamus. IL-1 also stimulates CRF neurons under these conditions, although it is not known whether the subpopulation of activated CRF neurons subsequently affects GnRH release. Numerous studies support a synergistic role for vasopressin with CRF, and in some cases appears to take over the function of CRF in different species, in situations of chronic stress, or when CRF itself is not available.

Chapter summary

The development and evolution of sexual reproduction has dominated over non-sexual reproduction in the metazoans because it acts to increase the fitness of the populations. The neuroendocrine model for the regulation of reproduction has been best studied in a variety of vertebrate species. Among invertebrates, insects have been the most studied models where the regulatory mechanisms for moulting and reproduction are intrinsically linked. In vertebrates, gonadotrophin-releasing hormone (GnRH) is the main hypothalamic-releasing factor that regulates the release of the gonadotrophins from the pituitary gland. GnRH is present in multiple forms throughout vertebrates and appears to play a role with reproduction in many invertebrate species as well. The regulation of the gonadotrophins by GnRH is achieved by modulation of the amplitude and frequency of the GnRH pulse frequency. Depending upon the species the different GnRH paralogues may be responsible for gonadotrophin release. The two fundamental gonadotrophins are follicle-stimulating hormone (FSH) or gonadotrophin-I, and luteinizing hormone (LH) or gonadotropin-II. These pituitary hormones act on the gonads to mature the gametes. The actions of gonadotropins on the gonads also regulate the synthesis and release of three principle steroids – oestrogens, androgens and progestins – that act to prepare the organism for reproductive competence. Seasonal regulation of the reproductive system is achieved primarily by melatonin from the pineal gland and prolactin from the lactotrophs of the anterior pituitary gland. Stress-inducing events can suppress the reproductive capabilities of vertebrates, by direct action of CRF on GnRH, the gonadotrophins and by glucocorticoid actions at the hypothalamic, pituitary and, in some cases, at the gonadal level.

11

Behaviour, learning and memory

Introduction

Over the course of the last 10 chapters we have been examining aspects of neuroendocrinology from a homeostatic and an information-flow perspective. But we have focused almost entirely upon physiological mechanisms that occur within an organism in response to a particular stimulus. Behaviour, which involves the physical orientation of an organism in time and space, is also a means of regulating homeostasis and receiving and transmitting information. Behaviour may be described as a series of distinct movements over a temporal and spatial framework, or it may be described relative to the function it serves. Similar or identical behaviours may have one meaning in one situation and a completely different meaning in a different situation. This is frequently the situation in mating behaviour. For example, the vocalization by a male may be perceived by a female as being part of the courtship, but it may be perceived as an aggressive call by a conspecific male. Social events play a significant role at regulating the organismal physiology. Some species may manipulate their social surroundings to promote secretion of the reproductive hormones that lead to the long-term success of a species.

Basic behavioural circuits

In Chapter 3, we raised the possibility that once an organism developed a cell system that had an ion-coupling ability, no matter how rudimentary, then it could facilitate niche and

Neuroendocrinology: An Integrated Approach   David A. Lovejoy
© 2005 John Wiley & Sons, Ltd

habit selection and ultimately adaptation. Among the simplest metazoans showing behaviour might be some sponge larvae whose negative phototaxism allows them to 'swim' away from light in order to settle on the substrate. However, once a nervous system is in place, then the complexity of potential behaviours available to the organisms increases considerably. Comparatively simple triploblastic metazoans such as the platyhelminthes can modify their behaviours in response to repeated stimuli, thus showing evidence of learning.

Learning is fundamental to complex behaviour. The ability to learn from experience modulates any given behaviour in a particular situation (Fig. 11.1). It ensures the survivability of an individual and increases the efficiency of reproductive success. In order to achieve this, if an individual receives some neurological reward for a behaviour, there is greater probability the behaviour will be repeated again. Learning, however, implies memory. In order to modify a particular behaviour to a stimulus, there needs to be a link of that stimulus with a physiological response. The onset of behaviour in an organism is the result of the integration of sensory input with other physiological systems. In the simplest system, the subsequent physiological pathways can give feedback to facilitate or depress the initial sensory input, depending upon the nature of the stimulus (Fig. 11.2).

A stimulus, then, might be classified as noxious when it acts to challenge the homeostatic integrity (Chapter 9) of the organism and subsequently elicits a stress or defensive response. Sudden changes in temperature or salinity might be considered noxious-type stimuli. Alternatively, a stimulus may be beneficial to an organism and have a reward potential, such as food, for example. On the other hand, a given stimulus might be neutral in that there is no overt physiological response. A novel neutral response (e.g. touch) may be initially construed as having an inherent positive or negative value and an appropriate response given. However, repeated exposure to such a stimulus can lead to habituation when eventually no response occurs.

The marine nudibranch (Mollusca), *Aplysia californica*, has been used as a model to understand simple learning circuits (Fig. 11.2). It has about 20 000 neurons in its central nervous system, but possesses a number of reflex behaviours that can be modified over time. Habituation may be considered the simplest form of implicit learning. It is a non-associative type of learning in which the organism learns that the novel stimulus is neutral in nature. Sensitization to a response involves the enhancement of synaptic transmission, whereas habituation involves an attenuation of synaptic transmission. Long-term memory

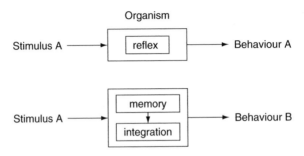

Figure 11.1 *Learning is fundamental to complex behaviour. An organism will modify its behaviour to a stimulus if it can remember previous encounters.*

(a)

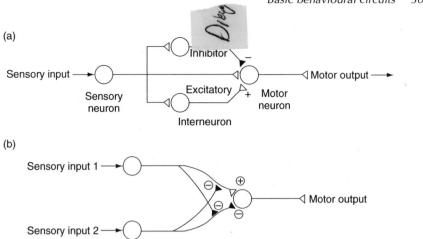

(b)

Figure 11.2 *Simple learning circuits (a) repeated stimulation leads to habituation of response by a facilitation of the inhibitory interneuron; (b) two sensory pathways converge on a single motor output pathway.*

typically involves the synthesis of new proteins, such as cytoskeletal and adhesion proteins (Chapter 2), that are required for synaptic contacts, and the formation of new synaptic contacts (Fig. 11.3). For example, 5-HT neurons in *A. californica* induce a PKA-mediated long-term potentiation of K^+ channels that acts, in part, to sensitize the gill-withdrawal reflex.

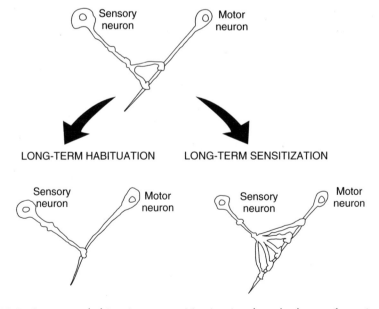

Figure 11.3 *Long-term habituation or sensitization involves the loss or formation of new synapses. Modified after Kandel et al. (1995), Simon & Schuster.*

Memory

If learning is fundamental to more complex behaviours, then memory is fundamental to the learning process. The more complex the ability to store specific memories, then the more complex the range of behavioural responses become. In both invertebrates and vertebrates, long-term memory for an event can be enhanced or attenuated by subsequent events occurring minutes to hours after the initial event. This suggests that the formation of memories occurs slowly over time. This process is called memory consolidation. It has been suggested that there may be a biological significance to delay memory consolidation until the significance of an experience can be evaluated. This would allow highly negative or positive experiences to be retained, so that the organism can anticipate the event the next time it occurs.

Numerous studies have shown that emotional arousal improves memory. In vertebrates and particularly mammals, the cerebral cortex has been implicated as being fundamental in the subjective aspects of emotion. However, the neocortex has relatively few connections with the hypothalamus. Both the amygdala and the substantia innominata (p. 313) have extensive and reciprocal connections in the cerebral cortex. Thus, these structures may represent the main interface between the visceral and autonomic centres of the hypothalamus and brainstem and the cortex (Fig. 11.4).

Motivation: Reward and fear

The onset of a behaviour is facilitated if there is motivation to elicit that behaviour. Whether a behaviour has a positive or negative value must ultimately be encoded in the organism's central nervous system as such. If the organism cannot attach a value to a stimulus, then most stimuli will remain relatively neutral and the animal will be limited in its ability to evolve the behaviour. The encoding of stimuli as possessing positive and negative values increases the motivation for the organism to either indulge or avoid the stimulus. As the central nervous system becomes more complex, the value of the stimulus

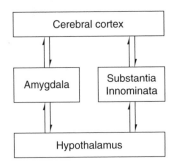

Figure 11.4 *Integrative centres of the brain to link higher order processing of the cerebral cortex with autonomic and visceral processing of the hypothalamus and lower brainstem structures.*

becomes multidimensional as more neurological and physiological systems become involved. The resulting array of behaviours then increases in complexity.

Reward

One of the initial studies on the understanding of reward circuitry was the electro stimulation finding by Olds and Milner in 1954. Subsequent mapping of the brain circuitry showed that stimulation in the region of the medial forebrain bundle, a bundle of axons that travels in a rostral–caudal axis from midbrain to the rostral basal forebrain and the ventral tegmental area of the mesolimbic system, was responsible for drug reinforcement in laboratory animals. In comparison to other neurohormones such as 5-HT, acetylcholine and norepinephrine, the brain has relatively few dopaminergic projections. These are divided more or less equally between the nigrostriatal pathway and the mesocorticolimbic projections that originate in the ventral tegmental area of the midbrain. It is the ventral tegmental neurons that are involved in reward and motivation (p. 310).

Recent observations have indicated that nicotine, like cocaine, activates the mesocorticolimbic dopamine system involved in reinforced behaviour patterns. The relevant reward target of nicotine also corresponds to the mesolimbic dopamine cells. These dopaminergic cells are located in the ventral tegmental area and project to various terminals: amygdala, lateral septum, hippocampus and particularly the nucleus accumbens. The activation of dopaminergic systems along this pathway by nicotine and cocaine, for example, may act as a reinforcement to continue the use (or abuse) of these drugs (Chapter 12). Ventral tegmental neuron projections activate cells in the nucleus accumbens that can subsequently activate the opioid- (i.e. enkephalin) based pathways to simulate the reward and the subjective experience of reward. This pathway is activated for a number of different stimuli that have reward potential including feeding and reproduction, for example.

The neural circuitry underlying reward behaviour is complex with several different neural loci being implicated. This may reflect that reward itself may have several components such as hedonic and incentive values, as well as in terms of probability, timing, quantity and quality and, moreover, may involve one or more sensory modalities of which each may possess subcentres for reward as well as integrative centres. The neural circuitry associated with reward behaviour and experiences involve the amygdala and interconnections with the nucleus accumbens (part of the striatum), the midbrain dopaminergic system including the substantia nigra and ventral tegmental area, the basal forebrain cholinergic system and the prefrontal cortex.

The sex steroids, for example, can have a significant effect on reward-motivated behaviours. Oestradiol activates the dopamine reward system located in the nucleus accumbens. Moreover, the major oestradiol-binding sites in the brain are generally similar through the major actinopterygian and sarcopterygian/tetrapod groups suggesting that much of this system is conserved in vertebrates. Oestradiol and progesterone can induce a number of motivated behaviours. For example, oestradiol-treated rats will bar press or cross an electric grid to gain access to the males. Testosterone has a rewarding effect in males. Testosterone injected into rats at a given location will induce these males to return to that site more frequently than to others.

Fear

If reward acts to potentiate a behaviour associated with a positive stimulus, then fear promotes avoidance of a noxious stimulus. The survival of an individual and ultimately the population is enhanced, if they have developed the ability to adequately react to threat and to anticipate the presence of aversive stimuli and danger. Fear behaviours are also complex and include neural circuits associated with the perception and recognition of danger, the learning and remembering of dangerous experiences and the coordination of defensive behaviours to the environmental threat.

The amygdala has been associated with the recognition of negative and unpleasant emotions such as fear, although it also appears to play a role in processing positive emotional experiences. However, the amygdala does have a central role in fear conditioning. The basolateral complex of the amygdala receives extensive information from the neocortex, thalamus and hippocampus (Fig. 11.5). It is, therefore, in a position to

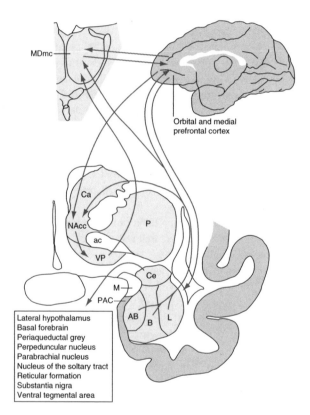

Figure 11.5 *Connections of the basolateral complex and central nucleus of the amygdala to other regions of the brain. AB – accessory basal nucleus; B – basal nucleus; L – lateral nucleus; M – medial nucleus of the amygdale; Ce – central nucleus of the amygdale; VP – ventral pallidum; P – putamen; Ca – caudate; PAC – periamygdaloid complex. NAcc nucleus accumbens. Reprinted from Baxter and Murray (2002) by the permission of Nature Publishing Group.*

receive memory and associative input regarding the nature of a particular stimulus. There are extensive projections to the central nucleus of the amygdala as well. The basolateral amygdala may permanently encode memories for the hedonic value of aversive stimuli. Conditioned approach and avoidance to a specific stimulus appear to involve the central nucleus of the amygdala and may involve the modulation of nigrostriatal dopamine projections.

As an interface between the neocortex and hippocampus, the amygdala plays a central role in the integration of the neuroendocrine regulation of a number of physiological processes through extensive projections throughout the brain. During the perception of a potentially dangerous event where a fear response occurs, the amygdala is poised to initiate a number of physiological responses. For example, it projects to the parabrachial nucleus in the brainstem to increase respiration. The amygdala also projects to the ventral tegmental area, locus coeruleus and dorsal lateral tegmental nucleus to activate dopamine, norepinephrine- and acetylcholine-based pathways to increase arousal and vigilance. Projections to the paraventricular nucleus of the hypothalamus act to stimulate CRF release and activate the HPA axis (p. 262 and Chapter 9). In addition, sympathetic activation occurs via amygdala projections to the lateral hypothalamus, and indirectly through a number of other sites associated with arousal (Fig. 11.6).

The hippocampus may also play a role in fear responses, although its exact nature of the role remains unclear. The hippocampus receives significant visuospatial, olfactory and auditory sensory information. For fear conditioning, the hippocampus may consolidate the memory before it is stored elsewhere, likely the neocortex.

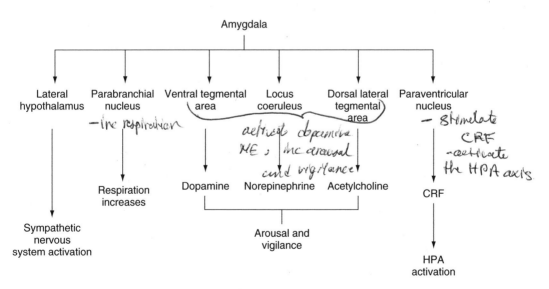

Figure 11.6 *Projections from the amygdala that regulation physiological systems associated with arousal.*

Stress and the modulation of learning and behaviour

Adrenal stress hormones can act to facilitate the storage of a memory if they are given within a particular time interval after the event. Although certain levels tend to facilitate the memory, higher concentrations can attenuate the memory experience. A number of psychiatric disorders such as depression and anxiety-related (mood) disorder have been associated with the dysregulation of the HPA axis.

Neurohormonal pathways

Epinephrine and glucocorticoids can improve the retention of memory. Glucocorticoids can pass readily across the blood–brain barrier, and can gain access to the amygdala. Epinephrine, on the other hand, cannot pass through the blood–brain barrier. One possibility is that peripheral epinephrine activates neurons of the nucleus of the solitary tract that subsequently project to the locus coeruleus (Fig. 11.7). The locus coeruleus contains the principal norepinephrine projections for the forebrain and, in addition, projects directly to parts of the amygdala. During stress, locus coeruleus neurons discharge at a higher rate, and there is an increase in norepinephrine in the amygdala during these periods suggesting that this circuit is responsible for the β-adrenergic-mediated pathway. During emotional arousal, 5-HT, dopamine, norepinephrine and acetylcholine are all released centrally in a much higher concentration than under normal circumstances. This suggests that there is an activation of these circuits during emotionally charged events. However, only β-adrenergic and muscarinic acetylcholine receptor antagonists have been shown to block the emotion-potentiating effects on memory.

The pathway mediating the cholinergic responses is less clear. Cholinergic projections from the basal forebrain to the cerebral cortex have been implicated in cortical plasticity. The substantia innominata is a heterogenous region situated under the anterior commissure in

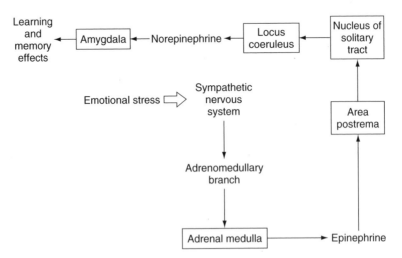

Figure 11.7 *Peripheral activation of the amygdala by the sympathetic nervous system.*

the forebrain, and includes the nucleus basalis. The nucleus basalis is the single major source of cholinergic innervation of the entire cerebral cortex. About 90% of the cholinergic neurons of the nucleus basalis project to widespread regions of the cerebral cortex. Thus, the nucleus basalis may be analogous to the raphe nuclei and locus coeruleus that supply the majority of the serotonergic and noradrenergic innervation respectively to the cortex. Afferents to the substantia innominata/nucleus basalis regions arise mainly from the amygdala, insular and temporal cortex and from the pyriform and entorhinal cortices. The basolateral amygdala is reciprocally connected to the substantial innominata suggesting that it is anatomically situated to receive and modulate acetylcholinergic pathways.

Lesioning of the basolateral amygdala, but not the central nucleus of the amygdala, can block the memory-enhancing effects of adrenal glucocorticoids. A similar situation occurs with the disruption of the stria terminalis, which is a major output pathway of the amygdala. The amygdala, in emotionally arousing situations, when under the influence of peripheral stress hormones facilitates the long-term memory consolidation in other brain regions where memories are actually stored (e.g. neocortex).

The basolateral amygdala facilitates long-term potentiation of the perforant path input to the dentate gyrus. The basolateral amygdala does not project directly to the medial septum and locus coeruleus, which are the main sources of norepinephrine; thus if the basolateral amygdala acts to potentiate the consolidation of memories in hippo-campal regions by adrenergic and acetylcholinergic pathways, then it may be an indirect mechanism.

CRF, glucocorticoids and hippocampal function

The hippocampal function is influenced by glucocorticoids by modulating neuronal excitability. Glucocorticoids can affect hippocampal-dependent behaviour such as spatial memory. This mechanism may also play a role in ageing, as some studies indicate that glucocorticoid levels are correlated with a reduction of hippocampal volume and memory deficits in aged rats. The hippocampus, in turn, has an inhibitory action on the HPA axis. Thus as a function of ageing, or chronic HPA activation, the inhibitory actions on the HPA axis become attenuated leading to enhanced HPA activation and a greater potential for mental dysfunction (Chapter 9).

The organism's response to stress can impair learning and memory in adulthood. This is likely caused by the loss of neurons in the hippocampus. For example, CRF administered to the brains of ten-day-old rats for several months leads to a 17% decrease in hippocampal neurons. The loss was most pronounced in the CA3 area of the hippocampus. Twelve-month-old rats have more neuronal loss than eight-month-old rats. A decline in the performance in the water maze, and less time investigating novel objects occurred in the CRF-treated animals indicating a deficit in some mental functions.

Glucocorticoids have affinity for both the Type I and Type II receptors whereas mineralocorticoids only have affinity for the Type I receptors (Chapters 6 and 9) (Fig. 11.8). In aldosterone-sensitive tissues, such as the kidney, the glucocorticoid-bound Type I receptor is enzymatically digested by 11-hydroxysteroid dehydrogenase, such that the confounding glucocorticoid signal is removed. In many regions of the brain, however, the Type I receptor is not coupled to the enzyme and, therefore, glucocorticoids signals through both receptors. Glucocorticoids have a ten-fold higher affinity for the Type I

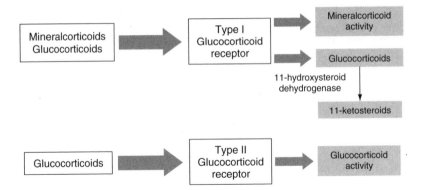

Figure 11.8 *Receptor activation and specificity by glucocorticoids and mineralocorticoids. Glucocorticoids have higher affinity for both receptor subtypes, but in some tissues get degraded when bound to Type I receptors.*

receptor than the Type II receptor and, therefore, will be selectively bound to the Type I receptor in the presence of mineralocorticoids. The Type II receptor is found in most cell types of the body; however, the Type I receptor is only found in brain, the epithelial cells of the kidney, colon and exocrine glands, and reflects the role the mineralocorticoids play in sodium and water readsorption (Chapter 6).

In the brain, the Type I receptor is found only in hippocampus, septum and amygdala. Both Type I and II receptors are, therefore, found in the hippocampus. Low glucocorticoids activate the Type II receptors and high concentrations of the steroid activate both receptors. Low concentrations of glucocorticoids will excite hippocampal neurons whereas high concentrations will decrease neuronal excitation. Activation of the Type I receptor has been linked to long-term potentiation, whereas activation of the Type II receptor appears to favour long-term depression of the neuronal activity. However, the molecular actions of the glucocorticoids are complex and little is known about the interaction of the Type I and Type II receptors when both are activated. Glucocorticoids can induce transcription through the ligand-activated receptor by binding to glucocorticoid responsive elements (GRE) in the promoter. However, they can also repress transcription by binding negative GREs. The activated Type II receptor can also bind other transcriptional factors such as AP-1 or NFκb to suppress their action or can facilitate the action of STAT 5. Some studies also suggest that the Type I and II receptors can heterodimerize to exert a distinct complement of actions.

Hormonal facilitation of behaviour

The onset of particular behaviours is dependent upon the physiological situation the animal finds itself in. Thus, the hormonal feedback mechanisms from virtually all physiological processes will act to modulate the behavioural circuits in the brain.

Sexual behaviours

A number of interacting hormone systems regulate courtship and reproductive behaviours. The onset of many of these behaviours are brought about by sex steroids but can be attenuated by stressful stimuli. There are a number of significant structural differences in the brains of males and females (Chapter 7) (Fig. 11.9). These sexually dimorphic forebrain nuclei are induced during early periods in development and include preoptic nucleus, medial bed nucleus of the stria terminalis, and medial amygdala. The medial preoptic area is important for male sexual behaviour. Pathways from the medial preoptic area including projections to the retrorubal field or ventral lateral periaqueductal field play particularly important roles. Amygdala lesions reduce the motivation to gain access to the females and this also reduces the male's sexual performance in the presence of the females. Disruption of the medial preoptic nucleus, bed nucleus of the stria terminalis and medial amygdala will interfere with male sexual behaviour. Female animals exposed to high levels of testosterone in the womb will show an increase in masculine behaviours. Exposures to testosterone and a decrease in oestradiol can also lead to an increase in body weight.

Sex steroids regulate male and female sexual behaviour and also singing in birds, territorial behaviours and spatial abilities in mammals. Sexual behaviours that are under the control of steroid hormones are not necessarily the same for all species of animals. For example, rodent behaviours are closely linked to steroid levels whereas in primates the behaviour is more independent.

Sexual behaviours can be induced by a number of hormonal events. Lordosis is the stereotyped response that female rodents display as a receptive behaviour in the presence of males. It can be triggered by initially priming the circuits with systemic administration of oestradiol and progesterone then centrally administering oxytocin. The ventromedial hypothalamus appears to play a role in eliciting lordosis. Oestradiol infusion into this region will lower the threshold for lordosis. Oestradiol, in the ventromedial hypothalamus of parthenogenic (female only) species of whiptail lizards (*Cnemidophorus inoratus*), can elicit sexual receptivity via the induction of oxytocin receptors. Also progesterone will induce oxytocin receptors in oestradiol-primed rats. However, a number of other hormones

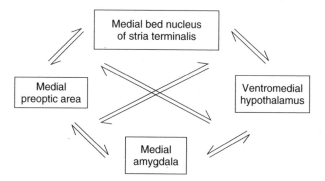

Figure 11.9 *A core group of sexually dimorphic interconnected nuclei that have been implicated in both sexual and aggressive behaviours.*

such as endorphins, GnRH, substance P, CCK and dopamine can also influence sexual behaviour. In rats, male stereotypical sexual behaviour includes pelvic thrusting, mounting, neck gripping and ejaculation. These behaviours are potentiated by testosterone. Testosterone has an organizational effect on the brainstem and spinal cord sites that are essential for penile erection. Testosterone appears to enhance neuronal survival in these sites by the activation of neurotrophic factors. Testosterone can also facilitate substance P expression in the brain. Tyrosine hydroxylase neurons (Chapters 5 and 9) in the medial amygdala are elevated during mating when testosterone is elevated. Both substance P and tyrosine hydroxylase neurons are associated with male sexual behaviours. Androgens are necessary for crowing and strutting behaviour in male quails (*Coturnix japonica*) and probably in most avian species. In the rough skinned newt, testosterone and vasotocin regulate male sexual behaviours. Arginine vasotocin or GnRH injections will stimulate sexual behaviour in both male and female newts. This system can be inhibited by glucocorticoids or the HPA activation. Corticosterone can inhibit androgen secretion and reproductive behaviour. In newts, corticosterone may reverse the neurophysiological effects of arginine vasotocin.

Aggressive behaviours

Many aggressive behaviours are sexually dimorphic and are also linked to the sex steroids. Castration of male rats at birth, which results in reduction in the level of circulating androgens, is associated with a reduction in inter-male aggressive behaviours as the males get older. Restoration of testosterone by injection will potentiate these behaviours. Similarly, injecting male hormone to newborn female rodents cause the females to behave more aggressively. However, castration of a male rodent more than a few days after birth does not cause a reduction in the proclivity for aggressive behaviour suggesting that the critical period for aggressive behaviours occurs during the same critical period as required for normal masculinization (Chapter 7). Thus, likely testosterone acts to lower the threshold for fighting, thereby establishing a biological readiness for normal aggressive behaviour and in facilitating the expression of aggression in the appropriate social settings. Aggression in rodents appears to involve the medial preoptic nucleus and anterior hypothalamus, medial amygdala and medial bed nucleus of the stria terminalis where the latter is particularly important. Testosterone appears to exert its effects on aggression, in part, by modulating vasopressin receptors.

Females will also fight when provoked, indicating that the relevant circuitry is present. In the spotted hyena, *Crocuta crocuta*, the females are particularly aggressive and have been used as a model to understand the role of androgens in aggression. Female hyenas are both larger and more aggressive than males as a result of being exposed to higher concentrations of testosterone and its metabolites in the womb. Females also have external male-like genitalia. Females exhibit rougher play than males. Androstenedione secreted by the ovary is changed to testosterone within the placenta thereby directly affecting the foetus. Testosterone concentrations are about the same in males and females but androstenedione levels remain high in females.

Scent marking

Scent marking is associated with both sexual and territorial behaviours. Central infusion of vasopressin can facilitate scent marking by Syrian hamsters. The bed nucleus of the stria terminalis and medial amygdala has been implicated in this behaviour. Female Syrian hamsters, in contrast to most species, tend to be more dominant and there is greater flank marking than males. Oestradiol, by increasing vasopressin gene expression, facilitates the likelihood of flank-marking behaviour. Vasopressin levels are higher in the medial amygdala, bed nucleus of the stria terminalis and lateral septum in males than in females for many mammal species. The amount of vasopressin expression in the bed nucleus of the stria terminalis is determined by androgens during the critical developmental period.

Social behaviours

Social behaviours include a number of affiliative and pair-bonding behaviours that are essential to establish the cohesiveness of a population. Voles have been utilized as a model for understanding the neuroendocrinology of social behaviours. The effects of oxytocin and vasopressin play a crucial role on the social behaviour of male and female voles. Both female and male voles injected with arginine vasopressin or oxytocin show increased social contact and partner preference compared to control groups. In contrast, males and females injected with an arginine-vasopressin antagonist show little social contact. However, when the antagonist was combined with oxytocin there was an increase in social contact but not partner preference. When an oxytocin antagonist was administered, there was little social contact. Administration of the oxytocin antagonist and arginine vasopressin results in an increase in social contact but no partner preference in both female and male voles. Partner preference was not exhibited with either of the antagonists suggesting that both arginine vasopressin and oxytocin are required for partner preference.

The V1aR vasopressin receptors facilitate affiliation and pair-bond formation through its reinforced actions in the ventral pallidum of the ventral forebrain. The ventral pallidum is associated with reward and conditioned place performance. In a particularly interesting study, transgenic voles with an overexpression of the V1a vasopressin receptor were created by targeting various regions of the brain using a viral vector containing the V1a receptor cDNA. Three groups of male voles between the ages of two to five months were used. In the experimental group the vector was introduced in the ventral pallidum area. One control group had the vector administered into the caudate putamen and the second control group received a non-receptor (*LacZ*) gene in either the ventral pallidum or the caudate putamen. A partner preference test was performed and the males were placed with a non-oestrous female. Normally, under non-oestrous conditions males do not form a partner preference. However, the group where the receptor was overexpressed in the ventral pallidum displayed high levels of affiliative behaviour compared to the control groups. It was also found that high levels of anxiety increased pair bonding in male voles.

Social preferences are sexually dimorphic in prairie voles. The stress of swimming and injections of corticosterone administered intraperitoneally were compared in males and female voles paired with the opposite sex. Male voles under swim stress and/or corticosterone administration facilitated partner preference for the familiar partner. However, females injected with corticosterone show no partner preference. Furthermore, when males and female voles are adrenalectomized, thus eliminating corticosterone, males did not form partner preferences, whereas females did. Some studies suggest the role of oxytocin and vasopressin may help explain some forms of autism. For example, some studies have reported that the plasma concentration of oxytocin in autistic children is half that observed in healthy same-aged subjects.

Vocalization

In many situations it is not clear what the purpose of a vocalization of a given species is. It may be associated with courtship, aggression, or perhaps a number of other aspects. The neuroendocrine regulation of vocalizations has been probably the best studied in avian species. In the zebra finch, testosterone potentiates the recognition of a conspecific song. Songbirds sing during the spring when the high vocal centre (HVC) nucleus enlarges as testosterone concentration becomes elevated (Fig. 11.10). Many neuropeptides are synthesized in the circuitry underlying song production. Testosterone and testosterone conversion to oestradiol induce synaptogenesis in the neuronal circuitry required for song production. Song production may involve vasotocin expression facilitated by testosterone. In male starlings (*Sturnus vulgaris*) testosterone is high in the spring when calling is used in part to attract mates. Many of the brain nuclei that regulate song contain high densities of adrenergic receptors. Testosterone can regulate the density of α_2-adrenergic receptor in the brain. Although many birds sing when the song nuclei are largest and testosterone is highest, starlings sing when testosterone is high or low. During the breeding season of starlings, the song nuclei, including the HVC, robust nucleus of the archistriatum and area X, were largest, testosterone was highest and the density of α_2-adrenergic receptor was lowest. The reverse pattern occurs outside the breeding season.

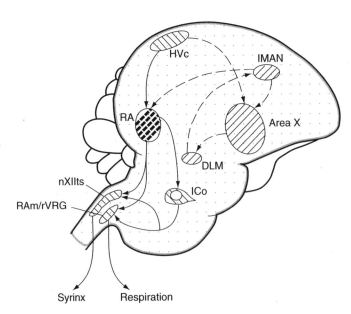

Figure 11.10 *Neural circuitry associated with song recognition in oscine songbirds. Reprinted from Ball et al. (2002) by the permission of Elsevier Science (USA).*

In frogs, arginine vasotocin potentiates the motivation to call. In green tree frogs (*Hyla cinerea*) arginine vasotocin can increase the probability of calling but does not affect either the latency period or how often they were observed calling. Corticosterone can inhibit calling in arginine vasotocin-treated males only at high doses. Lower concentrations do not appear to affect calling behaviour. Corticosterone also reduces androgen levels. Endogenous androgen levels are inversely correlated with the latency to begin calling suggesting a potentiating effect on calling by androgens. Plasma levels of dihydroxytesto-sterone are significantly increased in southern Leopard frog (*Rana sphenocephala*) males when exposed to a prerecorded chorus of conspecifics. Vocalization in the African clawed frog (*Xenopus laevis*) is sexually dimorphic. The elaborate singing of the males is induced by testosterone. Testosterone induces cell proliferation in the larynx in males and prevents the muscle fibre loss that occurs naturally in females. A number of neural sites also regulated by testosterone are associated with the control and regulation of the song. A vocal motor pattern generator in the tegmentum, sensory region of the thalamus, the preoptic region and the striatum are involved.

An analogous situation occurs in fishes that utilize electric fields for perception. The brown ghost (*Apteronotus*), for example, employs electric chirps as a mating call. These calls are regulated in part by the prepacemaker nuclei of the hypothalamus. This region is intensely innervated by CRF-immunoreactive fibers suggesting a role for CRF and chirping behaviour in this species.

Parental behaviour

A number of parental behaviours are similar to affiliative and pair-bonding behaviours (Fig. 11.11). Both oxytocin and vasopressin have been implicated in the regulation of these behaviours. Central infusion of vasopressin will increase parental behaviour in prairie voles. Testosterone concentrations modulate vasopressin receptors in the brain. Eliminating

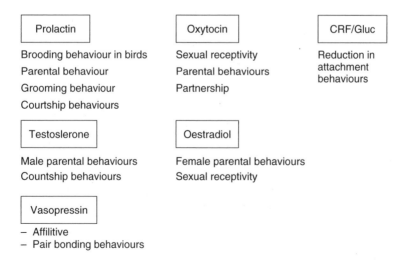

Figure 11.11 *Key hormones associated with courtship, mating and pair-bonding.*

testosterone and lowering central vasopressin concentrations will reduce male parental behaviour in voles. Castration reduces vasopressinergic expression in voles. Oxytocin can also elicit maternal behaviour. High oxytocin leads to maternal attachment whereas low oxytocin can lead to withdrawal. Central but not peripheral infusion of oxytocin will elicit partnership in prairie voles. Oxytocin can also stimulate female aggression. Centrally infused oxytocin will also stimulate parental care in male mice and may also be elevated in the expectant fathers.

In the monogamous prairie vole, *Microtus ochrogaster*, oxytocin receptors are more numerous in several brain regions including the bed nucleus of the stria terminalis compared to the non-monogamous mountain vole, *Microtus montanus*. There is greater male parental care among the monogamous species. The greater amount of time they spend with pups is correlated with a greater the number of oxytocin receptors. High concentrations of corticosterone will reduce attachment behaviours in voles. Oestradiol will increase oxytocin-expressing cells in the bed nucleus of the stria terminalis. This region appears to play a role with social behaviours and formation of partner preference. Oxytocin has been implicated in a number of behaviours associated with sexual arousal, pair bonding and sexual satisfaction. Oxytocin is also involved with parturition and lactation. Oxytocin can either elicit sexual receptivity or parental behaviour depending upon the site of action.

A role for prolactin in parental behaviour in both sexes has been documented in a number of mammalian orders including primates, ungulates, rodents and lagomorphs, and in birds. A large body of physiological evidence suggests that several brain regions may contain prolactin receptors through which prolactin mediates its influence on behaviour and pituitary hormone secretion. Infusions of ovine prolactin into the preoptic region of oestrogen-primed, ovariectomized virgin rats induces maternal behaviour. Injections of rat prolactin in the substantia nigra induces grooming behaviour. The behavioural effects of prolactin are probably due to either the prolactin generated by the anterior pituitary, which is then released into the brain via uptake across the choroid plexus and possibly circumventricular organs, or due to prolactin expressed and released in specific regions within the brain. Prolactin is found in a number of regions of the brain that have been implicated with behaviour including the bed nucleus of the stria terminalis, medial preoptic area, prefrontal cortex, septal nucleus, dorsal hippocampus, midline thalamic nucleus, central grey, dorsal raphe nuclei, locus coeruleus, nucleus of the solitary tract and medial amygdala. Prolactin receptors are present in the preoptic area, ventromedial hypothalamus, bed nucleus of the stria terminalis, suprachiasmatic nucleus and central grey. High concentrations of oestradiol are required for the expression of maternal behaviours. Suckling increases prolactin secretion in both mother and offspring from both the pituitary and hypothalamus. Decrease in attachment between a rat pup and mother will decrease prolactin and increase glucocorticoids in the pup. Prolactin infused into the lateral ventricle of female rats after being primed with oestradiol will induce the rat to respond with maternal behaviour such as pup retrieval and licking. Prolactin administration into the medial preoptic region will also elicit this behaviour whereas lesions to this region will destroy this behaviour.

Prolactin also elicits brooding behaviour in both sexes of birds. In turkeys, prolactin infusions into the brain can increase brooding and nest-making. Nest deprivation decreases prolactin. In doves, prolactin increases food regurgitation to neonates. In ring

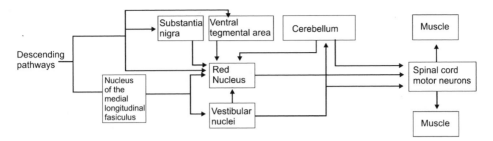

Figure 11.12   *Pathways associated with spinal cord motor control in fishes.*

doves, prolactin concentrations in males and females increase during the period of enhanced parental care. At the beginning of the rearing period, the female does most of the regurgitation, whereas toward the end of the rearing period the male does more of the regurgitation. Prolactin has also been noted to rise during the critical rearing period in penguins.

Locomotion

A CRF-mediated role on locomotor activity was established shortly after the peptides discovery in 1981, and has received much attention. However, amphibians and fishes may be particularly appropriate models for investigating the mechanisms of CRF on the neural circuitry. CRF can stimulate locomotory behaviours in urodele amphibians where the peptide's actions can be modified by the presence of opioids. Recently, it was found that in the brainstem of the roughskin newt (*Taricha granulosa*) discharges of neurons of the raphe region, associated with walking and swimming behaviours, can be modified by injections of CRF into the lateral ventricle.

The presence of urotensin-I in the nucleus of the medial longitudinal fasciculus (nMLF) suggests that it plays a role in the modulation of spinal cord motor circuits (Fig. 11.12). In rainbow trout (*O. mykiss*), orthodromic driving of spinal motor and interneurons by stimulation of the nMLF induced FOS immunoreactivity throughout the motor column in the spinal cord. Moreover, the startle response in trout activates many of the nMLF neurons. Electrical stimulation of the midbrain in decerebrate carp (*Cyprinus carpio*) produced bilateral or unilateral rhythmic movements of the tail. The lowest threshold currents required to elicit this behaviour occurred in the nMLF, MLF and the red nucleus. The nuclei of the origin of the descending pathways were identified by microinjecting L-glutamic acid where the smallest volume injected to obtain the required behaviour occurred in the nMLF. Thus, taken together, these studies suggest that CRF- or urotensin-I-sensitive or expressing nMLF neurons may project to spinal cord neurons to regulate the activities of individual central pattern generators.

Galanin modulation of neurological circuits

To regulate cognitive processes, Galanin and its receptors are distributed in brain regions, including the basal forebrain, hippocampus and cerebral cortex. The effects of galanin on cognition have been related mainly to inhibitory effects on acetylcholine transmission at the terminal level within the ventral hippocampus and the media septum-diagonal band. Intracerebral administration of galanin can impair learning and memory processes in a variety of tasks whereas the galanin receptor antagonists can block the inhibitory actions of galanin on memory tasks. By using the transgenic mice (GAL-tg) that overexpress galanin, the overexpression of galanin is associated with a reduction in the number of identifiable neurons producing acetylcholine in the horizontal limb of the diagonal band. Behavioural phenotyping indicated that GAL-tg mice displayed normal general health and sensory and motor abilities; however, GAL-tg mice showed selective performance deficits on the Morris spatial navigational task and the social transmission of food preference olfactory memory test. A substantial amount of galanin neurons within the ventral hippocampus most likely coexist with norepinephrine neurons derived from locus coeruleus. The effects of galanin on acetylcholine release, which are due to activation of galanin-receptors, appear to be indirectly mediated possibly via norepinephrine transmission.

Behavioural, neurobiologic and neuropathologic studies of patients with Alzheimer's disease (AD) has suggested that galanin plays a crucial role in the pathology of AD. The cholinergic basal forebrain (CBF) neurons provide the major cholinergic innervation of the cortex and hippocampus and are associated with cognitive function. In AD, CBF neurons undergo extensive degeneration that correlates with the duration of disease and degree of cognitive impairment. The extensive galaninergic fibre network that courses through the basal forebrain in humans hyper-innervates the remaining CBF neurons in AD. Because of the inhibitory action of galanin on the release of acetylcholine in the hippocampus, it was suggested that the overexpression of galanin may down-regulate the function of the remaining CBF neurons, further exacerbating cholinergic dysfunction in AD. On the other hand, galanin can evoke an increase in excitability in cholinergic neurons from the rat basal forebrain nucleus diagonal band of Broca. Thus, galanin may play a compensatory role by augmenting the release of acetylcholine from remaining CBF neurons, and thus, may serve to delay the progression of AD pathology linked to a reduction in central cholinergic tone.

An integrated approach to behavioural modulation

It may be evident to many readers that learning is not an isolated mechanism. The memory and encoding of emotions and stimulus–response events are channelled through a common set of neurological structures that also receive input from neuroendocrine factors associated with stress, reproduction, diuresis and feeding. The level of integration and the strength of signal between environmental stimuli and physiological responses of the milieu interieur dictates how the memory will be encoded and how the organism will behave in a similar situation the next time a similar stimulus is perceived.

Because reproductive, avoidance and aggressive behaviours possess a number of similar features in vertebrates, we may postulate then that the neurological basis of these behaviours are intrinsically linked at some part in the brain. For example, head-bobbing behaviour in anoles can signify aggression between males or courtship between males and females. Immobility is one of the characteristics of both receptive behaviour and fear. Central administration of CRF-like peptides can induce a period of immobility followed by an attenuation of exploratory behaviour. However, electrical stimulation of the midbrain central grey will also facilitate lordosis and lesions in the central grey will disrupt it. GnRH infusions into the central grey will potentiate lordosis behaviour, whereas immunoneutralization will inhibit the response. Infusions of the GABA receptor antagonist, bicuculline, or antisense oligonucleotides to GABA-synthesizing enzymes into the central grey reversibly reduce typical female sexual behaviours such as proceptivity and lordosis in the rat. In the central grey, anxiolytic drugs such as diazepam can not only facilitate lordosis, but also reduce the fear response in rats suggesting that both mechanisms are linked. Indeed, a fear response must be inhibited before sexual receptivity can occur.

An example of the interaction of such circuits may be associated with the urotensin-I/urocortin and GnRH-II in the midbrain. The nuclei in which they are found (nMLF or EW) may, therefore, regulate motor behaviours associated with reproductive activity and stress. Classically, studies suggest that cells of the central grey synapse onto neurons within the reticular formation of the medulla, which subsequently send their axons into the spinal cord to control the motor neurons. However, the role of the nMLF and EW nuclei in the regulation of these behaviours has not been investigated. For example, the nMLF extends fibres to all levels of the spinal cord. The presence of urotensin-I in the nMLF suggests that it plays a role in the modulation of spinal cord motor circuits. In rainbow trout, orthodromic driving of spinal motor neurons and interneurons by stimulation of the nMLF induced FOS immunoreactivity throughout the motor column in the spinal cord. Moreover, the startle response in trout activates many of the nMLF neurons. Electrical stimulation of the midbrain in decerebrate carp produces bilateral or unilateral rhythmic movements of the tail where the lowest threshold currents required to elicit this behaviour occurred in the nMLF.

Neurodegeneration and trauma

The integrity of the nervous system is ultimately responsible for the formation of the synaptic circuits required to carry out complex behaviours. A number of hormonal systems have an indirect effect on learning and behaviour by either protecting neuronal function or triggering neuronal degeneration. As we have discussed previously, often this neuroprotective or neurodegenerative effect is dependent upon the concentration of the chemical factor. These hormones can act to modulate the development of the nervous system in embryonic and juvenile animals, or can affect their function in adult animals.

We have discussed the role of galanin in reward behaviour; however, many studies support an important role of galanin in seizure activity. Galanin suppresses hippocampal excitability by post- and pre-synaptic actions. It hyperpolarizes hippocampal neurons, inhibits excitatory glutamate neurotransmission, and when applied intracerebroventricularly it suppresses or blocks kindling-, kainate-, bicuculline- and pentylenetetrazole-induced seizures. The latency of the first spike-wave discharge during the recording of electroencephalogram (EEG) is significantly increased and the duration of the generalized seizures is significantly decreased after galanin administration whereas these effects can be attenuated by galanin receptor antagonists. Furthermore, in a model of self-sustaining status epilepticus

(SSSE), when galanin was injected into the hilus of the dentate gyrus ten minutes after the end of perforant path stimulation, the seizure was suppressed more profoundly and made irreversible by galanin than by other peptides. It was also found that during SSSE the galanin-immunoreactive fibres in the hippocampus were depleted; however, late in the course of SSSE, galanin-immunoreactive interneurons appeared in the dentate hilus. This depletion of galanin might be expected to have a proconvulsant effect, and appears to result from excessive stimulation by seizures. Recently, studies reported that, in mice with a targeted disruption of the galanin gene (GalKO), there was an increased propensity to develop status epilepticus after perforant path stimulation or systemic kainic acid, whereas in mice that overexpress the galanin gene (GalOE), it showed increased resistance to seizure induction. Furthermore, the depolarization-induced glutamate release from hippocampal slices was greater in GalKO and lower in GalOE, suggesting that alterations of physiological and seizure responses in galanin transgenic animals may be mediated through modulation of glutamate release.

Alzheimer's disease is a neurodegenerative disease leading to a drastic disruption in cognitive function. A reduction in acetylcholine binding to muscarinic receptors has been shown to be associated with the development of AD. When animals were injected with the muscarinic receptor antagonist, scopolamine, they develop spatial memory impairment. Human volunteers also showed deficits in spatial memory when given injections of scopolamine.

Recently a great deal of attention has been devoted to a newly discovered endogenous protective mechanism that is activated in response to traumatic brain injury. Experiments conducted in a murine-based model system have indicated that this mechanism is dependent primarily on the action of a cannabinoid, known as 2-arachidonyl glycerol (2-AG), which is synthesized in the hypothalamus. Specifically, 2-AG appears to be a key component in a series of molecular interactions that ultimately serve to antagonize the activity of several harmful endogenous inflammatory mediators released within the brain post-trauma. Inhibition of these inflammatory molecules suggests that 2-AG may confer its beneficial effects by limiting the secondary brain damage normally induced by their release. In general, traumatic brain injury is associated with a high incidence of morbidity and mortality at least in part because no effective drug-based treatment is currently available. The induction of primary neurological trauma is rapidly followed by the release of endogenous inflammatory mediators such as TNFα and reactive oxygen species responsible for augmenting the initial damage (Chapter 7). Consequently the effect to these molecules is referred to a secondary damage. In general, minimization of secondary damage is associated with enhanced repair and recovery from the primary trauma. 2-AG may specifically act to decrease the severity of this secondary response. An *in vitro* assay demonstrating the preferential interaction of 2-AG with the cannabinoid receptor CB1 involved subjecting mice to closed head injury and injecting 1-AG in conjunction with progressively larger dose of a CB1 receptor antagonist. The neuroprotective role of 2-AG diminishes in a dose-dependent manner through the addition of receptor antagonist. Of note is that the fact that closed head injury was inflicted only on one cerebral hemisphere leaving the other half as a control against which to gauge the effects. 2-AG levels in the affected hemisphere were escalated tenfold by four hours post-trauma and remained elevated after 24 hours at sixfold levels. As expected, the uninjured hemisphere exhibited no elevation of 2-AG.

Production of synthetic 2-AG then enabled an evaluation of criteria such as its influence on oedema and the rate of neurological recovery post-trauma, upon intravenous administration. Oedema is defined as an influx of serous fluid into tissues in this case the brain is in danger because it elevates intracranial pressure. The dangerous rise in pressure is maximal around 24 hours post-injury. Even at the lowest dose of intravenously injected synthetic 2-AG oedema was reduced by 50%. Improved recovery rates were observed upon 2-AG additions. Assays monitoring the ability of 2-AG levels to confer hippocampal protection also demonstrated a positive correlation.

Chapter summary

Regardless of the organism, the onset of new behaviours and the modification of established behaviours require both learning and memory. A stimulus to an organism may be described as being positive, negative or neutral. Positive stimuli act to promote behaviours to facilitate interaction with the stimulus whereas negative stimuli act to induce behaviours that will avoid future interaction with the stimulus. Neutral stimuli are those that do not have a behaviour-modifying ability. In vertebrates, regions of the brain act to induce a physiological reward in positive stimuli whereas fear centres promote the opposite effect in the transduction of negative stimuli. The amygdala is a key region of the brain that integrates sensory and associative information to regulate the onset of both reward- and fear-potentiated behaviours. It may also play a role in memory consolidation in conjunction with the hippocampus and other sites, before the memory is stored. Many behaviours that are sexually dimorphic, including courtship, aggression and sexual behaviour, are regulated by the sex steroid milieu of the organism. The development of the brain circuitry of these behaviours appears to be achieved *in utero* or perinatally, in response to changes in circulating sex steroids. In the adult, sex steroids may act to facilitate or inhibit a number of these behaviours by interaction with vasopressin and oxytocin-sensitive regions of the brain. In mammals, emotional arousal associated with activation of the HPA axis can enhance some behaviours but depress the incidence of others.

12

Pheromones and chemo-attractants

Introduction

We now turn our attention to chemical signalling molecules that act outside an individual to coordinate the actions of other individuals within a population. The term 'pheromone' was first proposed in the late 1950s to describe secreted substances from one individual that subsequently acted on a second individual of the same species to elicit a specific action. Hormones, as we have seen, are defined as those chemicals that coordinate physiological actions within an individual. The number of physiological actions pheromones can have on individuals are vast, and in some species, notably insects, they can act to coordinate the individuals of a population such that the population or colony begins to perform as a superorganism. We might consider this as a higher level of organismal evolution. However, for most organisms including humans, pheromones act to modulate the actions of individuals with a group or a population.

Pheromones may be either specific and dedicated chemicals where they are only released to the exterior and act only on other individuals of the same species or organism belonging to different species; or, they may consist of generalized chemical substances where they have a hormonal action inside the organism but are released via sweat, saliva or urine and have a secondary pheromonal effect external to the organism. Pheromones are predominantly volatile chemicals in that they are quickly dispersed into the medium (water, air) into which they are released. This chemical attribute is necessary to ensure that as many individuals as possible are targeted. However, a number of pheromones are not volatile and require contact with a sensory organ before they are affective.

Neuroendocrinology: An Integrated Approach   David A. Lovejoy
© 2005 John Wiley & Sons, Ltd

Evolution of pheromones

Theoretically, pheromones are as old as the first chemotactic factors that evolved in the earliest cells. As we have discussed in Chapter 2, cell-to-cell signalling was a requirement for the evolution of the metazoans. Thus, the first organisms already had an exocrine ability. Although the first organisms were cells, by definition, any chemical that was secreted by the cell that had the ability to modulate the physiology or actions of another cell can be termed an exocrine factor. Many of these exocrine factors became paracrine and later endocrine factors once multicellularity developed. The first pheromones were likely metabolic waste products and, indeed, many pheromone-like molecules derived from such waste products are still used by numerous species in most extant taxa.

The first true pheromones may have been involved primarily with reproductive function in sexually reproducing species (Chapter 10). For example, the GnRH-like peptide mating factors of the single-cell fungal species, *Candida albicans* and *Saccharomyces cerevisiae*, qualify as sex pheromones. Species that evolved this ability would possess a great selective advantage over others that could not, as it would tend to remove many of the random elements from sexual interaction. By following a pheromonal gradient in the environment an individual could locate a potential mate. Pheromonal detection to coordinate the reproductive activities of one individual to another has likely evolved independently in several groups although the basic mechanism has likely been around since shortly after the evolution of the first sexually reproducing species.

The evolution of pheromones has been thought to progress through three discrete stages (Fig. 12.1). In the early stage of the evolution of pheromones, the male of a particular species may implement a type of 'chemical espionage' in order to detect the stage of the reproductive cycle of the female. A number of metabolic products, associated with the various stages of female reproduction that are ultimately released into the environment, may be perceived by the male. Such chemicals could evolve into a selective male attractant molecule analogous to a cellular chemotactic factor. In this situation, it may not be clear if the male is using the chemical factor to determine the reproductive competence of the female, or if the female is utilizing the chemical to regulate male behaviour. Regardless, however, this ability by itself would act to increase the efficiency of reproduction within a species. Eventually, under selection pressure, the female may actively secrete the pheromones. Then in the final stage in the evolution of pheromones the female pheromones may directly regulate the male reproductive cycle to maximize the survival of the offspring. In some organisms, where this event is tightly coupled, the male effectively becomes a physiological extension of the female, creating a 'superhermaphrodite', so to speak. For example, there are some species of fish where the male is highly degenerative and remains attached to the female during life, where its reproductive ability is regulated by the female. However, there are a number of other situations where the male secretes the attractants and regulates the female reproductive cycle (p. 340).

In physiologically advanced metazoans, the development and a greater reliance of complex pheromonal signalling systems would be expected in species where there is a lack of sensory input from other special sense modalities. Physical conditions in the environment, such as light conditions, or the size of the spatial range that a species occupies, may act to direct the development of an organism's sensory systems towards

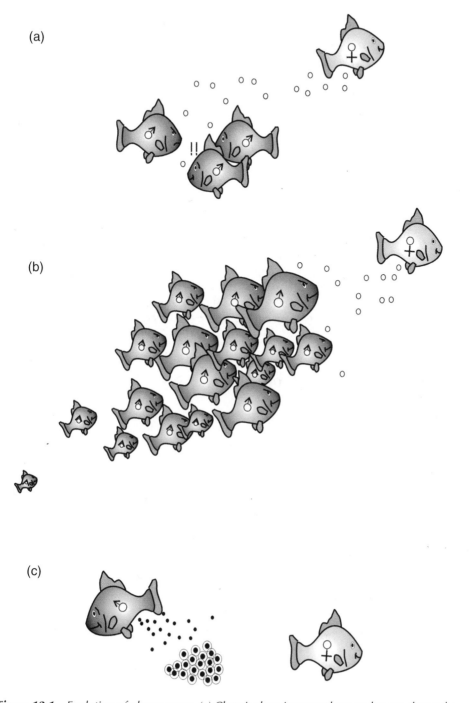

Figure 12.1 *Evolution of pheromones. (a) Chemical espionage where males can detect the reproductive state the female is in; (b) sex attractants: males are attracted to females who are reproductively ready; (c) pheromones from one sex regulate the reproductive readiness of the other sex.*

olfaction and pheromone detection and away from the development of other special senses, such as visual or auditory senses. Thus for species living in habitats with limited light, for example, in ocean depths, turbid water conditions or nocturnal habitats, vision has a limited use. Pheromonal systems can, therefore, be used for communication between individuals. Species ultimately need to develop a long-distance sensing mechanism, and thus species that have evolved effective long-distance perception abilities such as visual, echo-location (sonar), electroreceptive or auditory systems may be expected to possess less well-developed pheromonal release and detection systems.

Classification of pheromones

Pheromones may be classified in a number of different ways (Fig. 12.2). Releasing pheromones include those that elicit the rigid stereotyped responses typical of insects and some lower vertebrates. Signalling pheromones may be classified as those that stimulate more complex behavioural responses typical of higher vertebrates and mammals. Priming pheromones, on the other hand, are those that have been shown to produce physiological changes in the receptive individuals. An example of a priming pheromone might be the crowding pheromone of locusts that acts to induce the maturation of gregarious phase individuals.

Pheromones in invertebrates

All invertebrate species probably utilize some form of pheromonal messager at some point or another in their life cycle. However, insects have been particularly well studied as a result of the applied aspects of insect control. Many pesticides have been developed to target pheromonal systems, and this has acted to progress our knowledge about insect pheromone physiology.

Numerous chemical classes of pheromonal signals, including sterols, terpenes, eicosanoids, long-chain fatty acids and possibly alkaloid-like substances, are utilized by invertebrates. However, the pheromonal messages given off by an individual at any given time are usually not individual chemicals, but rather blends or 'cocktails' of pheromones and related

Type	Action	Example
Signalling pheromones	Complex behaviours	Reproductive pheromones of vertebrates
Priming pheromones	Physiological changes in receptive individuals	Locust crowding pheromone
Releasing pheromones	Stereotyped behaviours	Insect sex pheromones

Figure 12.2 *Types of pheromones and their actions.*

pheromonal metabolites. Although individual constituents of the cocktail may be shared by other species, the blend itself is species-specific. The constituents of the blend can act synergistically on the receiver. For example, the female pine beetle (*Dendroctonus brevicomis*) releases the pheromone exo-brevicomin and a terpene derived from the damaged bark of Ponderosa pine, on which it feeds. This combination attracts both males and females to the tree. Then the newly arriving males secrete a new pheromone, frontalin. The combination of the three pheromones is considerably more potent than each of the individual constituents. This cocktail release of pheromones may be likened to the mixture of releasing factors that get released into the portal system by the hypothalamus to generate complex physiological responses associated with the induced release of several pituitary hormones (Chapter 4). Insects also possess numerous components of their integument that act as recognition cues. The outer covering of insects consists of a variety of water-repellent lipids. In the social insects (bees, ants, wasps and termites), the mixture is characteristic and may help individuals distinguish between nest mates, and individuals from another colony.

Pheromonal detection and perception systems

Depending on the invertebrate lineage, the neurological processing of pheromonal signals occurs in different parts of the brain. Among arthropods, the signals may be processed in the olfactory lobe in crustaceans, but in the antennal lobe in insects. In molluscs, much of the processing appears to occur in the procerebral lobe.

In many insect species, the olfactory receptor cells are compartmentalized into cuticular structures called sensilla and are arranged along the length of each antenna. These sensilla are separated into two main classes depending on their response profile to olfactory stimulation (Fig. 12.3). Pheromonal olfactory receptor cells respond to sex and other pheromones, whereas general olfactory receptor cells respond to non-pheromonal odorants. Each is found in morphologically distinct sensilla. Like vertebrates (p. 338), each of the two types of olfactory receptor cells have separate neurological pathways into the brain. In moths, for example, the general olfactory receptor cells send axons to glomeruli in the main antennal lobe, whereas the pheromonal olfactory cells project their axons to a cluster of large sexually dimorphic glomeruli called the macroglomerular complex. Generally, the sensory neurons sharing the same receptor project to only one of the glomeruli, thus each glomerulus has a certain specificity for a given pheromone or odorant (Fig. 12.4). The strength of the stimulus, which reflects the environmental concentrations of the pheromone, is encoded by the discharge frequency of the receptor neurons. Each glomerulus is essentially a dense aggregation of synaptic neuropil with an intricate set

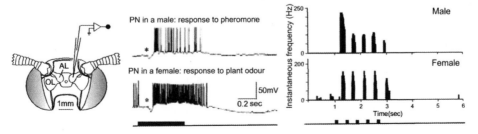

Figure 12.3 *Discrimination between pheromonal and non-pheromonal odours in a moth. Reprinted from Christensen and Hildebrand (2002) by the permission of Elsevier Science Ltd.*

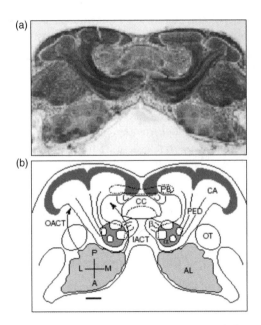

Figure 12.4 *Organization of the insect brain showing regions of pheromonal and olfactory processing. (a) Horizontal section through the brain of a scarab beetle,* Pachnoda marginata*; (b) AL, antennal lobe (note clusters of glomeruli in AL in top panel), PB protocerebral bridge, CA calyces of mushroom bodies, CC, central complex, OT optic tubercle, PED peduncle. IACT and OACT inner and outer antennocerebral tracts. Reprinted from Hansson (2002) by the permission of Elsevier Science Ltd.*

of local synaptic connections. These, in turn, project to higher neurological processing centres that integrate and produce a complex output signal that creates a neurological representation of the temporal and spatial distribution of the chemical. This is particularly important for the receiving individual to separate the specific chemical signal from the general perception of other chemicals in the environment. In many cases, where there is a blend or cocktail of pheromones and other odorants that are used in varying concentrations, a specific response to the complex combination can be made.

Classification of insect pheromones

Insect pheromones can be divided into five basic types (Fig. 12.5). Sex pheromones include both the sex attractants that are typically used over a long distance. Once the individuals come closer, then the courtship pheromones may be used for oviposition and fertilization. The courtship pheromones may comprise higher concentrations of the sex attractants or may be a separate pheromone specialized for courtship. The sex attractants tend to be produced primarily by the female although the lepidopterans (butterflies and moths) and some other groups are exceptions in that it is the males that are the primary producers of the sex attractants. Aggregation pheromones, on the other hand, are generally produced by both sexes and play several roles. The efficiency of mating can be improved by increasing the local concentration of both sexes. This is particularly important in species that are short-lived. Aggregation pheromones can act to promote a defensive reaction

Sex pheromones	Sex attractants
	Courtship pheromones
	Sexual inhibitors
Aggregation pheromones	Improved efficiency of mating
	Defensive reactions
	Exploitation of food resource
Dispersion pheromones	Reduce competition
	Seek out new resources
	Maintain local resources
Trail marking pheromones	Discovery of new resources
	Exploratory behaviour
Alarm pheromones	Defensive reactions
	Protection of colony

Figure 12.5 *Types of insect pheromones and their actions.*

providing security from predation, or these pheromones may be released in response to a particular food source to maximize the utilization of that food source. As a regulatory mechanism, when insect densities become too great, then dispersion pheromones may be given off. This can be used to encourage the species to seek out new resources. These pheromones will also act to maintain distance between colonies of the same species. Thus such pheromones act to ensure that the resources are not depleted in local areas and competition among populations of the same species is reduced. Trail-marking pheromones are typically volatile short-lived chemicals. In ants, for example, they consist of metabolic waste products secreted by the poison glands. Airborne pheromone trails are also types of trail-marking pheromones. Alarm pheromones are volatile chemicals that are quickly dispersed throughout a colony and are found in many species. A number of these pheromones appear to be derived from antipredator defence systems and are typically released, in addition to aggregation pheromones, in the presence of a predator.

In a number of insect species, reproduction may be achieved only by an alpha female or queen. In some cases, pheromones may be released to inhibit the reproductive ability of lower-ranked females. This can also occur in non-insect species, notably the naked mole rat. In the queenless ant species, *Dinoponera quadriceps*, the alpha female will chemically mark a challenging female. This results in the apparent punishment of the challenging female by low-ranking females.

Synthesis and storage of pheromones

In most insects, pheromones are synthesized in specialized cells or tissues associated with the epidermis. In insects, all pheromones are released by exocrine glands. They can occur in a number of different locations on the body depending upon the species. In lepidopteran species they may be present as sacs between the abdominal segments, mandibular regions as in honey bees, hindgut and genitalia in cockroaches or hind tibiae in aphids, for example. A number of the pheromones in insects have been initially derived from existing chemicals such as host odours or cuticular waxes. They serve as the foundation for the synthesis of pheromones. Many pheromone precursors are also obtained in the diet.

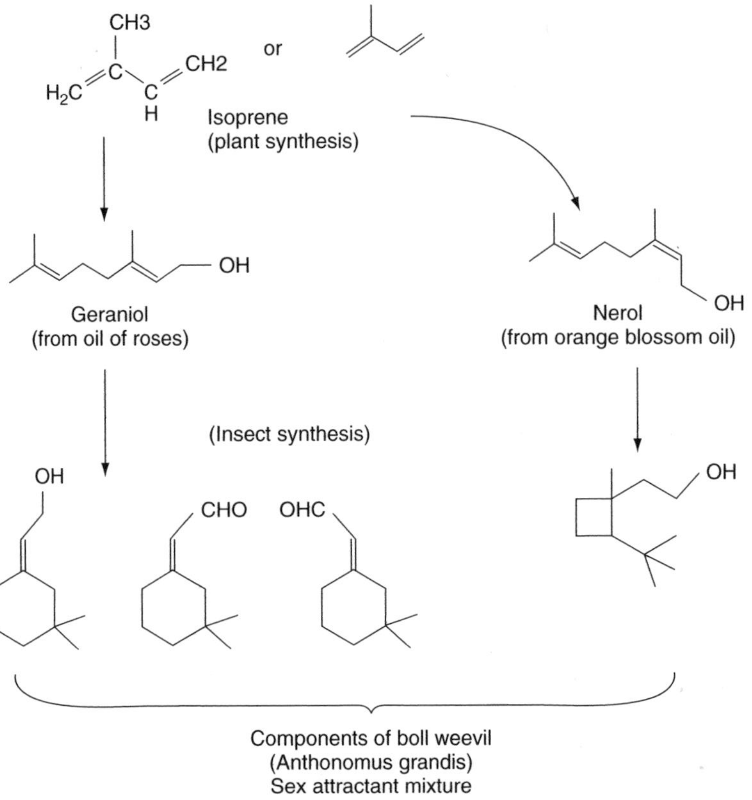

Figure 12.6 *Synthesis of boll weevil sex attractants from isoprenoid components in plants.*

The isoprenoids are a family of biologically active compounds with well over 20 000 known variants (Fig. 12.6). These chemicals are related by their construction from a repeating isoprene (C5) motif that leads to a number of products including dolichol, ubiquinone and steroids. As we saw in Chapter 2, the initial steps of this biosynthetic pathway evolved early in cell history and thus elements of this pathway are present in all kingdoms of living organisms. In vertebrates, much of the products of the isoprenoid pathway are directed into steroid biosynthesis. However, insects do not possess the enzyme squalene synthase and, therefore, cannot synthesize steroids *de novo*, although they can synthesize the precursors of steroids and modify steroids that they have taken in during feeding. Because the isoprenoid products are not directed towards steroid synthesis, many of these chemicals in insects are utilized as chemical messengers both internally and as pheromones. They have been utilized, for example, for the synthesis of juvenile hormone (JH), alarm pheromones in aphids and in termite defence secretions.

Pheromone regulation

The synthesis of pheromones is directed by a number of higher order neuroendocrine or endocrine factors. In ticks, for example, dopamine has been determined to be one of the

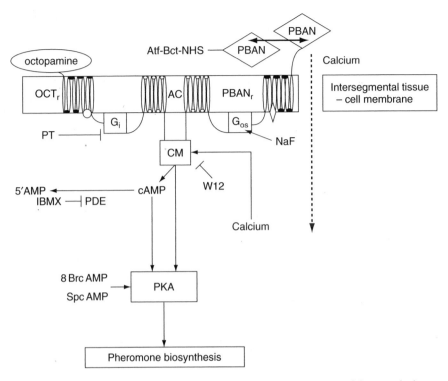

Figure 12.7   *Control of pheromone production in the moth. Reprinted from Rafaeli (1999) by the permission of European Society for Comparative Endocrinology.*

hormonal regulatory mechanisms to stimulate the production of pheromones after they have taken a blood meal. However, one of the best studied is the pheromone biosynthesis-activating neuropeptide (PBAN) which is a 33 or 34 amino acid peptide belonging to the pyrokinin-myotropin (FXPRL-NH$_2$) family of peptides and is produced by the neurosecretory cells in the suboesophageal ganglion. The structure of this neuropeptide has been characterized in several moth species. PBAN has a direct stimulatory ability on the production and stimulation of pheromone production. PBAN actively circulates in the haemolymph during active reproductive periods. The PBAN receptor possesses two affinity sites with differential responses to either low or high levels of PBAN, which can modulate either cAMP or Ca^{2+} mediated pathways, depending upon the level of binding site activation (Fig. 12.7). In the silkworm, *Bombyx mori*, the sex pheromone bombykol, (E,Z)-10,12-hexa-decadien-1-ol, is synthesized from acetyl CoA via a fatty acid intermediate. This synthesis is under direct control by PBAN.

Pheromones in vertebrates

The identification and characterization of vertebrate pheromones has lagged in comparison to the identification of insect pheromones. In insects, glands containing high concentrations of pheromonal substances are relatively easy to obtain and the constituents purified. In vertebrates, and mammals in particular, the putative pheromones are part of a complex biological cocktail consisting of both pheromonal and many non-pheromonal substances as typically found in sebaceous gland secretions, saliva, urine or faeces. Moreover, the physiological or behavioural manifestation of vertebrate pheromones may be much more subtle than insect pheromones, and the establishment of the appropriate assay conditions can be problematic.

Sensory systems associated with the detection of pheromones

There are two basic olfactory systems that have evolved in vertebrates to process volatile chemicals in the environment. The main olfactory system is used primarily to detect food sources or prey and odours associated with predators. These chemicals are initially detected in the main olfactory sensory neurons in the olfactory epithelium. The main olfactory epithelium contains the largest known family of G-protein-coupled receptors in mammals. These neurons project to specific clusters of glomeruli in the main olfactory bulb that ultimately provide a spatial map of the pheromonal gradient to the individual. In comparison to insects, which have relatively few glomeruli and have been identified and mapped, vertebrates, and mammals in particular, may have several thousand glomeruli. Our understanding of the neural processing of vertebrate pheromones is, therefore, far from complete. However, neurons of the olfactory bulb appear to relay the information to the olfactory cortical structures that include the olfactory tubercle, anterior olfactory nucleus, piriform cortex and the entorhinal cortex. These structures form an integrated unit along with the amygdala and to a lesser extent, the hippocampus and bed nucleus of the stria terminalis (Chapter 11).

The accessory olfactory system appears to be primarily involved in the detection of a particular set of mostly non-volatile and some volatile chemicals that have been implicated in a number of behaviour-modifying functions. The accessory olfactory system appears to be present in most vertebrates. As with the insects, the receptors utilized by the accessory olfactory system are morphologically distinct from their counterparts in the main olfactory system. Depending upon the vertebrate class, these receptors may be interspersed randomly or in clusters in the olfactory epithelium, or in the case of tetrapods, and particularly amniotes, these are found in the vomeronasal organ (Fig. 12.8).

The vomeronasal organ is not present in ray-finned fishes or in lungfish but does seem to be present in some aquatic salamanders and anurans. Although mudpuppies (*Necturus maculosus*) do not appear to possess such a system, *Amphiuma tridactylum* and *Siren intermedia* do possess functional vomeronasal and olfactory systems. Thus, in mudpuppies, members of the family Proteidae, the vomeronasal organ appears to be lost and represents a derived character for this lineage. This suggests that the vomeronasal organ originated in a species that represented the common ancestor for amphibians and amniotes.

Sensory neurons of the vomeronasal organ present in the nasal organ detect these pheromonal chemicals. This information is relayed to the accessory olfactory bulb and then to regions of the limbic system including the amygdala, bed nucleus of the stria terminalis, ventromedial hypothalamus and the preoptic area. In humans, the vomeronasal organ has largely been lost. It begins to develop during embryogenesis but is lost before birth.

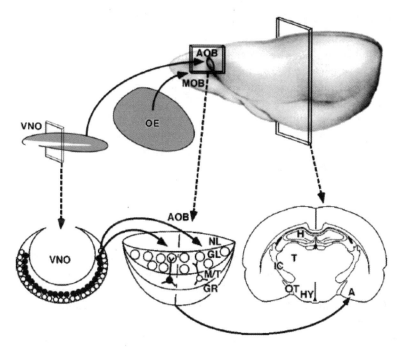

Figure 12.8 *Organization of the vomeronasal system in a rodent. AOB – accessory olfactory bulb; MOB – main olfactory bulb; VMO – vomeronasal organ; OE – olfactory epithelium. The layers of the AOB include nerve (NL), glomerular (GL) mitral/tufted (M/T) and granule cell (GR). Other abbreviations: A – amygdaloid complex; H – hippocampus; Hy – hypothalamus; IC – internal capsule; T – thalamus. Reprinted from Halpern and Martinez-Marcos (2003) by the permission of Elsevier Science.*

Cetaceans and aquatic crocodiles may have also lost the vomeronasal organ. The African clawed frog (*X. laevis*) is mostly aquatic and represents a phylogenetically older lineage of anurans. Along with the main olfactory epithelium and vomeronasal organ, it possesses a third olfactory organ, the middle chamber epithelium. The middle chamber epithelium possesses one class of sensory cell whose morphology is similar to that of the olfactory epithelium, and another class that has a structure like those sensory cells of the vomeronasal organ. The olfactory epithelium and vomeronasal organs in this species appear to be more specialized for the detection of airborne chemicals, whereas the middle chamber epithelium is adapted for the perception of water-borne chemicals.

Thus, regardless of the morphology of the organ system that detects pheromonal signals, the integration of the pheromonal response is ultimately transmitted to a series of neurological sites that are associated with motivation, learning and memory. Of the special sense, the olfaction and pheromonal detection system is unique in that it feeds directly into these sites. Environmental information arising from auditory, visual or vestibular sensory systems, for example, reach the bed nucleus of the stria terminalis, amygdala or hippocampus by a more indirect route. The direct interaction of pheromonal and olfactory senses into this region attests to their older evolutionary development.

Physiological actions of vertebrate pheromones

Pheromonal substances have been identified in all classes in vertebrates. However, phero-mones have been best studied in mammalian and fish species. Our understanding of the physiology of pheromone action in vertebrates is poor by comparison to what is known in invertebrates. This is due to the difficulty at the isolation and identification of the pheromonal signal combined with an appropriate physiological assay to detect the pheromonal action. Many of the vertebrate pheromones have a much longer latency period from the point of detection to a definable physiological change relative to insects and other invertebrates.

Amphibians, reptiles and birds

Pheromones are present in most lineages of amphibians, reptiles and birds. However, the comparatively few studies that are available indicate that these groups of vertebrates employ considerably less use of pheromones than a number of teleost and mammal species. In birds and amphibians, this may be due to the development of vocaliza-tions and auditory systems that are used for aggressive and courtship behaviours (Chapter 11). Also, in avian species there is considerable use of plumage for courtship displays.

There is little evidence for the use of pheromones in adult anurans. Much of the distal interaction among conspecifics appears to be achieved by the extensive use of vocalizations. During more proximal interactions, for example, courtship, tactile stimu-lation becomes the predominant method for oviposition and fertilization. However, given the variability of anuran morphologies, niche and habitat utilization, it is likely that pheromones are used in some species, particularly in species that are mostly aquatic (p. 338). Many amphibian species synthesize a bewildering spectrum of bioactive substances in their skin. Many of these chemicals appear to be used for defence (Chapter 13), but many may very well be used as pheromones. In urodele amphibians (newts and salamanders), however, a variety of pheromones have been found in chin, abdominal and cloacal glands. Urodeles are more aquatic than anurans and have less well-developed special senses. Despite the well-developed repertoire of auditory signals in birds, along with visual signals such as plumage, there is evidence of pheromonal substances in some avian lineages. In female mallard ducks, *Anas platyrhynchos*, diesters of 3-hydroxy C8, C10 and C12 acids are used. They are secreted by the uropygial glands only during the mating season and may play a role in courtship. Many snakes secrete a number of pheromonal substances. The female red-sided garter snake, *Thamnophis sirtalis parietalis*, for example, secretes a methyl ketone that, in conjunction with oestrogens, signals her receptivity to males. Once she mates, she releases a second pheromone to inhibit sexual behaviour in males. Some males have the ability also to secrete methyl ketone that also acts as a presumably female sex attractant to other males. This species typically mates in a large mass (mating ball) of females and males and thus one theory suggests that the pheromone-secreting male snakes have a greater opportunity to mate with the female as a number of the males are distracted and attempt mating with the pheromone-secreting male.

Fish

Spawning behaviour in externally fertilized fish generally differ from tetrapods in that it is induced by post-ovulatory prostaglandins and not by ovarian steroids. Prostaglandins also induce female sexual behaviours in externally fertilized amphibians, inhibit post-coital sexual behaviour in mammals and some reptiles and induce parturition behaviour in some marsupials. An ancestral prostaglandin-mediated mechanism may have originally evolved in external fertilizers to synchronize oviposition and sexual behaviour with the presence of ovulated oocytes. This has been subsequently modified in internal fertilizers to regulate other reproductive behaviours, such as coitus and parturition, which are responsive to reproductive tract stimulation. If so, then steroid-regulated female sexual behaviours is a phylogenetically younger development and, therefore, a derived character associated with internal fertilization.

A number of fish steroid and prostaglandin hormones function both internally and also as pheromones (Fig. 12.9). The sensitivity of olfactory hormones can be affected by season, gender and the presence of other steroids such as androgens. Thus pheromones can directly act not only to modulate behaviour, but also to regulate the sensitivity to other behaviour- and physiology-modifying pheromones and chemicals. The actual steroid and prostaglandin variants utilized as pheromones vary considerably among fish species.

Due to male–male sexual competition, many male fish have evolved a number of physiological and behavioural responses to the specific hormone and hormone metabolites released sequentially by females during the periovulatory period. In the black goby (*Gobius jozo*), the steroid etiocholanolone glucuronide is utilized to both attract females and induce them to oviposit. Other species may utilize two distinct pheromones to attract the female, then to oviposit.

Pheromonal systems in the goldfish have been particularly well studied and offer a model on the evolution and physiology of pheromones in fishes. There are at least two sets of pheromones in coordinating the male reproductive behaviour with that of the female in goldfish. There is initially a preovulatory steroidal pheromone similar to, or a metabolite of, the ovarian maturation inducing steroid 17α,20β-dihydroxy-4-pregnen-3-one. There is cocktail of C21 steroids released, and one or more act to stimulate the male to increase the milt volume. The perception of these steroids occur via the olfactory epithelium, then mediated via the medial olfactory tracts to increase gonadotropin release

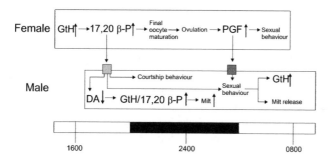

Figure 12.9 *Regulation of male reproductive physiology and behaviour by female pheromones in the goldfish. Modified after Stacey et al. (1994).*

from the pituitary gland. This mechanism may involve the reduction of the tonic dopamine inhibition of the gonadotropes. Exposure to this hormone not only increases milt volume and sperm motility but also enhances the fertilization behaviour of the male.

The female may also release a number of C19 steroids such as androstenedione and testosterone. C19 steroids can inhibit the males' response to the C21 steroids. Although both sexes release both types of steroids, males release far more of the C19 steroids. The blend of both types may reflect the stage of readiness of the female to ovulate such that the C21 to C19 ratio increased towards ovulation and, therefore, the males' milt production is timed to coordinate with the female. An alternative hypothesis suggests that the sensitivity of the male to C19 steroids may be related to the presence of other males nearby. After the oocytes are ovulated and enter the ovisac, then the reproductive tract begins to synthesize prostaglandin F2α or a similar variant. This acts internally to initiate female spawning behaviour. When the pheromone is released into the water and is perceived by males, they respond with a set of behaviours associated with sexual readiness.

Pheromones in mammals

Many, if not all, mammalian species use odours to identify potential mates and may release into their environment a variety of volatile and non-volatile chemicals via exocrine glands of the skin, microorganisms of the skin as well as through excretory products such as urine and faeces. In domestic swine, for example, androstenone is present in the male salvia and acts as an attractant to sows and facilitates receptive behaviour. Humans, apes and old world monkeys lack the functional genes responsible for the pheromonal signal transduction and tend to be relatively insensitive to vomeronasal pheromones. This loss of vomeronasal activity has been thought to coincide with the development of an acute trichromatic colour vision. However, the new-world Howler monkeys do possess a developed pheromonal system and trichromatic colour vision.

There are a number of structural similarities between mammalian pheromones and those of insects. Both farnesenes and 2-heptanone play a role in insect and mammalian signalling. Dehydro-exo-brevicomin, a pheromone, facilitates aggressive behaviour in the male mouse and is an attractant to the female mouse. It is structurally identical, except for the presence of a double bond, to the pheromone brevicomin in a bark beetle. The pheromone (Z)-7-dodecen-1-yl acetate has been found in insects as well as elephants. However, despite these similarities there is no strong evolutionary evidence that the biosynthetic pathway has been completely conserved in insects and vertebrates although it is likely that elements of the pathway have been conserved and there are alternate pathways that can be utilized to achieve the same molecular goal. Although it has been argued that elephants possess a relatively structured society and possess cognitive abilities that have been compared with those of primates and cetaceans, they utilize a variety of pheromone-regulated behaviours.

In rodents, pheromonal substances have been isolated, which regulate sexual attraction, oestrus induction, acceleration of puberty dominance and aggressive behaviours. Vaginal discharges stimulate sexual behaviour in the male hamsters. This causes a short-term

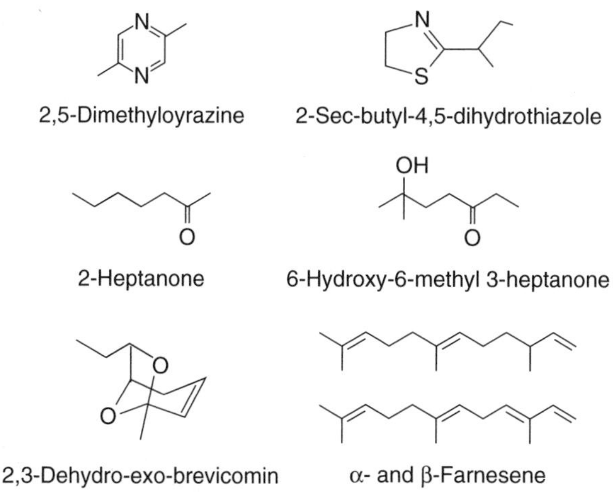

2,5-Dimethyloyrazine   2-Sec-butyl-4,5-dihydrothiazole

2-Heptanone   6-Hydroxy-6-methyl 3-heptanone

2,3-Dehydro-exo-brevicomin   α- and β-Farnesene

Figure 12.10 *Pheromonal substances found in the urine of female mice.*

increase in testosterone and an increase in sexual behaviour. This may involve an increase in aromatase in the brain and increase of conversion to oestrogens to induce the onset of sexual behaviours. Application of the vaginal discharges to the hind legs of a male hamster, for example, will cause other males to be sexually attracted to the treated male.

In mice, pheromones can act to regulate the timing of puberty, suppression of ovulation and maintenance of pregnancy. In mice, young females will attain puberty at an earlier stage when exposed to the urine of adult males than young females that are not exposed. The pheromone appears to be a small peptide about 6–8 amino acids long and is secreted in the urine (Fig. 12.10). Adult females can inhibit the onset of puberty in young females by secreting a different factor in their urine. These two processes can act to regulate the population of mice. In mice, a group of adult females can also show inhibition of ovulation. The active agent appears to be secreted in the urine. The presence of a male can disinhibit this inhibition. In mice, pheromones from a new male can inhibit the pregnancy in females. In novel males belonging to the same group, the effect occurs about 30% of the time. However, with males coming from outside of the group, then the effect occurs about 80% of the time. The mechanism appears to involve a decrease in the female prolactin levels, a resulting decrease in the activity of the corpus luteum and a resulting fall in plasma progesterone. This inhibits the implantation of the fertilized egg cell in the uterus.

Pheromonal associated mechanisms

A number of proteins have been identified that bind pheromonal-like chemicals to facilitate their actions. The lipocalins are carrier proteins that are expressed in the nasal mucosa of rodents. Male mice use a class of proteins called major urinary proteins (MUP) that bind small volatile molecules such as brevicomin- and thiazole-related chemicals. The MUPs allow for the slow release of small volatile chemicals. In the vomeronasal organ, a protein (vomeromodulin) has been identified and it appears to play a role in pheromonal transport.

Male mice display mating preferences for oestrous females with dissimilar major histocompatibility complex (MHC) proteins relative to their own. These proteins are excreted in the urine and act as recognition cues. One role of the MHC proteins as pheromonal substances is that it inhibits the mice from breeding with genetically similar individuals thus ensuring against too much inbreeding.

Neurological processing of pheromonal signals

The sexually dimorphic regions of the limbic system receive considerable input of olfactory signals. The medial nucleus of the amygdala receives olfactory input from two sources: the vomeronasal organ and the olfactory tract. Oestradiol enhances the acuity of olfactory cues for males. This information is relayed to the medial amygdala via the vomeronasal organ. Oestradiol and progesterone receptors are localized in sites that include a number of the sexually dimorphic sites as well as the ventromedial hypothalamus. Male rats treated with testosterone can distinguish between females that are in oestrous and those that are not. Oestrogens may play a role in the development of the main olfactory system to ultimately induce sex differences to play a role in sexual partner selection. Female mice can form a pheromonal memory of the male they mate with. The synaptic plasticity occurs in the accessory olfactory bulb.

Chapter summary

Pheromones are externally released hormones that act to coordinate actions among the individuals thereby creating cohesion within the population. Pheromones are found in all metazoan taxa and may be derived from several sources, such as *de novo* synthesis, waste metabolites and breakdown products of nutrients, or the result of commissural interaction among resident species such as bacteria. Pheromones may be used as sex attractants, for aggression, dispersion or for defence and alarm. The perception and neural circuitry associated with the integration of pheromonal signals appears to be analogous in insects and vertebrates. In moths, pheromonal and olfactory signals are differentiated by the detection of the former in sensilla along the antenna, which project to the main antennal lobe of the brain. Detection of pheromones occurs in a distinct subset of sensilla that instead send their axons to the macroglomerular complex of the brain. In vertebrates, the situation differs in that volatile signals are generally perceived by the olfactory organ which projects to the main olfactory bulb then to elements of the olfactory and limbic system, which include the olfactory tubercle, anterior olfactory nucleus, piriform cortex and the entorhinal cortex. Sensory neurons of the vomeronasal organ present in the nasal organ detect non-volatile and some volatile chemicals. This information is relayed to the accessory olfactory bulb and then to regions of the limbic system including the amygdala, bed nucleus of the stria terminalis, ventromedial hypothalamus and the preoptic area. The morphology of the pheromonal detection systems can vary considerably among species.

13

Xenobiotics and hormone mimics

Introduction

In the last chapter, we examined physiological and behavioural implications associated with the release and perception of chemical signals from one individual to another individual of the same species. In this chapter, we will focus on the chemicals produced by one species and their effect on a different species. Any living organism is essentially a biosynthetic factory that produces hundreds, if not thousands, of biologically active compounds that are released into the environment. Although a number of these compounds are used as receptor agonists for either endogenous or exogenous uses, many are simply metabolic waste products whose temporal existence is highly transient. Thus, their presence does not necessarily imply they have a usage. For many of these compounds, their effect in another species may be a matter of happenstance. However, regardless of whether these compounds have a known use in the species from which they found, a number of such compounds have significant biogenic properties.

Types of xenobiotics

All biogenic molecules can be classified as toxins or nutrients. Any compound acting like a nutrient at a particular concentration, regardless of its structure, is toxic if its concentration is increased sufficiently high enough. On the other hand, any toxic compound at a low enough dose can act as a nutrient. Thus, for any xenobiotic compound there can be a number of different actions depending upon its concentration. Recall from Chapter 1 that Paracelsus brought attention to the nutrient/toxin quality of drugs, minerals and nutrients. Sadly, each year there are a number of cases where people have been essentially poisoned by ingesting too much of a particular substance. In the last few years, vitamin A, vitamin B6, vitamin E and melatonin have induced toxic reactions in patients who believed that if some amount was good for you, then more is better. The number of hormones abused by professional athletes seems to grow each year. The overuse of these substances has been implicated in the increased incidence of stroke, heart attack, neurological problems and erratic behaviour in these individuals.

All signalling molecules, or molecules used for communication, are referred to as semiochemicals (Fig. 13.1). They can be divided into those chemicals that impart a physiologically relevant signal among individuals within a species, which are called pheromones (Chapter 12); and those chemicals that act as signalling between species, which are referred to as alleochemicals. Alleochemicals can be divided into three main groups. Kairomones are those alleochemicals that benefit the receiver but disadvantage the producer. Allomones benefit the producer by modifying the behaviour on the receiver, although the effect on the receiver is largely neutral. Synomones are those chemicals that have a mutual benefit on both the producer and receiver. For the most part, these are natural products associated with pheromonal signalling that another species has exploited to track down the species as prey, to avoid as a predator or to locate resources such as food sources.

In addition, there are a number of specific toxins and endocrine mimics produced by a given species, which upon ingestion produce a physiological response on the predator species (Fig. 13.2). The prey species, whether animal or non-animal, is essentially passive in their transmission of chemicals to the predator. Predator species may seek out these prey or food species for their nutrient value or as frequently the case with humans, for their psychotropic qualities. Predators can also utilize a number of chemical secretions to subdue their prey. Another group of xenobiotics include the waste products of a species. Here, where the population becomes particularly dense, the increased concentrations of

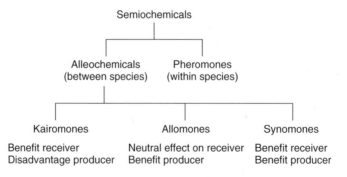

Figure 13.1   *Types of exocrine and xenobiotic signalling molecules.*

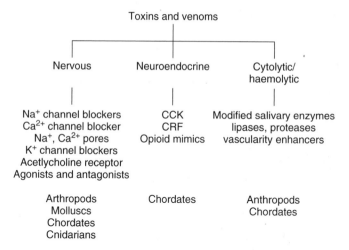

Figure 13.2   *Types of venoms and toxins and examples of major taxa where they are predominantly found.*

metabolic waste act in a noxious manner to ward off other species. These xenobiotics may be produced directly by the species, or indirectly by the species interaction with the environment. The industrial waste of humans is a particular good example of this. We will focus, however, on those xenobiotics that induce a neurological response (Fig. 13.3).

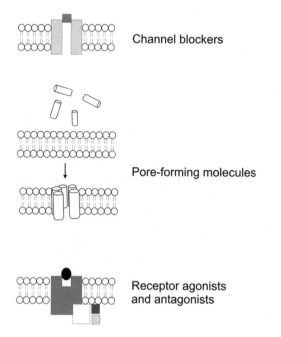

Figure 13.3   *Types of neural and neuroendocrine type toxins.*

Vertebrate toxins and defences

Virtually every metazoan species produces some metabolites that are toxic to another species. Such toxins may include alkaloids, biogenic amines, peptides and proteins, enzymes, mucus and neurotoxins. The toxins may arise from synthesis within the animal as an exocrine toxin with a specific defensive function, it may be a metabolic byproduct that induces a toxic effect in a predator if eaten. The toxin may also be obtained from food sources, where it is not synthesized by the animal. Every class of vertebrate possesses species that contain toxins. The Amphibia and most of the venomous fishes appear to utilize the toxins for defence. The venoms of the Reptilia and some insectivorous mammals, on the other hand, are used primarily for prey capture.

Venoms and toxins in fishes

Despite the large number of fish species, there are a comparatively few that are toxic. Among the elasmobranchs, the most venomous species are restricted to the family Batidae (rays). The venom, which is present in a caudal spine, is used for defence. Noxious substances have been reported in dorsal spines of other elasmobranchs and the sister class, Holocephali, but appear not to utilize neurotoxins. Among the ray-finned fishes, the most venomous species utilizing neurotoxins are found in a couple of orders. The order Scorpaeniformes includes the most toxic species of teleosts (Fig. 13.4). The stonefish (*Synanceia* sp.), soldierfish (*Gymnapistes* sp.) and lionfish (*Pterois* sp.) venoms have been the best characterized. The active ingredient in the toxins appears to be primarily a neural and neuromuscular toxin that can inhibit both acetylcholine and adrenergic transmission by the formation of pores in the nerve endings. These toxins as a result

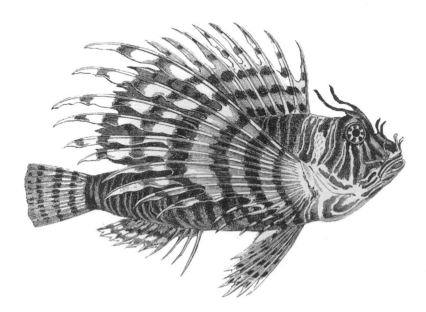

Figure 13.4   Lionfish.

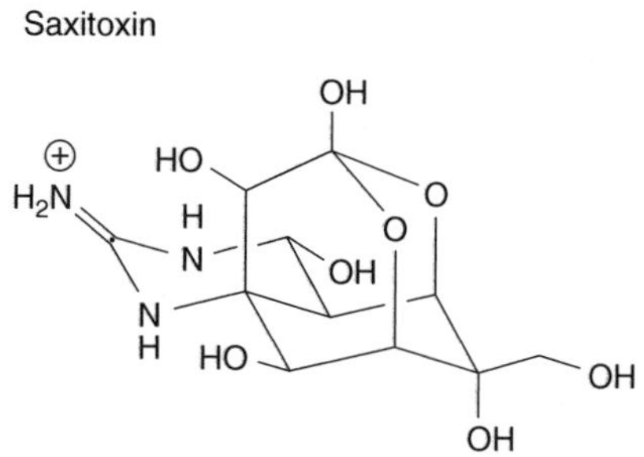

Saxitoxin

Tetrodotoxin

Figure 13.5   *Structure of tetrodotoxin.*

inhibit nerve transmission. The formation of these pores may also lead to an increase in intracellular Ca^{2+} resulting in cellular necrosis. However, composition and specificity of the toxin reaction differs considerably among these species. Some studies indicate that there is little specificity of the pore-forming toxins on nerve endings, whereas toxins from the lionfish may be specific for muscarinic and adrenergic receptors. The order Tetraodontiformes (sunfishes, boxfishes and porcupine fishes) also includes the puffer fishes. Several of these species contain lethal levels of tetrodotoxin, a Na^+ channel blocker that inhibits neural transmission (Fig. 13.5). The Batrachordiformes (toadfishes) possess poisonous spines and are capable of inflicting a painful, but not fatal, wound. The venom in these species appears to be cytolytic with no neurotoxic properties.

Toxins in the amphibia

The Amphibia have probably the most toxic and greatest assortment of different bioactive components in their skin. Most are relatively harmless to humans. Amphibians are relatively defenceless on land, thus the evolution of potent concoctions of toxins allowed their colonization of many regions. Among the most toxic are the poison-arrow frogs of the family Dendrobatidae (Fig. 13.6). There are about 160 known species that inhabit the neotropical regions of Central and South America. Virtually all toxins found in this group of frogs are taken in from dietary sources, primarily ants, beetles and millipedes. At least 500 different alkaloid-type (nitrogenous organic compounds) toxins have been identified. The identified toxins include a variety of chemical classes such as decahydraquinolines, izidines, coccinellines and spiropyrrolizines, many of which reflect the diet of the animal to a certain degree. The coccinellines, for example, are toxic products produced by fat body of coccinellid beetles (ladybug beetles) and stored in the haemolymph (Fig. 13.7). Over 50 different alkaloids have been isolated and identified in ladybug beetles. Once ingested by the frog, these chemicals remain in the tissues. Depending upon the toxin, they may act as ion channel blockers, analgesics and hormone mimics. *Phyllobates terribilis* appears to be the most toxic of the poison-arrow frogs. Batrachotoxin is one of the dominant toxins found in this and in other poison-arrow frogs. It is an alkaloid that prevents the closing of sodium channels in nerve and muscle cells. This leads to irreversible depolarization, producing cardiac arrhythmias, fibrillation and cardiac failure, not to mention a significant disruption of synaptic transmission. A single frog may contain up to 1900 mg of

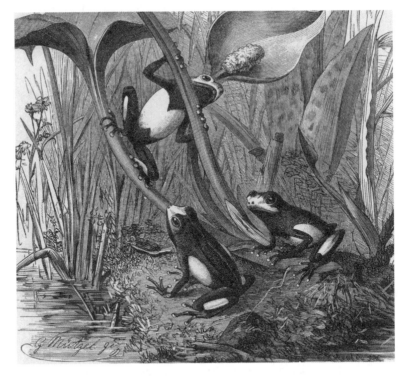

Figure 13.6   *Poison-arrow frogs (*Dendrobates *sp.).*

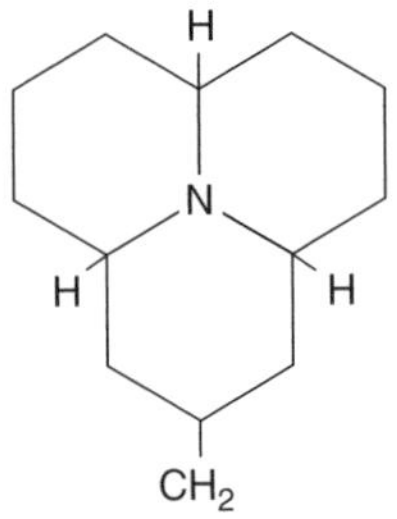

Figure 13.7   *Coccinelline.*

batrachotoxin where about 200 mg is enough to kill an adult human. Anecdotal reports indicate that just to touch the animal is enough to trigger a toxic response. The indigenous peoples of South America have exploited the toxins in these frogs for use in hunting, hence the name of poison-arrow frogs.

The tree frogs (Hylidae) also possess a number of toxins found in the skin or in exocrine glands. Although these species are considerably less toxic than the Dendrobatidae species, the toxins nevertheless induce a strong noxious physiological response in the predator species. Unlike the Dendrobatidae, they synthesize their own toxins. Rather interestingly, many of the toxins are highly modified neuropeptides. Toxins from hylid species may include a variety of different peptides such as immunomodulatory peptides, opioids (dermorphins and deltorphins) and antimicrobial peptides. They also possess a number of modified neuropeptides including variants of tachykinins, bradykinins, corticotrophin-releasing factor, caeruleins and bombesins. About 50 different bioactive compounds have been isolated from these frogs. In addition to the skin peptides, a number of biogenic amines and other classes of xenobiotics have been isolated. The monkey- and leaf-frogs of the Phyllomedusinae subfamily of the family Hylidae have large glands in pectoral and pelvic regions. The contents are released mechanically via pressure, for example, when a predator grasps them in their mouth. The main predators of these frogs appear to be arboreal snakes and some birds.

Many of the peptides in the Phyllomedusinae resemble those peptides in the brain that have been implicated in the inhibition of feeding, and the promotion of the neural stress response. In Chapter 4, we discussed the role of the blood–brain barrier and its role in restricting not only xenobiotics but a number of endogenous compounds, notably peptides that are produced outside the blood–brain barrier do not gain access to the brain and, therefore, disrupt normal neurological processing. However, a number of endogenously produced peptides by peripheral organs, which need to gain entry to the brain as they serve as endocrine feedback mechanism to modulate neurological and neuroendocrine system, can enter the brain via uptake mechanisms across the blood–brain barrier or via the circumventricular organs. Many of the peptides of the Phyllomedusinae species are highly modified to allow absorption across the buccal epithelium into the blood stream where they may be taken up by the area postrema where they act to inhibit ingestion. The area postrema has been implicated in the detection of some nutrients and toxins in the blood stream. The frog skin peptides may also play a role in taste aversion learning by predators who subsequently learn to avoid these frogs in the future. The ability of these peptides to cross the blood–brain barrier is also illustrated by the use of the frog secretions by the indigenous peoples of northern South America in hunting 'magic'. Although the author has not personally tried this, reports have indicated that before a hunt the hunters make burns in their skin, then rub the frog secretions into the burn. This results in a bout of sickness and vomiting, followed by a period of disorientation. After which the hunters report a feeling of well-being and a sharpened ability to hunt. Thus, the systemic administration of the toxin cocktail appears to gain entry into the brain.

The peptide sauvagine is a constituent of the skin glands in the Phyllomedusinae species. It was isolated in 1979 and shortly afterwards was shown to be a homologue of the CRF family. The primary structure of sauvagine is much different than that would be predicted from the rate of residue substitution based on a sequence comparison of the urotensins-I and the urocortins. It possesses only about 40% sequence similarity with the primary structure of rat urocortin and about 50% with urotensin-I. The primary structure of sucker and trout urotensin-I is much closer to rat urocortin than sauvagine is. Several phylogenetic lines of evidence suggest that sauvagine is a highly modified variant of urotensin-I and does not represent a separate vertebrate paralogue of urotensin-I or CRF.

Sauvagine-like peptides appear to be present only amongst the Anura. The evolution of the frogs and the Amphibia in general may explain, in part, the unusual sequence of sauvagine. The Amphibia separated from the rest of the vertebrate lineage over 360 million years ago well before any of the groups of living bony fish had evolved. Early amphibian radiations were concomitant with the coalescing of the major continents into the supercontinents of the Carboniferous period. This time was characterized by major shifts in climatic conditions, and extensive new habitats in the form of shallow seas and lowland marshes were formed. The environmental pressure evoked by these conditions may have been the impetus for the amphibian lineage to undergo major physiological adaptations to facilitate the evolution into the new semiterrestrial niches. Two such adaptations could impinge on the actions of CRF-related peptides: transition from an aquatic to terrestrial environment, and osmoregulation via the skin. Later, during the Jurassic–Cretaceous transition, the Anura underwent a second major radiation that coincided with the rise of angiosperms and the associated holometabolous insects. Exploiting the insects as a food source, this presumably led to a movement to more terrestrial habitats.

The presence of osmoregulatory peptides in the skin suggests a functional relationship with the osmoregulatory role of the skin. Most of the Amphibia are characterized by the high number of bioactive compounds in the serous glands of their skin. Sauvagine was originally isolated from the leaf frog, *Phyllomedusa sauvagei*, and the peptides' unusual structure may reflect, in part, the unusual adaptive physiology of fluid balance and osmoregulation of this species. This species belongs to one of the phylogenetically younger subfamilies of tree frogs (Hylidae). In most frogs, after metamorphosis, urea excretion is the primary mode of nitrogenous waste removal. Typically, however, the relative toxicity of urea is reduced by the excretion of high quantities of body water. Although this does not represent a concern for those species close to water, it does pose a physiological problem for terrestrial species. *P. sauvagei* is one of several species of frogs producing uric acid, which has evolved to live in semi-arid conditions. Uricotelic frogs have high rates of water uptake across their ventral surface and *P. sauvagei* is also one of few species of frogs that drink water to replenish body fluids.

Toxins and venoms in reptiles

Unlike amphibians, where toxins are used primarily for defence, toxins and venoms of reptiles are utilized primarily for prey capture. Reptile species that utilize toxins tend to be limited to the squamates (snakes and lizards). As many as 1300 of the 3200 species of snakes are venomous. Squamate toxins can be divided into two basic classes. Haemolytic (or cytolytic) toxins include proteases and lipases that frequently are modified salivary gland enzymes. Some species incorporate acetylcholinesterase in their toxins, which acts to hydrolyze acetylcholine at the bite site, thus disrupting the physiological response to the bite. The neurotoxins are usually polypeptide channel blockers and receptor antagonists. However, it is primarily species of the Elapidae that utilize neurotoxic venoms. Many species use a combination of toxins along with other agents to increase the efficacy of the toxins. The pit viper, for example, uses a cocktail of haemolytic toxins and other factors. It includes an epidermal growth factor-like hormone mimic to increase vascular permeability to increase efficacy of toxins. The green mamba (*Dendroaspis augusticeps*) is a particularly venomous species of snake. A number of components have been isolated from its venom, including 57- and 59-amino acid peptide trypsin inhibitors as well as a polypeptide toxin, dendrotoxin that blocks KV1.1, KV1.2 and KV1.6 potassium channels. The trypsin inhibitors act to inhibit the proteolytic breakdown of the dendrotoxin in the blood stream of the prey. This extends the action of the dendrotoxin.

A number of species utilize toxins that interact with various ion channels of the nervous system. The cobra (*Naja naja*) utilizes the α-bungarotoxin which acts on the muscarinic acetylcholine receptors M1, M2 and M4 to induce muscle paralysis and other effects on the central nervous system. Helothermine is a 25.5-kDa polypeptide toxin isolated from the Mexican beaded lizard (*Heloderma horridum horridum*). The toxin is a promiscuous ligand that can inhibit at least three pharmacologically distinct Ca^{2+} currents. The evolutionary origin of this toxin may have occurred before the separation of the snakes and lizards. The Australian king brown snake utilizes a 24-kDa polypeptide toxin with some structural similarity to helothermine. However, the king brown snake toxin appears to inhibit the current through cyclic nucleotide-gated ion channels. For example, the toxin can antagonize the cGMP-dependent currents of rat olfactory cyclic nucleotide-gated channels. The toxins in the Mexican beaded lizard and the Australian king brown snake may have had a common evolutionary origin where one toxin was utilized as a cyclic nucleotide-gated ion channel blocker and the other as muscarinic receptor blocker. This may not be unexpected given that there is structural similarity among the ion channel receptors (Chapter 5). An alternative hypothesis is that the common ancestor for both toxins was a non-toxin polypeptide, however this seems less likely.

Although it is likely that the ancestor of the snakes, as it diverged from a lizard-like reptile, possessed some type of toxin, the utilization of toxins in snakes is thought to have played a role in their success as a lineage. A venomous species has the advantage over a non-venomous species in that its contact with prey is limited, and it reduces potential injury to the snake. Many species will bite the prey, inject the venom, then let go. They can then follow the prey and eat at their leisure after the prey is immobilized. In ectothermic species where the ability to supply energy demands may be limited, then the use of venoms to subdue the prey becomes an energetically efficient mechanism for prey capture.

In many parts of the world, the healing properties of some snakes and the venom they contain are prominent in the local folklore. The European asp, for example, is still exploited for its apparently energizing and healing properties. In some parts of north eastern Europe, these snakes are captured and preserved in an alcoholic beverage. As the author has found out, this may mean flavouring a locally produced vodka or whiskey with one of two of the asps, by keeping the snakes in each bottle of the drink. The author's experience with drinking this concoction, during a trip to that part of the world, led to a bout of intense illness followed by a night of wild dreams and hallucinations, then more sickness the following morning. In fairness, however, the nutrient quality of the drink may have been lost by being too enthusiastic to down the beverage.

Toxins and xenobiotics in invertebrates

Both lophotrochozoan and ecdysozoan species produce a dazzling array of toxins and xenobiotics bioactive in other organisms. As invertebrates make up over 95% of the animals species on this planet, we have only barely begun to understand the nature of these biogenic molecules.

Lophotrochozoan species

Among the Lophotrochozoa, the molluscs and annelids have been the best studied in regards to toxins and venoms. The Polychaeta, a class of primarily marine annelids, possesses the most potent neurotoxins of the annelids. The fanged bloodworm, *Glycera dibranchiata*, and a related species *Glycera convolulata* contain a neurotoxin that triggers acetylcholine release by binding to presynaptic membranes. This appears to induce the formation of ion permeable channels that are selective to Na^+ and K^+ and possibly Ca^{2+} and Mg^{2+} that ultimately leads to neurotransmitter release by depolarizing the membrane.

Perhaps some of the most impressive of the venomous invertebrates are the predatory gastropods of the *Conus* genus. Numerous distinct biogenic substances with estimates running as high as 50 000 are produced among these species. Like the anurans, these biogenic compounds include a number of different chemical classes (Fig. 13.8).

Among the best well studied are the conotoxins. The conotoxins are small peptides with a high level of cysteines. Although there is considerable variation among the non-cysteine amino acids, the position of the cysteines show a high level of conservation among paralogues and orthologues (Fig. 13.9). There are several families of conotoxins classified on the basis of their cysteine placements. These peptides have been shown to act as specific Na^+, K^+ or Ca^{2+} channel, NMDA receptor antagonists and nicotinic acetylcholine inhibitors. For example, the conopeptide, SO-3, is a 25-residue peptide with three cysteine bridges that has strong analgesic properties in mice. It may act by inhibiting N-type Ca^{2+} channels. On the other hand, the venom from *Conus anemome* contains a peptide factor that binds neuropeptide Y (NPY). It is unclear what its function is, but one possibility is that it inhibits NPY activity thus lowering the threshold for sympathetic activation and an increased dissemination of the *Conus* toxin constituents. The *Conus* lineage has developed diverse actions of the conopeptides by varying the placements of the cysteines and the number of amino acids in the chain. By this process, the conopeptides can be created in a seemingly endless pattern of three-dimensional structures to fit the binding pocket of theoretically any receptor or protein. We might think of this as an example of a very exquisite biological mechanism for manufacturing receptor and ion channel mimics.

Ecdysozoans

Among the ecdysozoan species, the arthropods, and notably the arachnids (spiders, mites, ticks and scorpions), have developed a variety of toxins mostly for the purpose of predation. However, venoms are also found in numerous insect and centipede species. There are a number of similarities among the venoms used by these organisms, which likely reflect their common evolutionary origins. In many parts of the world, beverages steeped in some of these species have been used as health elixirs, although there are a number of cases of poisoning and deaths associated with such preparations.

Although a number of these toxins are cytolytic pore-forming toxins, a number of species utilize neurotoxins. The Chinese bird spider (*Selenocosmia hainana*) utilizes a 33-amino acid peptide with three sets of cysteine bonds that can block a number of Na^+ channel subtypes. A number of the tarantula toxins, on the other hand, inhibit several types of K^+ channels. The toxin C119 from the scorpion, *Centruroides limpidus limpidus*, is also an inhibitor of Na^+ channels and can have a significant neurodepressant effect in rats when injected into the brains.

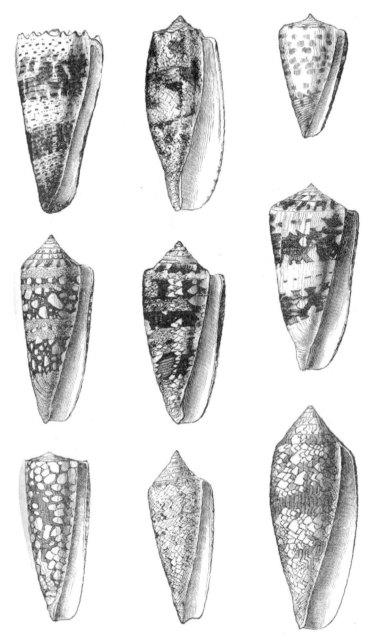

Figure 13.8   Examples of Conus gastropods. From Figuier (1888).

A number of components of insect toxins have been isolated. Both dopamine and nor-epinephrine have been detected in the venom of wasps and honeybees, and epinephrine has been found to be a minor component of bee venom. The pompilidotoxins derived from the venom of the solitary wasp slow Na^+ activation thus acting to facilitate synaptic

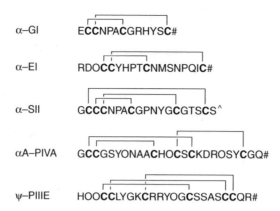

α–GI   ECCNPACGRHYSC#

α–EI   RDOCCYHPTCNMSNPQIC#

α–SII   GCCCNPACGPNYGCGTSCS^

αA–PIVA   GCCGSYONAACHOCSCKDROSYCGQ#

ψ–PIIIE   HOOCCLYGKCRRYOGCSSASCCQR#

Figure 13.9 *Examples of some conotoxins. Modified after Olivera (1997). [Note that 'O' stands for hydroxyproline.]*

transmission. The toxins and venoms produced by the various species may be highly specific for the prey that the insect predator has adapted to. For example, the endoparasitic larvae of the wasp, *Pimpla hypochrondriaca*, utilize a unique polypeptide toxin that does not appear to possess orthologies to any known polypeptide toxins in other species. The adult of this species lays its egg in the pupa of a fly which subsequently secretes a number of agents to paralyse the pupa and prevent it from developing further while the wasp larva feeds on it. Other wasp species are specialized to lay their larvae on a paralysed bee (Fig. 13.10). The tropical ant, *Paraponera clavata*, is also a predator of insect larvae, and utilizes an insect-specific neurotoxin, poneratoxin, which blocks voltage-gated Na^+ channels, blocking synaptic transmission and paralyzing the larva.

A number of insect species have evolved the ability to produce steroid variants that help to ward off vertebrate predators. In the last chapter we discussed the sterol variants synthesized by insects as pheromones. Further development of the biosynthetic enzymes have led to some species producing exact replicas of the steroids found in vertebrates. Some water beetles synthesize and store a number of corticosteroid variants that act as a defence against fish, frogs and small mammal predators. Other species synthesize the sex steroids, oestradiol and testosterone, perhaps as contraceptive method to inhibit the growth of certain populations of predators.

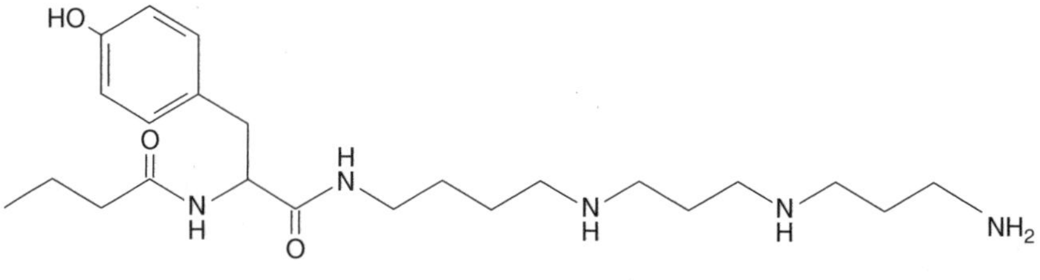

Figure 13.10 *Philanthotoxin, a wasp venom.*

Poriferans and radiates

Recently, both the poriferan (sponges) and cnidarian (sea anemones, jellyfish) have been shown to synthesize a number of bioactive compounds. One might find the number of biogenic compounds that are synthesized by sponge species somewhat surprising. On the other hand, this is one of their main forms of defence. Some of the selective pressures driving the evolution of xenobiotic synthesis in sponges may be similar to that for plants and fungi (p. 358).

Many of these compounds are derived from the isoprenoid synthesis pathway and have been utilized as mimics for 5-HT receptors. In the Jamaican sponge, *Smenospongia aurea*, a number of compounds have been isolated, including at least eight indole alkaloids. At least three of these could displace high affinity antagonists from the human 5-HT2a and 2c subtypes. In addition, alkaloids that could specifically block somatostatin and VIP action in rats have been isolated from the sponge *Xestospongia*. The species *Dysidea herbacea* synthesizes a unique amino acid called dysiherbaine that acts as an agonist for both kainate and AMPA glutamate receptors. The peptide, when injected directly into mouse brain, can induce seizures.

The Cnidaria are characterized by the presence of nematocytes, stinging cells containing venom that play a role in predation and defence. All four classes of cnidarians – Cubozoa (box jellyfish), Scyphozoa (jellyfish), Anthozoa (corals and anemones) and Hydrazoa (hydra-like animals) – possess venoms, although the Cubozoa possesses some of the most poisonous and sometimes lethal species. Cnidarians have a combination toxins in the venom, and these vary from species to species. Currently, cytolytic pore-forming polypeptide toxins, muscarinic receptor and NMDA blockers as well as a number of K^+, Na^+ and Ca^{2+} channel blockers have been identified. Some of the toxins found in cnidarians show considerable specificity for insect Na^+ channels, notably two of the toxins from the sea anemone, *Bunodosoma granulifera*, BgII and BgIII. The natural predators of this species are large crustaceans. Thus the highly specific actions on the insect Na^+ channels likely reflect the phylogenetic relationship of insects and crustaceans and the structural similarity among their respective Na^+ channels.

Toxins and hormone mimics in plants

Plants originated in the Silurian Period about 400–505 million years ago. They have the shortest evolutionary history and are the only kingdom to have completely evolved on land. The rise of the insects was attributable to the advanced colonization of land by plants. The terrestrial evolution of plants occurred in the absence of predators, similar to the situation postulated for the Ediacaran assemblage of species (Chapter 2). The radiation of insects became the first major predatory force that had the potential to affect the survival of plants as a group. Thus, plants that developed a defence against insects could be selected for.

Plant defences fall into three categories. Nutritional defences include nitrogen or amino acid balances that are unfavourable to insects. Physical defences can include the growth of external cuticles and epidermal hairs that make the plants mechanically difficult to hold, manipulate and consume. Plants have also developed a bewildering array of sub-stances that repel or poison an insect. Thus, many of the original chemical defences developed by plants may have had an effect not only on insects but other animals due to the structural similarity of the molecular components in biochemical and endocrine path-ways. Later, with the increased colonization of vertebrates in terrestrial habitats, plants with defences against these more complex organisms with herbivorous diets were selected for. In addition, a number of compounds produced by plants can act as hormone mimics simply due to chance.

In many situations, compounds that have evolved in plants to protect them from grazing by animal species may be particularly toxic to humans. Many toxic species found in one part of the world have been exported to other regions by human activity. The tropical seaweed, *Caulepa taxifola*, for example, has been introduced to the Mediterranean Sea, where it has undergone a massive invasion of new habitats. This species produces caulerpenyne that can cause a depression of the after depolarization of neurons by inhibiting the basal and Na^+ induced activity of a Na^+/K^+ ATPase and a Ca^{2+} dependent K^+ channel. This seaweed has been the cause of a number of poisoning cases in humans who have eaten it by mistake.

Alkaloids are among the largest group of identified bioactive compounds found in plants. Well over 10 000 different alkaloids have been identified. Tubocurarine (Fig. 13.11) is the active ingredient of curare (Chapter 1), a mixture that may include as many as 30 different ingredients. This compound, prepared from the extracts of several plant species from the rainforests of the Amazon and Orinoco, has likely been used since times of antiquity by the indigenous peoples of this region for hunting purposes. Curare induces death by acting as an antagonist to the nicotinic receptors, thus preventing acetylcholine transmission at these sites. The nightshade, *Atropa belladonna*, a species of plants belonging to the Solanaceae, the same group as tomatoes, has been known for over two thousand years as both a medicinal herb and as a toxin. Hyoscyamine is the primary

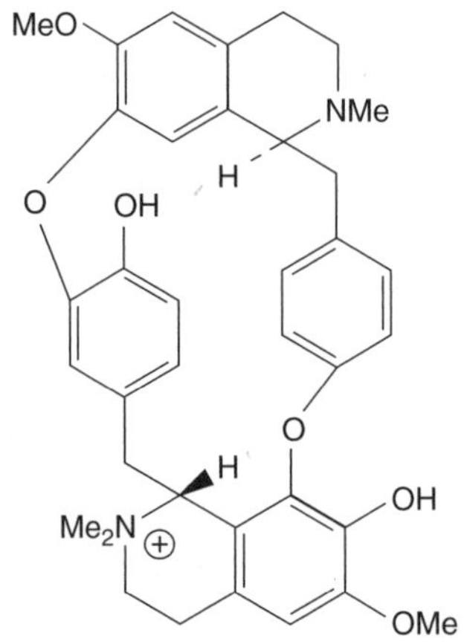

(+)-Tubocurarine

Figure 13.11   *Tubocurarine.*

active ingredient and it antagonizes the muscarinic receptor thus inhibiting acetylcholine transmission in the parasympathetic nervous system. For this reason it has been useful historically as a herbal therapeutic as a sedative or to treat gastrointestinal problems.

Many of these compounds have been used as pharmacological therapeutics in medicine. Our knowledge of plant–animal interactions in the environment can lead to the development of many additional useful compounds. There is some evidence that the therapeutic uses of plants are not limited to humans, however. Tanzanian chimpanzees ingest the leaves of the *Aspilia* plant that contains the chemical thiarubine. This chemical has been implicated in the prevention of infection by some parasites and microorganisms of the gastrointestinal tract. Chimpanzees that ingest this plant have considerably reduced incidence of such infections.

Neurotransmitter and neuromodulator mimics

Many of the basic biosynthetic pathways found in eukaryotic species evolved well before the divergence of plants, fungi and animals, and thus all three kingdoms have a considerable capacity to manufacture bioactive compounds that are similar or identical to compounds found in other kingdoms. Both melatonin and 5-HT have been found in St Johns wort, a plant that has been used to treat depression. The role of these hormones has not been clear in plants. In St Johns wort, 5-HT was in higher concentrations in flower buds at the tetrad stage of microspore development and higher melatonin concentrations were found during uninucleate microsporogenesis. The regeneration potential of isolated anthers was highest in the same stage that had the highest levels of melatonin.

Caffeine (Fig. 13.12) is probably the most consumed psychostimulant. It is consumed as a series of plant extracts as coffee (*Coffea arabica*), black or green tea (*Camellia sinensis*), cocoa (*Theobroma cacao*), guarana (*Paullinia cupana*), mate (*Ilex paraguariensis*) and kola (*Cola nitida*). Caffeine belongs to a class of compounds called methylxanthines. Its primary mode of action is the antagonism of the adenosine receptors. High doses of caffeine can induce a stress-like neuroendocrine effect with increased ACTH, TSH β-endorphin and cortisol concentrations. At millimolar concentrations, methylxanthines can inhibit the phosphosdiesterase enzymes; however, it is unlikely that these concentrations would be achieved under normal caffeine intake regimens.

The opium poppy (*Papaver somniferum*) has probably been exploited for its narcotic properties since Neolithic times. More than 30 different alkaloids have been identified in opium, including morphine, codeine, noscapine and papaverine. The opioid substances

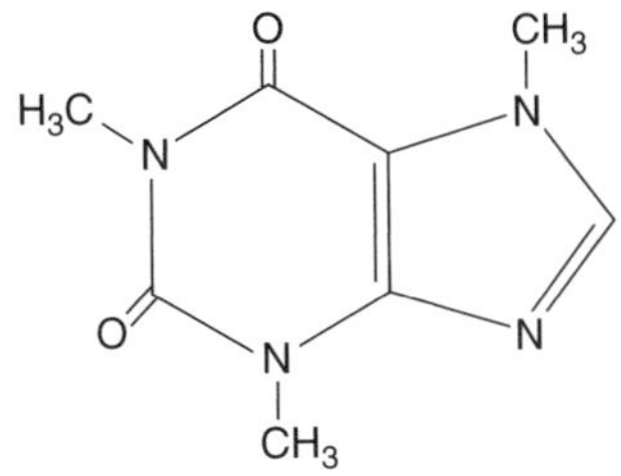

Figure 13.12 *Caffeine.*

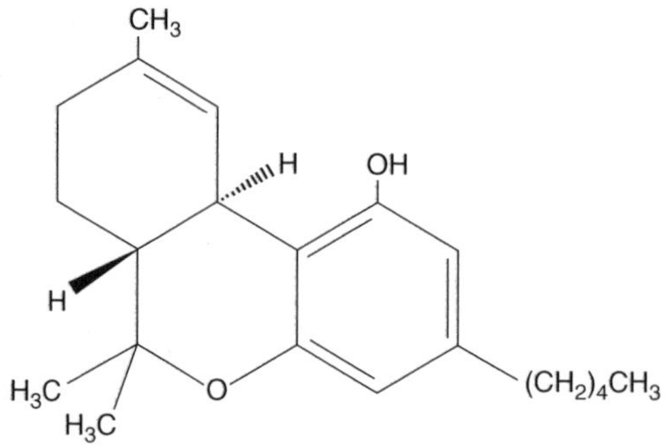

Figure 13.13   *Δ9-Tetrahydrocannabinol, the active ingredient in* Cannabis.

interact with the μ, κ and δ opioid receptor. Morphine inhibits both CRF and GnRH, leading to both a decrease in HPA and HPG activation. Increases in plasma prolactin occur and may be associated with an activation of dopaminergic systems.

The pharmacological uses of *Cannabis sativa* have been documented for almost 5000 years. Around 200 AD Galen (Chapter 1) reported that hemp was commonly being used in cakes and other foods to help lighten the atmosphere at parties. The active ingredient of *Cannabis*, tetrahydrocannabinol (Fig. 13.13), binds to the endocannabinoid receptors in vertebrates (Chapters 5 and 9). Both of these potent plant substances led the way for the isolation and characterization of endogenous hormones in vertebrates, endorphins and cannabinoids respectively, and for the characterization of specific receptors in the brain.

The primary active ingredient in the tobacco plant (*Nicotiana tabacum*) is nicotine, but other active ingredients include nornicotine, anabasine, cotinine and a host of others. Although nicotine is in the highest concentrations, all components appear to play an effect to achieve the psychoactive effects of nicotine. Nicotine initially stimulates the nicotinergic acetylcholine receptors; however, prolonged use of nicotine results in the desensitization of the receptor. Nicotine appears to affect the mesolimbic dopamine cells by binding to their nicotinic cholinergic sites found on the somata and dendrites. This mechanism, in turn, modulates the release of dopamine that mediates the effect of reward. Self-administration of nicotine increased dopamine release in both the ventral tegmental area (VTA) and NAS and nicotine dependence in rats is attenuated by nicotinic receptor antagonists. Nicotine induced FOS immunoreactivity in cholinergic projections from the pedunculo-pontine nuclei, and laterodorsal tegmental nuclei to the VTA. Neurons in the PPTg have a higher expression of FOS than in LDTg, suggesting that the projection for the PPTg to VTA has greater rewarding effects that that of the LDTG. The PPTg may be the primary target or reward signal.

Cocaine is the main ingredient in the plant *Erythroxylon coca*. Some of the other psychoactive ingredients include metabolic variants of cocaine and truxillin. Cocaine acts to block the reuptake mechanisms for dopamine, norepinephrine and epinephrine, thus increasing the amount of these neurotransmitters at synapses. Because of this specificity there is sympathetic activation with cocaine use. Cocaine also has a secondary effect by antagonizing voltage-gated Na^+ channels.

Steroid mimics

The most intensely studied of the hormone mimics are those that possess steroid-like activity. These hormones are among the greatest concern due to their lipophilic activity, are stored in adipose tissue and can bioaccumulate. Moreover, many readily pass through the blood–brain barrier allowing the potential to affect all neural and neuroendocrine processes. Red clover contains alkaloids that mimic oestrogen. Cattle eating red clover suffer from reproductive disturbances. Steroid-synthesizing pathways are well established among a number of plant lineages. A number of species can manufacture phytoecdysteroids that mimic the natural moulting hormones of insects. They are stored in the leaves and act to disrupt the normal development of the insects that feed on them. In sedges, a compound with the same structure as JH in insects is produced. Insects that feed on these plants show a disruption of growth and reproductive ability. Plants can also make a compound that interferes with JH production in insects. This substance, precocene, is processed by the insects' corpora allata and kills the cells. As a result, JH is not produced.

This effect is not limited to insects. 'Phytoestrogen' is a generic term referring to endocrine mimics in plants having oestrogenic activity. The best characterized of the phytoestrogens are the isoflavonoids (Fig. 13.14). Isoflavonoids almost entirely restricted to the Leguminosae/Fabaceae family (peas, beans, clover). Hundreds of different isoflavonoids have been identified. Many have physiologically active oestrogen-like effects. The isoflavonoids, daidzein and coumestrol, from clover have sufficient activity to modulate the reproductive activity of grazing animals. This may have developed due to the evolutionary coexistence with herbivores and plants where there was a need to reduce grazing pressure in order for the plants to survive.

Isoflavones show a number of oestrogenic-like effects in humans. Soy isoflavones have been implicated with decreased plasma testosterone and androstenedione levels in human males. Phytoestrogen-free diets can increase prostate weight. Although increased intake of isoflavones have been implicated with higher bone mineral density in post-menopausal

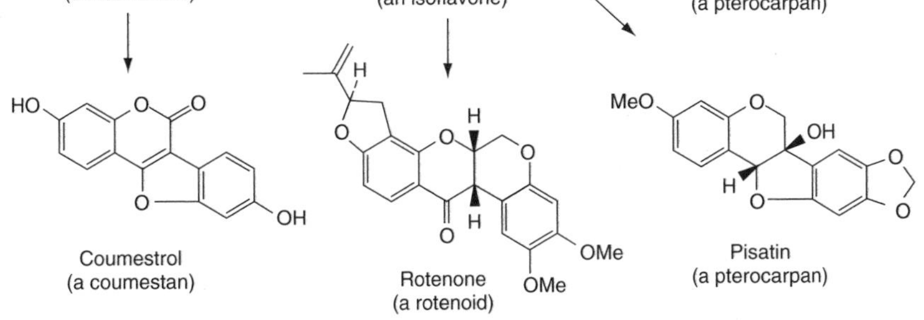

Figure 13.14 *Biosynthetic pathway for isoflavones.*

women, this does not seem to occur in pre-menopausal women and may be associated with a decrease in bone density. Moreover, an increased cardiovascular disease risk in women has been implicated with high isoflavone diets. Isoflavones may also be associated with aberrant menstrual cycles. A number of hormonal profiles have been shown to change. Decreased plasma progesterone and oestradiol concentrations have been documented as well as changes in the T3/T4 ratio. Testosterone and androstenedione levels may also be affected in women. Little is known of the actions of the isoflavones on the foetus. These molecules are likely to cross both the placenta and the blood–brain barrier, and could conceivably have an affect on the developing brain.

Hormone mimics from anthropogenic sources

A wide range of anthropomorphically produced chemicals released into the environment have the capacity to disrupt the endocrine and nervous systems in metazoans (Fig. 13.15). This leads to abnormalities in growth, development, reproduction and behaviour. Pesticides

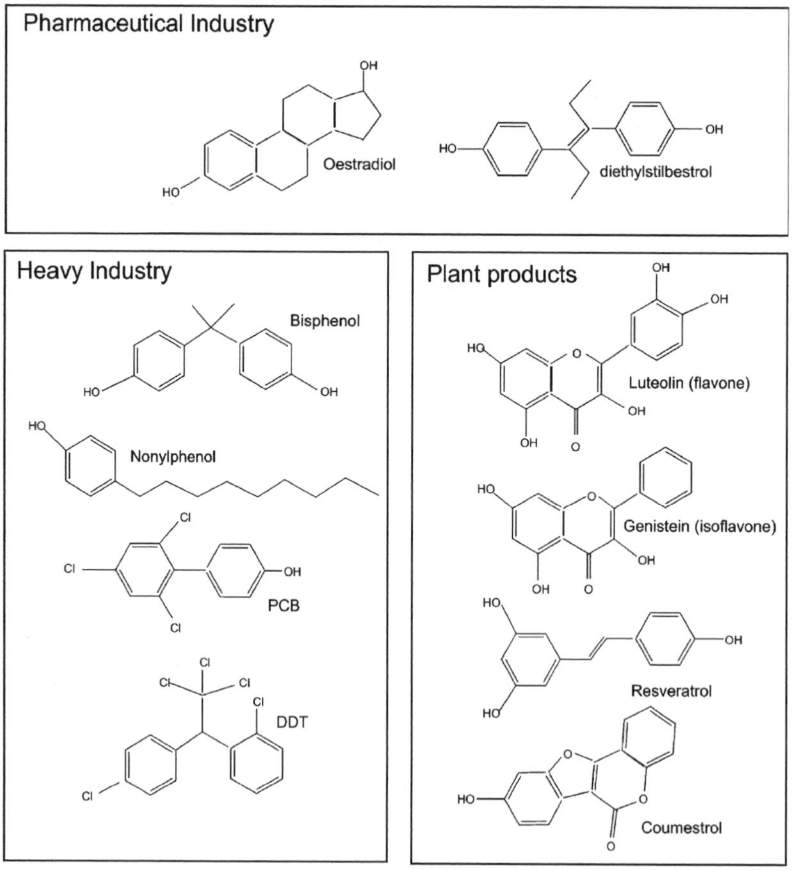

Figure 13.15   *Structures of some hormone mimics and their source. From McLachlan (2001).*

that mimic oestrogens have been shown to alter sexual and reproductive behaviours in birds. In mammals, polychlorinated biphenyls (PCB) and DDT-derived compounds interact with steroid hormone receptors, thyroid hormone receptors and the aryl hydrocarbon receptor. Nonylphenyl can act as an oestrogen agonist, androgen antagonist and can alter gonadotropin synthesis and secretion.

In a number of amphibians and ray-finned fish, there is considerable plasticity in the reproductive development in adults. The presence of exogenous steroids or steroid-like mimics can have significant effects on behaviour and development. In some rivers, industrial waste has induced full or partial sex reversal in 100% of the male fish. Nonylphenol decreases gonadotropins and increases vitellogenin production in the livers of male rainbow trout (*O. mykiss*). Naphthylene and β-naphthaflavone on the other hand can increase steroidogenesis in testes. In the killifish, bisphenol A and nonylphenol can induce vitellogenin synthesis in the male liver. In guppies, DDE and the fungicide vinclozolin have been implicated with reduced male colouration, reduced spermatogenesis, induced altered courtship behaviour and decreased testes size.

There is a worldwide decline in amphibians. A number of these chemicals that mimic steroid, thyroid and possibly retinoic acid hormones can disrupt metamorphosis in frogs, leading to developmental abnormalities. Methroprene and atrazine have been identified as possible thyroid hormone disruptors. In the frog, *Rana pipiens*, 1 µM of dibutylphthalate induce formation of ovaries in 7% of males. Xenopus exposed to DDT and DDE can reduce male colouration and promote female colouration in males. Male frogs generally absorb more of the xenobiotic than female frogs. Bisphenol A or methoxychlor can increase vasotocin to produce antidiuretic effect and decrease the diuretic effect of mesotocin (Chapter 6).

Tributyl tin is a component of an antifouling agent that is applied to ships' hulls. It can accumulate in the ganglia of gastropods and has been implicated with the imposition of male characteristics on female molluscs (imposex). It appears to inhibit the actions of the cytochrome P450-dependent aromatase, thus increasing the levels of androgens and may also involve the actions of a neuroendocrine factor. Although the factor has not been conclusively determined, the neuropeptide APGWamide has been shown to induce imposex in *Llyanassa obsoleta* and therefore tributyl tin may also be acting as an agonist on the APGWamide receptor.

A number of pesticides developed to control insects were developed specifically to interfere with the endocrine system to, for example, disrupt the mechanisms of ecdysterone or JH receptors. However, as we have seen in previous chapters, there is considerable functional similarity between the steroids of arthropods and those of vertebrates.

Chapter summary

Xenobiotics include all biologically active substances that act on a particular individual but are produced outside that individual. Thus, xenobiotics fall into the categories of semiochemicals, venoms and toxins, and metabolic products, which may not have a defined function but are biologically active on other species. All signalling molecules are referred to as semiochemicals. Pheromones are those that signal between individuals within a species, whereas alleochemicals are those that are involved in signalling between species. Alleochemicals are divided into three main groups – kairomones, allomones and synomones. These chemicals may be used as a defence against predators, or grazers, in the case of plant species. They may also be used to lure prey species to a predator. Venoms and toxins are produced by species within all major taxa of the metazoa, and many plant species. The neurologically active toxins act as either agonists or antagonists of neurotransmitter and receptor interactions, or may disrupt normal synaptic communication by specific agents that act on the presynaptic or post-synaptic membranes. Many other toxins, found notably in species of amphibians and some insects, are highly modified hormones that when taken in modify the behaviour of are predator species. Many of the waste products, primarily from anthropogenic activities, mimic hormones in other species and act to disrupt their behaviour, physiology and life cycle, thus threatening the long-term survival of these species.

Glossary

Agonist   A ligand that activates a receptor. An inverse agonist is a ligand that stimulates a receptor into having an opposite response relative to the agonist.

Alkaloid   A heterogenous group of nitrogen containing organic compounds.

Antagonist   A ligand that inhibits a receptor from transducing a signal. A partial antagonist is a ligand that does not completely inhibit the receptor, and therefore has partial activity. A partial antagonist may also be considered a partial agonist.

Autocrine   The action of a chemical signalling molecule being secreted from a particular cell binds to a receptor on that same cell to modify its action in some manner.

Autotrophic   An organism that can synthesize its own food sources directly from an energy source such as light or chemical energy. Plant cells, obtaining energy directly from photosynthesis, are autotrophic.

Chemical ecosystem   The theory that in any complex biological system, molecules are selected by their ability to interact favourably with some molecules and resist degradation by enzymes. They become part of a dynamic equilibrium in a manner analogous to an organismal ecosystem.

Chemotaxis   Locomotion induced by chemical substances.

Dextro   An isomer with a right-handed orientation.

Dimerization   The process of two proteins combining during a transduction process. If the proteins are identical, then it is referred to as homodimerization. If the protein units are different, then it is referred to as heterodimerization.

Dynamic equilibrium   An equilibrium achieved through the active interaction of the components.

Entropy   A tendency for an organized system to move away from order and toward randomness.

Eukaryote   Cells characterized by having organelles derived from a symbiotic relationship with other cells.

Exocrine   Secretions external to the organism.

Hermaphrodite   An organism that possesses functional male and female reproductive organs during the course of their lifetime.

Neuroendocrinology: An Integrated Approach   David A. Lovejoy
© 2005 John Wiley & Sons, Ltd

Heterotrophic   An organism that cannot synthesize its own food materials and must obtain them from the ingestion and digestion of other organisms.

Homeostasis   The process of maintaining a balance in physiological systems.

Homeotherm   An organism that can regulate its own internal temperature.

Hydrophilic   The tendency to be attracted toward water. For complex molecules, this means that they can be dissolved in an aqueous solution.

Hydrophobic   The tendency for a molecule not be dissolved in an aqueous solution. Instead, these molecules will dissolve favourably in solutions that are more lipid-like.

Intracrine   Signalling systems that reside entirely within a cell and are associated with organelle to organelle signalling, or intramolecular interaction within the cytosol for example.

Ionotropic receptor   A receptor that utilizes an ion channel to transduce the ligand receptor interaction.

Isomer   A structurally similar variant of a particular biomolecule.

Last universal common ancestor   The last hypothetical ancestor between prokaryotes and eukaryotes.

Levo   An isomer with a left-handed orientation.

Metabotropic receptor   A receptor system that imparts a structural modification on an accessory protein to transduce the receptor-ligand interaction.

Neurosecretion   Secretion of biogenic and signalling molecules from cells of a neural origin.

Organelle   Structural components within a cell bounded by a lipid bilayer membrane.

Orthologue   A protein or gene present in a particular species that has the same genetic origin as a protein or gene in another species.

Paracrine   Secretion and diffusion of bioactive molecules from one type of cells that effect the action of a different type of cell in the local vicinity. Paracrine secretion does not use the vascular system for transport.

Paralogue   Structurally similar proteins or genes that have arisen from a gene duplication.

Phototaxism   Locomotion to or away from a light source.

Pinocytosis   Uptake of fluids by a cell, using endocytosis.

Poikilotherm   Organisms that cannot internally regulate their internal temperature.

Prokaryote   Cells characterized by naked DNA without a nucleus, a double lipid bilayer membrane, and a lack of organelles (i.e. bacteria).

Protocell   Hypothetical abiotic structures that existed before the first true cells.

Prebiotic synthesis   Synthesis of biogenic compounds before life had evolved.

Stereoisomers   Left and right oriented versions of the same molecule (e.g. L-alanine and D-alanine).

Symbiosis   Organisms sharing resources for the mutual benefit of both organisms.

Thermophilic   Organisms with a tolerance for high ambient temperatures.

References

1 History of neuroendocrinology and neurohormones

General

Boostin, D.J. (1983) The discovers. *A History of Man's Search to Know His World and Himself.* Random House, New York, 745 pages.

Duffin, J. (2000) History of Medicine. *A Scandalously Short Introduction.* University of Toronto Press, Inc., Toronto, 432 pages.

Locy, W.A. (1915) Biology and its Makers. 3rd Edition, Holt, Rinehart and Winston, Inc., New York.

Nordenskiold, E. (1928) *The History of Biology: A Survey.* Tudor Publishing Co., New York, 629 pages.

Wells, H.G., Huxley, J. and Wells, G.P. (1938) *The Science of Life*, Cassell and Company, Ltd, London, 1575 pages.

Ancient science

Aristotle (1951) *De Anima.* In the version of William of Moerbeke and the commentary of St Thomas Aquinas. Translated by Foster, K. and Humphries, S., Routledge & Kegan Paul Ltd, London, 504 pages.

Armstrong, K. (2002) *Islam: A short history*, The Modern Library, Modern Library, New York, 230 pages.

Bennett, D. (2000) Medical practice and manuscripts in Byzantium Soc. *Hist. Med.* 13, 279–291.

Science in the renaissance

Debus, A.G. (1978) *Man and Nature in the Renaissance*, Cambridge University Press, Cambridge, 159 pages.

Sarton, G. (1957) Six wings. *Men of Science in the Renaissance*, Indiana University Press, Bloomington, Indiana, 318 pages.

Neuroendocrinology: An Integrated Approach   David A. Lovejoy
© 2005 John Wiley & Sons, Ltd

Science in the 19th and 20th centuries

Coleman, W. (1971) *Biology in the Nineteenth Century: Problems of Form, Function and Transformation*, Cambridge University Press, Cambridge, 187 pages.
Harris, G.W. (1948) Neural control of the pituitary gland. *Phys. Rev.* 28, 139–179.
Klavdieva, M.M. (1995) The history of neuropeptides I. *Front. Neuroendocrinol.* 16, 293–321.
Olmstead, J.M.D. (1939) Claude Bernard. Cassell and Company, Ltd, London, 318 pages.

2   Origin of life and the first signalling molecules

General

Dyson, F. (1999) *Origins of Life*, 2nd Edition, Cambridge University Press, New York, 100 pages.
Lahav, N., Nir, S. and Elitzur, A.C. (2001) The emergence of life on Earth. *Prog. Biophys. Mol. Biol.* 75, 75–120.
Loewenstein, Werner R. (1999) *The Touchstone of Life: Molecular Information, Cell Communication and the Foundations of Life*, Oxford University Press, New York, 366 pages.
Maynard Smith, John and Szathmáry, Eörs (1999) *The Origins of Life: From the Birth of Life to the Origins of Language*, Oxford University Press, 180 pages.
Morgan, D.E. (2004) *Biosynthesis in Insects*, Royal Society of Chemistry, Cambridge, 199 pages.
Nisbet, E.G. and Sleep, N.H. (2001) The habitat and nature of early life. *Nature*, 409, 1083–1091.
Willis, Christopher and Bada, Jeffrey (2000) *The Spark of Life*, Perseus Publishing, Cambridge, MA, 291 pages.

Prebiotic synthesis of organic compounds

Brinton, K.L., Engrand, C., Glavin, D.P., Bada, J.L. and Maurette, M. (1998) A search for extraterrestrial amino acids in carbonaceous Antarctic micrometeorites. *Orig. Life Evol. Biosph.* 28, 413–424.
Clark, B.C. (2001) Planetary interchange of bioactive material: probability factors and implications. *Orig. Life Evol. Biosph.* 31, 185–197.
Deamer, D.W. (1997) The first living systems: A bioenergetic perspective. *Microbiol. Mol. Biol. Rev.* 61, 239–261.
Dworkin, J.P., Deamer, D.W., Sandford, S.A. and Allmandola, L.J. (2001) Self-assembling amphiphilic molecules: Synthesis in simulated interstellar/precometary ices. *Proc. Natl. Acad. Sci. USA* 98, 815–819.
Podlech, J. (2001) Origin of organic molecules and biomolecular homochirality. *Cell Mol. Life Sci.* 58, 44–60.
Segre, D., Ben-Eli, D., Deamer, D.W. and Lancet, D. (2001) The lipid world. *Orig. Life Evol. Biosph.* 31, 119–145.
Weber, A.L. (2001) The sugar model: Catalysis by amines and amino acid products. *Orig. Life Evol. Biosph.* 31, 71–86.

Origin of genetic material

Dennis, P.P., Omer, A., Lowe, T. (2001) A guided tour: Small RNA function in Archaea. *Mol. Microbiol.* 40, 509–519.

Joyce, G.F. (1989) RNA evolution and the origins of life. *Nature* 338, 217–224.
Lee, D.H., Granja, J.R., Martinez, J.A., Severin, K. and Ghadri, M.R. (1996) A self-replicating peptide. *Nature* 382, 525–528.
Orgel, L.E. (1992) Molecular replication. *Nature* 358, 203–209.
Schwartz, A.W. and Chittenden, G.J. (1977) Synthesis of uracil and thymine under stimulated prebiotic conditions. *Biosystems* 9, 87–92.

Eukaryote and prokaryote divergence

Margulis, Lynn (1998) *Symbiotic Planet: A New Look at Evolution*, Basic Books, New York, 147 pages.
Poole, A., Jeffares, D. and Penny, D. (1999) Early evolution: Prokaryotes, the new kids on the block. *Bioessays* 21, 880–889.
Sandman, K. and Reeve, J.N. (2000) Structure and functional relationships of archaeal and eukaryal histones and nucleosomes. *Arch. Microbiol.* 173, 165–169.

Adsorption of organic materials on mineral surfaces

Edwards, M.R. (1996) Metabolite channeling in the origin of life. *J. Theor. Biol.* 179, 313–322.
Edwards, M.R. (1998) From a soup or a seed? Pyritic metabolic complexes in the origin of life. *Trends Evol. Ecol.* 13, 178–181.
Ferris, J.P., Hill, A.R., Jr, Liu, R. and Orgel, L.E. (1996) Synthesis of long prebiotic oligomers on mineral surfaces. *Nature* 381, 59–61.
Hazen, R.M., Filley, T.R. and Goodfriend, G.A. (2001) Selective adsorption of L and D-amino acids on calcite: Implications for biochemical homochirality. *Proc. Natl. Acad. Sci. USA* 98, 5487–5490.
Mitsuzawa, S. and Watanabe, S.I. (2001) Continuous growth of autocatalytic sets. *Biosystems* 59, 61–69.

3   Rise of metazoans and the elaboration of signalling systems

General

Gee, Henry (1996) *Before the Backbone: Views on the Origin of the Vertebrates*, Chapman & Hall, London, 346 pages.
Maynard, Smith J. and Szathmary, Eors (1995) *The Major Transitions in Evolution*, Oxford University Press, Oxford, 346 pages.
Margulis, L., Schwartz, K.V. (1988) *Five Kindoms*, 2nd Edition, WH Freeman and Company, New York, 376 pages.
Weivel, Ewald R., Taylor, C. Richard and Bolis, Liana (1998) *Principles of Animal Design*, Cambridge University Press, Cambridge, 314 pages.

Precambrian explosion

Gould, S.J. (1989) *Wonderful Life: The Burgess Shale and the Nature of Discovery*, W.W. Norton & Company, New York, 346 pages.
McMenamin, Mark A.S. (1998) *The Garden of Ediacara: Discovering the First Complex Life*, Columbia University Press, New York, 295 pages.

Miyata, T. and Suga, H. (2001) Divergence pattern of animal gene families and relationship with Cambrian explosion. *Bioessays* 23, 1018–1027.

Ohno, S. (1998). The notion of the Cambrian Pananimalia genome and a genomic difference that separated vertebrates from invertebrates. In *Progress in Molecular and Subcellular Biology*, Ed. Muller, W.E.G, Vol. 21, Springer-Verlag, pp. 97–117.

Evolution of the nervous system

Albert, J. (1999) Computational modeling of an early evolutionary stage of the nervous system. *Biosystems* 54, 77–90.

Lawn, I.D., Mackie, G.O. and Silver, G. (1981) Conduction system in a sponge. *Science* 211, 1169–1171.

Leys, S.P. and Degnan, B.M. (2001) Cytological basis of photoresponsive behavior in a sponge larva. *Biol. Bull.* 201, 323–338.

Symmetry and development

Bosch, T.C.G. (2003) Ancient signals: peptides and the interpretation of positional information in ancestral metazoans. *Comp. Biochem. Physiol. B* 136, 185–196.

Hobmayer, B., Rentzsch, F., Kuhn, K., Happel, C.M., Cramer, von Laue C., Snyder, P., Rothbacher, U. and Holstein, T. (2000) WNT signalling molecules act in axis formation in the diploblastic metazoan *Hydra. Nature* 407, 186–189.

Schutze, J., Skorokhod, A., Muller, I.M. and Muller, W.E. (2001) Molecular evolution of the metazoan extracellular matrix: Cloning and expression of structural proteins from the demosponges *Suberites domuncula* and *Geodia cydonium. J. Mol. Evol.* 53, 402–415.

Steele, R. (2002) Developmental signaling in hydra: What does it take to build a 'simple' animal. *Dev. Biol.* 248, 199–219.

Takahashi, T., Koizuma, O., Arimura, Y., Romanovitch, A., Bosch, T.C.G., Kobayakawa, Y., Mohri, S., Bode, H.R., Yum, S., Hatta, M. and Fujisawa, T. (2000) A novel peptide Hym355 positively regulates neuron differentiation in hydra. *Development* 127, 997–1005.

Evolution of hormone systems

Chan, S.J., Oliva, A.A., La, Mendola J., Grens, A., Bode, H. and Steiner, D.F. (1992) Conservation of the prohormone convertase gene family in metazoa. Analysis of the cDNAs encoding a PC3-like protein from hydra. *Proc. Natl. Acad. Sci. USA* 89, 6678–6682.

De Petrocellis, L., Melck, D., Bisogno, T., Milone, A. and Di Marzo, V. (1999) Finding of the endocannabinoid signalling system in hydra, a very primitive organism: Possible role in the feeding response. *Neuroscience* 92, 377–387.

Lagna, G. and Hemmat-Brivanlou, A. (1999) A molecular basis for SMAD specificity. *Dev. Dyn.* 214, 269–277.

Morishita, F., Nitagai, Y., Furukawa, Y., Matshshima, O., Takahashi, T., Hatta, M., Fujisawa, T., Tunamoto, S. and Koizuma, O. (2003) Identification of a vasopressin-like immunoreactive substance in hydra. *Peptides* 24, 17–26.

Perovic, S., Krasko, A., Prokic, I., Muller IM. and Muller, W.E. (1999) Origin of neuronal-like receptors in the metazoa: Cloning of a metabotropic glutamate/GABA-like receptor from the marine sponge *Geodia cydonium. Cell Tissue Res.* 296, 395–404.

Pires-daSilva A. and Sommer, R.J. (2002) The evolution of signalling pathways in animal development. *Nat. Rev. Gen.* 4, 39–49.

Genome evolution

Lundin, L.G., Larhammar, D. and Hallbook, F. (2003) Numerous groups of chromosomal regional paralogies strongly indicate two genome doublings at the root of the vertebrates. *J. Struct. Funct. Genomics* 3, 53–63.
Suga, H., Koyanagi, M., Hoshiyama, D., Ono, K., Iwabe, N., Kuma, K. and Miyata, T. (1999) Extensive gene duplication in the early evolution of animals before the parazoan-eumetazoan split demonstrated by G-proteins and protein tyrosine kinases from sponge and hydra. *J. Mol. Evol.* 48, 646–653.

4   Elaboration of neuroendocrine systems

General

Bentley, P.J. (1998) *Comparative Vertebrate Endocrinology*, 3rd Edition, Cambridge University Press, Cambridge, 526 pages.
Butler, A.B. and Hodos, W. (1996) Comparative vertebrate neuroanatomy. *Evolution and Adaption*, Wiley Liss Inc., New York, 514 pages.
Carpenter, M.B. (1991) *Core Text of Neuroanatomy*, 4th Edition, Williams and Wilkins, Baltimore, USA.
Gullan, P.J. and Cranston, P.S. (1994) *The Insects: An Outline of Entomology*, Chapman & Hall, Inc., London, 491 pages.
Kershaw, D.R. (1988) *Animal Diversity*, Chapman & Hall, Inc., London, 428 pages.

Metazoan phylogeny

Blair, J.E., Ikeo, K., Gojobori, T., Blair Hedges, S.B. (2002) The evolutionary position of nematodes. *BMC Evol. Biol.* 2, 7.
Bourlat, S.J., Nielsen, C., Lockyer, A.E., Littlewood, D.T. and Telford, M.J. (2003) *Xenoturbella* is a deuterostome that eats molluscs. *Nature* 424, 925–928.
Davis, G.K., Patel, N.H. (1999) The origin and evolution of segmentation. *Trends Gen.* 15, M68–M72.
Kotikova, E.A., Raikova, O.I., Reuter, M. and Gustafsson, M.K.S. (2002) The nervous and muscular systems in the free living flatworm *Castrella truncata* (Rhabdocoela): An immunocytochemical and phalloidin fluorescence study. *Tissue Cell* 34, 365–374.
Mineta, K., Nakazawa, M., Cebria, F., Ikeo, K., Agata, K. and Gojobori, T. (2003) Origin and evolutionary process of the CNS elucidated by comparative genomics analysis of planarian ESTs. *Proc. Natl. Acad. Sci. USA* 100, 7666–7671.

Hypothalamus and pituitary evolution

Kawamura, K., Kouki, T., Kawahara, G. and Kikuyama, S. (2002) Hypophyseal development in vertebrates from amphibians to mammals. *Gen. Comp. Endocrinol.* 126, 130–135.
Markakis, E.A. (2002) Development of the neuroendocrine hypothalamus. *Front. Neuroendocrinol.* 23, 257–291.

Hormone systems

Brownwell, P.H., Ligman, S.H. (1992) Mechanisms of circulatory homeostasis and response in *Aplysia. Experientia* 48, 818–827.

Buttarelli, F.R., Pontieri, F.E., Margotta, V. and Palladini, G. (2000) Acetylcholine/dopamine interaction in planaria. *Comp. Biochem. Physiol., C* 125, 225–231.

Buttarelli, F.R., Pontieri, F.E., Margotta, V., Palladina, G. (2002) Cannabinoid-induced stimulation of motor activity in planaria through an opioid receptor mediated mechanism. *Prog. Neuropsychopharmacol. Biol. Psychiatry* 26, 65–68.

Gustafsson, M.K.S., Halton, D.W., Kreshchenko, N.D., Movsessian, S.O., Raikova, O.I., Reuter, M. and Terenina, N.B. (2002) Neuropeptides in flatworms. *Peptides* 23, 2053–2061.

Hay-Schmidt, A. (2000) The evolution of the serotonergic nervous system. *Proc. R. Soc. Lond. B* 267, 1071–1079.

Itoh, M.T. and Igarashi, J. (2000) Circadian rhythm of serotonin levels in planarians. *Neuroreport* 11, 473–476.

McPartland, J., Di Marzo, V., De Petrocellis, L., Mercer, A. and Glass, M. (2001) Cannabinoid receptors are absent in insects. *J. Comp. Neurol.* 436, 423–429.

Nathoo, A.N., Moeller, R.A., Westlund, B.A. and Hart, A.C. (2001) Identification of neuropeptide-like protein gene families in *Caenorhabditus elegans* and other species. *Proc. Natl. Acad. Sci. USA* 98, 14000–14005.

Raikova, O.I., Reuter, M., Jonelius, U. and Gustafsson, M.K.S. (2000) The brain of the Nemeretodermatida (Platyhelminthes) as revealed by anti-5HT and anti-FMRFamide immunostainings. *Tissue Cell* 32, 358–365.

Whim, M.D., Church, P.J. and Lloyd, P.E. (1993) Functional roles of peptide co-transmitters at neuromuscular synapses in Aplysia. *Mol. Neurobiol.* 73, 335–347.

Blood brain barrier

Kastin, A.J., Pan, W., Maness, L.M. and Banks, W. (1999) Peptides crossing the blood-brain barrier: Some unusual observations. *Brain Res.* 848, 96–100.

Brain evolution

Nakazawa, M., Cebria, F., Mineta, K., Ikeo, K., Agata, K. and Gojobori, T. (2003) Search for the evolutionary origin of a brain: Planarian brain characterized by microarray. *Mol. Biol. Evol.* 20, 784–791.

Reichert, H. and Simeone, A. (2001) Developmental genetic evidence for a monophyletic origin of the bilaterian brain. *Philos Trans R. Soc. Lond. B Biol. Sci.* 356, 1533–1544.

Ruiz-Trillo, I., Ruitort, M., Littlewood, T.J., Herniou, E.A. and Baguna, J. (1999) Acoel flatworms: Earliest extant bilaterian metazoans, not members of the Platyhelminthes. *Science* 283, 1919–1923.

Sarnat, H.B. and Netsky, M.G. (2002) When does a ganglion become a brain? Evolutionary origin of the central nervous system. *Semin. Pediatr. Neurol.* 9, 240–253.

Younossi-Hartenstein, A., Jones, M. and Hartenstein, V. (2001) Embryonic development of the nervous system of the temnocephalid flatworm *Craspedella pedum. J. Comp. Neurol.* 434, 56–68.

Autonomic nervous system

Hartenstein, V. (1997) Development of the insect stomatogastric nervous system. *Trends Neurosci.* 20, 421–427.

5 Neurohormones and receptors: Structure, function and co-evolution

General

Strand, F. (1999) Neuropeptides. *Regulators of Physiological Processes*, MIT Press, Cambridge, MA 658 pages.

Steroid-thyroid receptor superfamily and their ligands

Ahuja, H.S., Szanto, A., Nagy, L. and Davies, P.J. (2003) The retinoid X receptor and its ligands: Versatile regulators of metabolic function, cell differentiation and cell death. *J. Biol. Regul. Homeost. Agents* 17, 29–45.
Baker, M.E. (2002) Albumin, steroid hormones and the origin of vertebrates. *J. Endocrinol.* 175, 121–127.
Bonneton, F., Zelus, D., Iwema, T., Robinson-Rechavi, M. and Laudet, V. (2003) Rapid divergence of the ecdysone receptor in *Diptera* and *Lepidoptera* suggests coevolution between ECR and USP-RXR. *Mol. Biol. Evol.* 20, 541–553.

Growth factors and receptor kinases

Carter-Su, C. and Smit, L.S. (1998) Signalling via JAK tyrosine kinases: Growth hormone receptor as a model system. *Recent. Prog. Horm. Res.* 53, 61–82.
Gu, J. and Gu, X. (2003) Natural history and functional divergence of protein tyrosine kinases. *Gene* 317, 49–57.

Glutamate, GABA and their receptors

Davenport, R. (2002) Glutamate receptors in plants. *Ann Bot. (Lond.)* 90, 549–557.
Gready, J.E., Ranganathan, S., Schofield, P.R., Matsuo, Y. and Nishikawa, K. (1997) Predicted structure of the extracellular region of ligand gated ion channel receptors shows SH2-like and SH3-like domains forming the ligand-binding site. *Protein Sci.* 6, 983–998.

Receptor-ligand evolution

Baker, M.E. (2003) Evolution of adrenal and sex steroid action in vertebrates: A ligand-based mechanism for complexity. *Bioessays* 25, 396–400.
Boulay, J.L., O'Shea, J.J., Paul, W.E. (2003) Molecular phylogeny within Type I cytokines and their cognate receptors. *Immunity* 19, 159–163.
Thornton, J.W., Need, E. and Crews, D. (2003) Resurrecting the ancestral steroid receptor: Ancient origin of estrogen signaling. *Science* 301, 1714–1717.

6 Osmoregulation, metabolism and energy production

General

Kacsoh, B. (2000) *Endocrine Physiology*, McGraw-Hill, New York, 741 pages.
Schulkin, J. (1999) *The Neuroendocrine Regulation of Behaviour*, Cambridge University Press, Cambridge, 323 pages.

Diuresis

Acher, R. (1999) Organismal versus molecular evolution: Insights from neurophysiological hormone systems. In *Recent Developments in Comparative Endocrinology and Neurobiology.* Eds Roubas, E., Wendelaar Bonga, S.E., Vaudry, H. and De Loof A. Shaker Publishing BV, Maastricht, pp. 8–12.

Acher, R., Chauvet, J. and Chavet, M.T. (1995) Man and the chimaera. Selective vs neutral oxytocin evolution. *Adv. Exp. Med. Biol.* 395, 615–627.

Fitzsimons, J.T. (1998) Angiotensin, thirst and sodium appetite. *Physiol. Rev.* 78, 583–686.

Salzet, M., Deloffre, L., Breton, C., Vieau, D. and Schoofs, L. (2001) The angiotensin system elements in invertebrates. *Brain Res. Rev.* 36, 35–45.

Te Brugge, V.A., Schooley, D.A. and Orchard, I. (2002) The biological activity of diuretic factors in *Rhodnius prolixus*. *Peptides* 23, 671–681.

Calcium regulation

Aboufatima, R., Chait, A., Dalal, A. and de Beaurepaire, R. (1999) Calcitonin microinjection into the periaqueductal gray impairs contextual fear conditioning in the rat. *Neurosci. Lett.* 275, 101–104.

Buervenich, S., Xiang, F., Sydow, O., Jonnson, E.G., Sedvall, G.C., Anvret, M. and Olson, L. (2001) Identification of four novel polymorphisms in the calcitonin/alpha-CGRP (CALCA) gene and an investigation of their possible associations with Parkinson's disease, schizophrenia and manic depression. *Hum. Mutat.* 17, 435–436.

Coast, G.M., Webster, S.G., Schegg, K.M., Zhang, J., Tobe, S.S. and Schooley, D.A. (2001) The *Drosophila melanogaster* homologue of an insect calcitonin-like diuretic peptide stimulates V-ATPase activity in fruit fly Malpighian tubule. *J. Exp. Biol.* 204, 1795–1804.

Dubrovsky, S.L., Murphy, J., Christiano, J. and Lee, C. (1992) The calcium secondary messenger system in bipolar disorders: Data supporting new research directions. *J. Neuropsychiatry Clin. Neurosci.* 4, 3–14.

Dubrovsky, S.L., Thomas, M., Hijazi, A. and Murphy, J. (1994) Intracellular calcium signalling in peripheral cells of patients with bipolar affective disorder. *Eur. Arch Psychiatry Clin. Neurosci.* 243, 229–234.

Furuya, K., Mikchak, R.J., Schegg, K.M., Zhang, J., Tobe, S.S., Coast, G.M. and Schooley, D.A. (2000) Cockroach diuretic hormones: Characterization of a calcitonin-like peptide in insects. *Proc. Natl. Acad. Sci. USA* 97, 6469–6474.

Koh, P.O., Undie, A.S., Kabbani, N., Levenson, R., Goldman-Rakic, P.S. and Lidow, M.S. (2003) Up-regulation of neuronal calcium sensor-1 (NCS-1) in the prefrontal cortex of schizophrenic and bipolar patients. *Proc. Natl. Acad. Sci. USA* 100, 313–317.

Mathe, A.A., Agren, H., Wallin, A. and Blennow, K. (2002) Calcitonin gene-related peptide and calcitonin in the CSF of patients with dementia and depression. *Prog. Neuropsychopharmacol. Biol. Psychiatry* 26, 41–48.

Nakamoto, H., Soeda, Y., Takami, S., Minami, M. and Satoh, M. (2000) Localization of calcitonin receptor mRNA in the mouse brain: Coexistence with serotonin transporter mRNA. *Mol. Brain Res.* 76, 93–102.

Vik, A. and Yatham, L.N. (1998) Calcitonin and bipolar disorder: A hypothesis revisted. *J. Psychiatry Neurosci.* 23, 109–117.

Energy and nutrition

Elekonich, M.M. and Horodyski, F.M. (2003) Insect allatotropins belong to a family of structurally-related myoactive peptides present in several invertebrate phyla. *Peptides* 24, 1623–1632.

Grill, H.J. and Kaplan, J.M. (2002) The neuroanatomical control of energy balance. *Front. Neuroendocrinol.* 23, 2–40.

7 Growth and development

General

Schulkin, J. (1999) *The Neuroendocrine Regulation of Behavior*, Cambridge University Press, Cambridge, 323 pages.

Sexual differentiation

Dorner, G., Docke, F. and Gotz, F. (1975) Male-like sexual behaviour of female rats with unilateral lesions in the hypothalamic ventromedial nuclear region. *Endokrinologie* 65, 133–137.

Gorski, R.A. (1985) Sexual dimorphisms of the brain. *J. Anim. Sci. Suppl.* 3, 38–61.

Gorski, R.A. (1993) Estradiol acts via the estrogen receptor in the sexual differentiation of the rat brain, but what does this complex do? *Endocrinology* 133, 431–432.

Jansson, J.O. and Frohmann, L.A. (1987) Inhibitory effect of the ovaries on neonatal androgen imprinting of growth hormone secretion in female rats. *Endocrinology* 121, 1417–1423.

LeVay, S. (1994) *The Sexual Brain*, MIT Press, Cambridge, MA, 172 pages.

Mong, J.A. and McCarthy, M.M. (1999) Steroid-induced developmental plasticity in hypothalamic astrocytes. Implications for synaptic patterning. *J. Neurobiol.* 40, 602–619.

Roof, R.L. (1993) The dentate gyrus is sexually dimorphic in prepubescent rats: Testosterone plays a role. *Brain Res.* 610, 148–151.

Regulation of growth

Aguila, M.C., Marubayashi, U. and McCann, S.M. (1992) The effect of galanin on growth hormone-releasing factor and somatostatin release from median eminence fragments in vitro. *Neuroendocrinology* 56(6), 889–894

Bole-Feysot, C., Goffin, V., Edery, M., Binart, N. and Kelly, P.A. (1998) Prolactin (PRL) and its receptor: Actions, signal transduction pathways and phenotypes observed in PRL receptor knockout mice. *Endocr. Rev.* 19, 225–268.

Chan, Y.Y., Grafstein-Dunn, E., Delemarre-van de Waal, H.A., Burton, K.A., Clifton, DK. and Steiner, R.A. (1996) The role of galanin and its receptor in the feedback regulation of growth hormone secretion. *Endocrinology* 137(12), December, 5303–5310.

Eigenmann, J.E., Patterson, D.F. and Froesch, E.R. (1984) Body size parallels insulin-like growth factor I levels but not growth hormone secretory capacity. *Acta Endocrinol. (Copenh)* 106, 448–453.

Favier, R.P., Mol, J.A., Koostra, H.S. and Rijnberk, A. (2001) Large body size in the dog is associated with transient GH excess at a young age. *Journal of Endocrionology* 170, 479–484.

Gerfen, C.R., Engber, T.M., Mahan, L.C., Susel, Z., Chase, T.N. and Monsma, F.J., Jr (1990) D1 and D2 dopamine receptor-regulated gene expression of strianigral and striatopallidal neurons. *Science* 250, 1429–1432.

Hansen, G.N., Hansen, B.L. and Scharrer, B. (1988) Diversity of prolactin systems in the insect *Leucophaea maderae*: Use of antiserum polyclonality for immunocytochemical detection of neuropeptide heterogeneity. *Cell Tissue Res.* 252, 557–563.

Kelley, K.M., Schmidt, K.E., Berg, K., Sak, K., Galima, M.M., Gillespie, C., Balogh, L., Hawayek, A., Reyes, J.A. and Jamison, M. (2002) Comparative endocrinology of the insulin-like growth factor binding protein. *J. Endocrinol.* 175, 3–18.

Liposits, Z., Merchenthaler, I., Reid, J.J. and Negro-Vilar, A. (1993) Galanin-immunoreactive axons innervate somatostatin-synthesizing neurons in the anterior periventricular nucleus of the rat. *Endocrinology* 132(2), 917–923.

Liu, B., Wakuri, H. and Mutoh, K. (1996) Prolactin in the cestodes, *Taenia solium* and *Taenia hydatigena*: An immunocytochemical study. *Okajimas Folia Anat. Jpn* 73, 25–35.

Lopez, FJ. and Negro-Vilar, A. (1990) Galanin stimulates luteinizing hormone-releasing hormone secretion from arcuate nucleus-median eminence fragments in vitro: Involvement of an alpha-adrenergic mechanism. *Endocrinology* 127(5), 2431–2436.

Moore, J.P., Jr, Cai, A., Maley, B.E., Jennes, L. and Hyde, J.F. (1999) Galanin within the normal and hyperplastic anterior pituitary gland: Localization, secretion, and functional analysis in normal and human growth hormone-releasing hormone transgenic mice. *Endocrinology* 140(4), 1789–1799.

Moore, J.P. Jr, Morrison, D.G. and Hyde, J.F. (1994) Galanin gene expression is increased in the anterior pituitary gland of the human growth hormone-releasing hormone transgenic mouse. *Endocrinology* 134(5), 2005–2010.

Nap, R.C., Mol, J.A. and Hawewinkel, H.A. (1993) Age-related plasma concentrations of growth hormone (GH) and insulin-like growth factor I (IGF-1) in Great Dane pups fed different dietary levels of protein. *Domest. Anim. Endocrinol.* 10, 237–247.

Parker, M.S. and Ourth, D.D. (1999) Specific binding of human interferon-gamma to particulares from hemolympth and protocerebrum of tobacco hornworm (*Manduca sexta*). *Comp. Biochem. Physiol. B* 122, 155–163.

Schmid, K.P., Maier, V., Huag, C. and Pfeiffer, E.F. (1990) Ultrastructural localization of prolactin-like antigenic determinants in neurosecretory cells in the brain of the honeybee (*Apis mellifica*). *Horm. Metab. Res.* 22, 413–417.

Swinnen, K., Broeck, J.V., Verhaert, P. and De Loof, A. (1990) Immunocytochemical localization of human growth hormone and prolactin-like antigenic determinants in the insects, *Locusta migratoria* and *Sarcophaga bullata*. *Comp. Biochem. Physiol. A* 95, 373–378.

Terakado, K., Ogawa, M., Inoue, K., Yamamotoa, K. and Kikuyama, S. (1997) Prolactin-like immunoreactivity in the granules of neural complex cells of the ascidian *Halocynthia roretzi*. *Cell Tissue Res.* 289, 63–71.

Veenstra, J.A., Romberg-Privee, H.M., Schooneveld, H. and Polak, J.M. (1985) Immunocytochemical localization of peptidergic neurons and neurosecretory cells in the neuroendocrine system of the Colorad potato beetle with antisera to vertebrate regulatory peptides. *Histochemistry* 82, 9–18.

Metamorphosis

Barron, M.G. (1986) Endocrine control of smoltification in anadromous salmonids. *J. Endocrinol.* 108, 313–319.

Carr, J.A. and Norris, D.O. (1990) Immunohistochemical localization of corticotropin-releasing factor- and arginine vasotocin-like immunoreeactivities in the brain and pituitary of the American bullfrog (*Rana catesbeiana*) during development and metamorphosis. *Gen. Comp. Endocrinol.* 78, 180–188.

Denver, R.J. (1988) Several hypothalamic peptides stimulate in vitro thyrotropin secretion by pituitaries of anuran amphibians. *Gen. Comp. Endocrinol.* 72, 383–393.

Denver, R.J. (1997) Environmental stress as a developmental cue: Corticotropin-releasing hormone is a proximate mediator of adaptive phenotypic plasticity in amphibian metamorphosis. *Horm. Behav.* 31, 169–179.

Denver, R.J. (1998) Hormonal correlates of environmentally induced in the western spadefoot toad, *Scaphiopus hammondii*. *Gen. Comp. Endocrinol.* 110, 326–336.

Kuenzel, W.J. (2003) Neurobiology of molt in avian species. *Poult. Sci.* 82, 981–991.

Kulczykowska, E., Sokolowska, E., Takvam, B., Stefansson, S. and Ebbesson, L. (2004) Influence of exogenous thyroxine on plasma melatonin in juvenile Atlantic salmon (*Salmo salar*). *Comp. Biochem. Physiol. B* 137, 43–47.

Kuhn, E.R., Geris, K.L., van der Geyten, S., Mol, K.A. and Darras, V.M. (1998) Inhibition and activation of the thyroid axis by the adrenal axis in vertebrates. *Comp. Biochem. Physiol. A* 120, 169–174.

Ageing

O'Neil, P.A. (1992) Neuroendocrinology and ageing. *Med. Lab Sci.* 49, 283–290.
Niimi, M., Takahara, J. and Kawanishi, K. (1992) Corticotropin releasing factor and galanin-containing neurons projecting to the median eminence of the rat. *Neurosci. Res.* 14, 295–299.

8   Biological rhythms

General

Elliott, J.A. (1976) Circadian rhythms and photoperiodic time measurement in mammals. *Fed. Proc.* 35, 2339–2346.

Melatonin

Dubocovich, M.L. (1995) Melatonin receptors: Are there three multiple subtypes? *Trends Pharmacol. Sci.* 16, 50–56.
Dubocovich, M.L. and Takahashi, J.S. (1987) Use of 2-[125I]iodomelatonin to characterize melatonin binding sites in chicken retina. *Proc. Nat. Acad. Sci. USA* 84, 3916–3920.
Goldman, B.D. and Nelson, R.J. (1993) Melatonin and seasonality in mammals. In *Melatonin: Biosynthesis, Physiological Effects and Clinical Applications*, Eds Hu, H.S. and Reiter, R.J. CRC Press, Boca Raton, FL, 225–252.
Larsen, P.J., Enquist, L.W., Card, J.P. (1998) Characterization of the multisynaptic neuronal control of the rat pineal gland using viral transneuronal tracing. *Eur. J. Neurosci.* 10, 128–145.
Reiter, R.J. (1991) Pineal gland: interface between the photoperiodic environment and the endocrine system. *Trends. Endocrinol. Metab.* 2, 13–19.
Sugden, D. (1989) Melatonin biosynthesis in the mammalian pineal gland. *Experientia* 45, 922–932.

Seasonal rhythms

Bole-Feysot, C., Goffin, V., Edery, M., Binart, N. and Kelly, P.A. (1998) Prolactin (PRL) and its receptor: Actions, signal transduction pathways and phenotypes observed in PRL receptor knockout mice. *Endocrine Rev.* 19(3), 225–268.
Curlewis, J.D. (1992) Seasonal prolactin secretion and its role in seasonal reproduction: A review. *Reproduction, Fertility and Development* 4, 1–23.
Dutt, A., Kaplitt, M.G., Kow, L.-M. and Pfaff, D.W. (1994) Prolactin, central nervous system and behavior: A critical review. *Neuroendocrinology* 59, 413–419.
Goldman, B.D., Matt, K.S., Roychoudhury, P. and Stetson, M.H. (1981) Prolactin release in golden hamster: Photoperiod and gonadal influences. *Biol. Reprod.* 24, 287–292.
Lincoln, G.A. and Short, R.V. (1980) Seasonal breeding: Natures contraceptive. *Recent Prog. Horm. Res.* 36, 1–52.
Heydon, M.J., Milne, J.A., Brinklow, B.R. and Loudon, A.S.I. (1995) Manipulating melatonin in Red deer: Differences in the response to food restriction and lactation on the timing of the breeding season and prolactin dependent pelage changes. *J. Exp. Zool.* 273, 12–20.

Kennaway, D.J., Gilmore, T.A. and Seamark, R.F. (1982) Effect of melatonin feeding on serum prolactin and gonadotropin levels and the onset of seasonal estrous cyclicity in sheep. *Endocrinology* 110(5), 1766–1772.

Lincoln, G.A. and Clarke, I.J. (1994) Photoperiodically-induced cycles in the secretion of prolactin in hypothalamo-pituitary disconnected rams: Evidence for translation of the melatonin signal in the pituitary gland. *J. Neuroendocrinol.* 6, 251–260.

Lincoln, G.A. and Clarke, I.J. (1995) Evidence that melatonin acts in the pituitary gland through a dopamine-independent mechanism to mediate effects of daylength on the secretion of prolactin in the ram. *J. Neuroendocrinol.* 7(8), 637–643.

Lincoln, G.A., Libre, E.A. and Merriam, G.R. (1989) Long-term reproductive cycles in rams after pinealectomy or superior cervical ganglionectomy. *J. Reprod. Fertil.* 85, 687–704.

Mrosovsky, N. (1995) A non-photic gateway to the circadian clock of hamsters. *Ciba Foundation Symposium* 183, Wiley and Sons, Chichester, pp. 154–174.

Mrosovsky, N. (1996) Locomotor activity and non-photic influences on circadian clocks. *Biol. Rev.* 71, 343–372.

Reiter, R.J. (1975) Exogenous and endogenous control of the annual reproductive cycle in the male golden hamster: Participation of the pineal gland. *J. Exp. Zool.* 191, 111–120.

Reiter, R.J. (1991) Pineal gland: Interface between the photoperiodic environment and the endocrine system. *Trends Endocrinol. Metab.* 2, 13–19.

Reiter, R.J. (1991) Pineal melatonin: Cell biology of its synthesis and its physiological interactions. *Endocrine Rev.* 12, 151–180.

Ruby, N.F., Nelson, R.J., Licht, P. and Zucker, I. (1993) Prolactin and testosterone inhibit torpor in Siberian hamsters. *Am. J. Physiol.* 264(1), Part 2, R123–R128.

Ruby, N.F. and Zucker, I. (1992) Daily torpor in the absence of the SCN in Siberian hamsters. *Am. J. Physiol.* 263(2) Part 2, R353–R362.

9   Stress, arousal and homeostatic challenge

General

Cridland, A. and Henry, J.L. (1988) Effects of intrathecal administration of neuropeptides on a spinal nociceptive reflex in the rat: VIP, galanin, CGRP, TRH, somatostatin and angiotensin II. *Neuropeptides* 11, 23–32.

Feldman, S., Conforti, N. and Saphiev, D. (1990) The preoptic area and bed nucleus of the stria terminalis are involved in the effects of the amygdala on adrenocortical secretion. *Neuroscience* 37, 775–779.

Gray, T.S. and Magnuson, D.J. (1987) Neuropeptide neuronal efferents from the bed nucleus of the stria terminalis and central amygdaloid nucleus to the dorsal vagal complex in the rat. *J. Comp. Neurol.* 262, 365–378.

Hypothalamo-pituitary–adrenal axis

Aubry, J.-M., Bartanusz, V., Jezova, D., Belin D. and Kiss, J.Z. (1999) Single stress induces long-lasting elevations in vasopressin mRNA levels in CRF hypophysiotrophic neurones, but repeated stress is required to modify AVP immunoreactivity. *J. Neuroendocrinol.* 11, 377–384.

Arnold-Reed, D.E. and Balment, R.J. (1994) Peptide hormones influence interrenal secretion of cortisol in the trout, *Oncorhynchus mykiss. Gen. Comp. Endocrinol.* 96, 85–91.

Bern, H., Pearson, D., Larson, B.A. and Nishiota, R.S. (1985) Neurohormones from fish tails: The caudal neurosecretory system. I. 'Urophysiology' and the caudal neurosecretory system of fishes. *Rec. Prog. Horm. Res.* 41, 533–552.

Boonstra, R., McColl, C.J. and Karels, T.J. (2001) Reproduction at all costs: The adaptive stress response of male arctic ground squirrels. *Ecology* 82, 1930–1946.

Boonstra, R., Hik, D., Singleton, G.R. and Tinnikov, A. (1998) The impact of predator: Induced stress on the snowshoe hare cycle. *Ecology Monographs* 79, 371–394.

Dunn, A.J. and Berridge, C.W. (1990) Physiological and behavioural responses to corticotropin-releasing factor administration: Is CRF a mediator of anxiety of stress responses? *Brain Res. Rev.* 15, 71–100.

Gillies, G.E., Linton, E.A. and Lowry, P.J. (1982) Corticotropin-releasing activity of the new CRF is potentiated several times by vasopressin. *Nature* 299, 355–357.

Hauger, R.L. and Dautzenberg, F.M. (1999) Regulation of the stress-response by corticotropin-releasing factor receptors. In *Neuroendocrinology in Physiology and Medicine*, Eds Conn, P.M. and Freeman, M.E., Humana Press, New Jersey, pp. 261–286.

Hauger R.L. and Aguilera, G. (1993) Regulation of pituitary corticotropin-releasing hormone (CRH) receptors by CRH: interaction with vasopressin. *Endocrinology* 133, 1708–1714.

Heinrichs, S.C., Lapsansky, J., Lovenberg, T.W., De Souza, E.B. and Chalmers, D.T. (1997) Corticotropin-releasing factor CRF1 but not CRF2 receptors mediate anxiogenic-like behaviors. *Regul. Pept.* 71, 15–21.

Hik, D.S., McColl, C.J., Boostra, R. (2001) Why are Arctic ground squirells more stressed in the boreal forest than in alphine meadows. *Ecoscience* 8, 275–288.

Hisano, S., Fukui, Y., Chikamoriaoyama, M., Aizawa, T. and Shibasaki, T. (1993) Reciprocal synaptic relations between CRF immunoreactive and TRH immunoreactive neurons in the paraventricular nucleus of the rat hypothalamus. *Brain Res.* 620, 343–346.

Kelsall, C.J. and Balment, R.J. (1998) Native urotensins influence cortisol secretion and plasma cortisol concentration in the euryhaline flounder, *Platichthys flesus*. *Gen. Comp. Endocrinol.* 112, 210–219.

Corticotrophin-releasing factor family

Baršyte, D., Tipping, D.R., Smart, D., Conlon, J.M., Baker, B.I. and Lovejoy, D.A. (1999) Rainbow trout (*Oncorhychus mykiss*) urotensin-I: Structural differences between urotensins-I and urocortins. *Gen. Comp. Endocrinol.* 115, 169–177.

Hsu, S.Y. and Hsueh, A.J. (2001) Human stresscopin and stresscopin-related peptide are selective ligands for the type 2 corticotropin-releasing hormone receptor. *Nat. Med.* 98, 605–611.

Lederis, K., Fryer, J.N., Okawara, Y., Schonrock, C. and Richter, D. (1994) Corticotropin-releasing factors acting on the fish pituitary: Experimental and molecular analysis. In *Fish Physiology*, Eds Sherwood, N.M. and Hew, C., Academic Press, San Diego, pp. 67–100.

Lewis, K., Li., C., Perrin, M.H., Blount, A., Kunitake, K., Donaldson, C., Vaughan, J., Reyes, T.M., Gulyas, J., Fischer, W., Bilezikjian, L., Rivier, J., Sawchenko, P.E. and Vale, W.W. (2001) Identification of urocortin III, an additional member of the corticotropin-releasing factor (CRF) family with high affinity for the CRF2 receptor. *Proc. Nat. Acad. Sci. USA* 98, 7570–7575.

Lowry, C.A., Deviche, P. and Moore, F.L. (1990) Effects of corticotropin-releasing factor (CRF) and opiates on amphibian locomotion. *Brain Res.* 513, 94–100.

Lowry, C.A. Rose, J.D. and Moore, F.L. (1996) Corticotropin-releasing factor enhances locomotion and medullary neuronal firing in an amphibian. *Horm. Behav.* 30, 50–59.

Lovejoy, D.A. (1996) Peptide hormone evolution: Functional heterogeneity within GnRH and CRF families. *Biochem. Cell Biol.* 74, 1–7.

Lovejoy, D.A. and Balment, R.J. (1999) Evolution and physiology of the corticotropin-releasing factor (CRF) family of neuropeptides in vertebrates. *Gen. Comp. Endocrinol.* 115, 1–22.

Reyes, T.M., Lewis, K., Perrin, M.H., Kunitake, K.S., Vaughan J., Arias, C.A., Hogenesch, J.B., Rivier, J.E., Vale, W.W. and Sawchenko, P.E. (2001) Urocortin II: A member of the corticotropin-releasing factor (CRF) neuropeptide family that is selectively bound by the type 2 CRF receptors. *Proc. Natl. Acad. Sci. USA* 98, 2843–2848.

Sawchenko, P.E. and Swanson, L.W. (1989) Organization of CRF immunoreactive cells and fibers in the rat brain: Immunohistochemical studies. In *Corticotropin-Releasing Factor: Basic and Clinical Studies of a Neuropeptide*, Eds De Sonza, E.B. and Nemeroff, C.B., CRC Press, Boca Raton, FL, pp. 29–51.

Swanson, L., Sawchenko, P., Rivier, J. and Vale, W. (1983) Organization of ovine corticotropin-releasing factor immunoreactive cells and fibers in the rat brain: An immunohistochemical study. *Neuroendocrinology* 36, 165–186.

Vaughan, J., Donaldson, C., Bittencourt, J., Perrin, M.H., Lewis, K., Sutton, S., Chan, R., Turnbull, A.V., Lovejoy, D., Rivier, C., Rivier, J., Sawchenko, P.E. and Vale, W. (1995) Urocortin, a mammalian neuropeptide related to fish urotensin I and to corticotropin-releasing factor. *Nature* 378, 287–292.

Galanin

Austin, M.C., Cottingham, S.L., Paul, S.M. and Crawley, J.N. (1990) Tyrosine hydroxylase and galanin mRNA levels in locus coeruleus neurons are increased following reserpine administration. *Synapse* 6(4), 351–357.

Bartfai, T., Bedecs, K., Land, T., Langel, U., Bertorelli, R., Girotti, P., Consolo, S., Xu, X.-J., Wiesenfeld-Hallin, Z., Nilsson, S., Pieribone, V. and Hökfelt, T. (1991) M-15, high-affinity chimeric peptide that blocks the neuronal actions of galanin in the hippocampus, locus coeruleus and spinal cord. *Proc. Natl. Acad. Sci. USA* 88, 10961–10965.

Bartfai, T., Fisone, G. and Langel, U. (1992) Galanin and galanin antagonists: Molecular and biochemical perspectives. *Trends Pharmacol. Sci.* 13, 312–317.

Ch'ng, J.L.C., Christofides, N.D. and Anand, P. (1985) Distribution of galanin immunoreactivity in the central nervous system and the response of galanin-containing neuronal pathways to injury. *Neuroscience* 16, 343–354.

Cimini, V. (1996) Galanin inhibits ACTH release in vitro and can be demonstrated immunocytochemically in dispersed corticotrophs. *Exp. Cell Res.* 228, 212–215.

Hao, J.X., Shi, T.J., Xu, I.S., Kaupilla, T., Xu, X.J., Hokfelt, T., Bartfai, T. and Wiesenfeld-Hallin, Z. (1999) Intrathecal galanin alleviates allodynia-like behavior after peripheral nerve injury. *Eur. J. Neurosci.* 11, 427–432.

Hokfelt, T., Wiesenfeld-Hallin, Z., Villar, M. and Melander, T. (1987) Increase of galanin-like immunoreactivity in rat dorsal root ganglion cells after peripheral axotomy. *Neurosci. Lett.* 83, 217–220.

Hooi, S.C., Maiter, D.M., Martin, J.B. and Koenig, J.I. (1990) Galaninergic mechanisms are involved in the regulation of corticotropin and thyrotropin secretion in the rat. *Endocrinology* 127, 2281–2289.

Kerr, B.J., Cafferty, W.B.J., Gupta, Y.K., Bacon, A., Wynick, D., McMahon, S.B. and Thompson, S.W.N. (2000) Galanin knock out mice reveal nociceptive deficits following peripheral nerve injury. *Eur. J. Neurosci.* 12, 793–802.

Khoshbouei, H., Cecchi, M. and Morilak, D.A. (2002) Modulatory effects of galanin in the lateral bed nucleus of the stria terminalis on behavioral and neuroendocrine responses to acute stress. *Neuropsychopharmacology* 27(1), 25–34.

Holmes, P.V., Blanchard, D.C., Blanchard, R.J., Brady, L.S. and Crawley, J.N. (1995) Chronic social stress increases levels of preprogalanin mRNA in the rat locus coeruleus. *Pharmacol. Biochem. Behav.* 50(4), 655–660.

Liu, H.X., Brumovsky, P., Schmidt, R., Brown, W., Payza, K., Hodzic, L., Pou, C., Godbout, C. and Hokfelt, T. (2001) Receptor subtype-specific pronociceptive and analgesic actions of galanin in the spinal cord: Selective actions via GalR1 and GalR2 receptors. *Proc. Natl. Acad. Sci. USA* 98(17), 9960–9964.

Reeve, A.J., Walker, K., Urban, L. and Fox A.J. (2000) Excitatory effects of galanin in the spinal cord of intact, anaesthetized rats. *Neurosci. Lett.* 295, 25–28.

Sweerts, B.W., Jarrott, B. and Lawrence, A.J. (1999) Expression of preprogalanin mRNA following acute and chronic restraint stress in brains of normotensive and hypertensive rats. *Brain Res. Mol. Brain Res.* 69(1), 113–123.

Sweerts, B.W., Jarrott, B. and Lawrence, A.J. (2000) Acute and chronic restraint stress: Effects on [125I]-galanin binding in normotensive and hypertensive rat brain. *Brain Res.* 873(2), 318–329.

Villar, M.J., Cortes, R., Theodorsson, E., Wiesenfeld-Hallin, Z., Schalling, M., Fahrenkrug, J., Emson, P.C. and Hokfelt, T. (1989) Neuropeptide expression in rat dorsal root ganglion cells and spinal cord after peripheral nerve injury with special reference to galanin. *Neuroscience* 33, 587–604.

Wiesenfeld-Hallin, Z., Xu, X.-J., Langel, U., Bedecs, K., Hokfelt, T. and Bartfai, T. (1992) Galanin-mediated control of pain: Enhanced role after nerve injury. *Proc. Natl. Acad. Sci. USA* 89, 3334–3337.

Proopiomelanocortin family

Kolk, S.M., Kramer, B.M., Cornelisse, L.N., Scheene, W.J., Jenks, B.G. and Roubos, E.W. (2002) Multiple control and dynamic response of the xenopus melanotrope cell. *Comp. Biochem. Physiol. B* 132, 257–268.

Lui, J.P., Robinson, P.J., Funder, J.W. and Engler, D. (1990) The biosynthesis and secretion of adrenocorticotropin by the ovine anterior pituitary is predominantly regulated by arginine vasopressin (AVP). *J. Biol. Chem.* 265, 14136–14142.

Stefano, G.B., Salzet-Raveillon, B. and Salzet, M. (1999) *Mytilus edulis* hemolymph contains pro-opiomelanocortin: LPS and morphine stimulate different processing. *Mol. Brain Res.* 63, 340–350.

Neuroanatomy of stress-related circuits

Moga, M.M. and Gray, T.S. (1985) Evidence for corticotropin-releasing factor, neurotensin, and somatostatin in the neural pathway from the central nucleus of the amygdala to the parabranchial nucleus. *J. Comp. Neurol.* 241, 275–288.

Palkovits, M. (2000) Stress-induced expression of co-localized neuropeptides in hypothalamic and amygdaloid neurons. *Eur. J. Pharmacol.* 405(1–3), 161–166.

Veening, J.G., Swanson, L.W. and Sawchenko, P.E. (1984) The organization of projections from the central nucleus of the amygdala to brain stem sites involved in central autonomic regulation: A combined retrograde transport-immunohistochemical study. *Brain Res.* 303, 337–347.

Pfieffer, M., Koch, T., Schorder, H., Klutzny, M., Kirscht, S., Kreiencamp, H.J., Hollt, V. and Schulz, S. (2001) Homo and heterodimerization of somatostatin receptor subtypes. Inactivation of sst(3) receptor function by heterodimerization with sst (2A). *J. Biol. Chem.* 276, 14027–14036.

Weissman, M.M. and Olfson, M. (1995) Depression in women: Implications for health care research. *Science* 269, 799–801.

10   Reproduction

Hypothalamo-pituitary-gonadal axis

Bauer-Dantoin, A.C., Weiss, J. and Jameson, J.L. (1995) Roles of estrogen, progesterone, and gonadotropin-releasing hormone (GnRH) in the control of pituitary GnRH receptor gene expression at the time of preovulatory gonadotropin surges. *Endocrinology* 136, 1014–1019.

Huhtaniemi, I.T., Warren, D.W. (1990) Ontogeny of pituitary–gonadal interactions. Current advances and controversies. *Trends Endocrinol. Metab.* 1, 356–362.

Kepa, J., Neeley, C.I., Jacobsen, B.M., Bruder, J.M., McDonnell, D.P., Leslie, K. and Wierman, M.E. (1994) Estrogen receptor mediated repression of rat gonadotropin releasing hormone (GnRH) promoter activity in hypothalamic cells. *Endocrine* 2, 947–956.

GnRH family

Lovejoy, D.A., Fischer, W.H., Ngamvongchon, S., Craig, A.G., Rivier, J.E., Nahorniak, C.S., Peter, R.E. and Sherwood, N.M. (1992a) A new form of gonadotropin-releasing hormone (GnRH) from dogfish shark brain provides insight into the evolution of GnRH. *Proc. Natl. Acad. Sci. USA* 89, 6373–6377.

Lovejoy, D.A. Stell, W.K. and Sherwood, N.M. (1992b) Partial characterization of four forms of gonadotropin-releasing hormone from the brain and terminal nerve of the spiny dogfish (*Squalus acanthias*). *Regul. Peptides* 37, 39–48.

Sherwood, N.M., Lovejoy, D.A. and Coe, I.R. (1993) Origin of mammalian gonadotropin-releasing hormones. *Endocrine Rev.* 14, 241–254.

GnRH expression and migration

Actions of stress on reproduction

Bingaman, E.W., Magneson, D.J. Gray, T.S. and Handa, R.J. (1994) Androgen inhibits the increases in hypothalamic corticotropin-releasing hormone (CRH) and CRH-immunoreactivity following gonadectomy. *Neuroendocrinology* 59, 228–234.

Burgess, L.H. and Handa, R.J. (1992) Chronic estrogen induced alternations in adrenocorticotropin and corticosterone secretion, and glucocorticoid receptor mediated functions in female rats. *Endocrinology* 131, 1261–1269.

Calogero, A.E., Weber, R.F.A. and D'Agata, R. (1993) Effects of rat prolactin on gonadotropin-releasing hormone secretion by the explanted male rat hypothalamus. *Neuroendocrinology* 57, 152–158.

Calogero, A.E., Weber, R.F.A., Raiti, F., Burello, N., Moncada, M.L., Mongioi, A. and D'Agata, R. (1994) Involvement of corticotropin-releasing hormone and endogenous opioid peptides in prolactin-suppressed gonadotropin-releasing hormone release in vitro. *Neuroendocrinology* 60, 291–296.

Caraty, A., Miller, D.W., Delaleu, B. and Martin, G.B. (1997) Stimulation of LH secretion in sheep by central administration of corticotrophin-releasing hormone. *J. Reprod. Fertil.* 111, 249–357.

Chen, M.-D., Ordog, T., O'Byrne, K.T., Goldsmith, J.R., Connaughton, M.A. and Knobil, E. (1996) The insulin hypoglycemia-induced inhibition of gonadotropin-releasing hormone pulse generator activity in the rhesus monkey: Roles of vasopressin and corticotropin-releasing factor. *Endocrinology* 137, 2012–2021.

Fischer, U.G., Wood, S.H., Bruhn, J., Roseff, S.J., Mortola, J., Rivier, J.E. and Yen, S.S.C. (1992) Effect of human corticotropin-releasing hormone on gonadotropin secretion in cycling and postmenopausal women. *Fertil. Steril.* 58, 1108–1112.

Haleem, D.J., Kennett, G. and Curzon, G. (1988) Adaptation of female rats to stress: Shift to male pattern by inhibition of corticosterone synthesis. *Brain Res.* 458, 339–347.

Ibanez, L., Potau, N., Marcos, M.V. and de Zegher, F. (1999) Corticotropin-releasing hormone: A potent androgen secretogogue in girls with hyperandrogenism after precocious pubarche. *J. Clin. Endocrinol. Metab.* 84, 4602–4606.

Karanth, S., Lysön, K., Aguila, M.C. and McCann, S.M. (1995) Effects of luteinizing hormone releasing hormone, alpha-melanocyte-stimulating hormone, naloxone, dexamethasone and indometh-acin on interleukin-2-induced corticotropin-releasing factor release. *Neuroimmunomodulation* 2, 166–173.

Lovejoy, D.A., Aubry, J.-M., Turnbull, A., Sutton, S., Potter, E., Yehling, J., Rivier, C. and Vale, W.W. (1998) Ectopic expression of CRF-binding protein: Minor impact on HPA axis regulation but induction of sexually dimorphic weight gain. *J. Neuroendocrinol.* 10, 483–491.

MacLusky, N.J., Naftolin, F. and Leranth, C. (1988) Immunocytochemical evidence for direct synaptic connections between corticotrophin-releasing factor (CRF) and gonadotrophin-releasing hormone (GnRH)-containing neurons in the preoptic area of the rat. *Brain Res.* 439, 391–395.

Nappi, R.E. and Rivest, S. (1995) Ovulatory cycle influences the stimulatory effect of stress on the expression of corticotropin-releasing factor receptor messenger ribonucleic acid in the paraventricular nucleus of the female rat hypothalamus. *Endocrinology* 136, 4073–4083.

Nappi, R.E., Petraglia, F., Guo, A.L., Criscuolo, M., Trentini, G.P. and Grenzzani, A.R. (1996) Estrous cycle- and acute stress-related changes of rat ovarian immunoreactive corticotropin-releasing factor. *Gynecol. Endocrinol.* 10, 75–82.

Norman, R.L. (1994) Corticotropin-releasing hormone effects on luteinizing hormone and cortisol secretion in intact female rhesus macaques. *Biol. Reprod.* 50, 949–955.

Rivier, C. and Rivest, S. (1991) Effects of stress on the activity of the hypothalamic-pituitary-gonadal axis: Peripheral and central mechanisms. *Biol. Reprod.* 45, 523–532.

Rivest, S. and Rivier, C. (1995) The role of corticotropin-releasing factor and interleukin-1 in the regulation of neurons controlling reproductive functions. *Endocrine Rev.* 16, 177–199.

Selye, H. (1939) Effects of adaptation to various damaging agents on the female sex organs in the rat. *Endocrinology* 25, 615–624.

Sirinathsinghji, D.J.S. (1986) Regulation of lordosis behaviour in the female rat by corticotropin-releasing factor, β-endorphin/corticotropin and luteinizing hormone-releasing hormone neuronal systems in the medial preoptic area. *Brain Res.* 375, 49–56.

Sirinathsinghji, D.J.S., Rees, L.H., Rivier, J. and Vale, W.W. (1983) Corticotropin-releasing factor is a potent inhibitor of sexual receptivity in the female rat. *Nature* 305, 232–235.

Tellam, D.J., Perone, M.J., Dunn, I.C., Radovick, S., Brennand, J., Rivier, J.E., Castro, M.G. and Lovejoy, D.A. (1998) Direct regulation of GnRH transcription by CRF-peptides in an immortalized neuronal cell line. *Neuroreport* 9, 3135–3140.

Tellam, D.J., Mohammad, Y.N. and Lovejoy, D.A. (2000) Molecular integration of hypothalamo-pituitary-adrenal axis-related neurohormones on the GnRH neuron. *Biochem. Cell Biol.* 78, 205–216.

Tilbrook, A.J., Canny, B.J., Stewart, B.J., Serapiglia, M.D. and Clarke, I.J. (1999) Central administration of corticotrophin releasing hormone but not arginine vasopressin stimulates the secretion of luteinizing hormone in rams in the presence and absence of testosterone. *J. Endocrinol.* 162, 301–311.

Vamvakopolous, N.C. and Chrousos, G.P. (1993) Evidence of direct estrogenic regulation of human corticotropin-releasing hormone gene expression: Potential implications for the sexual dimorphism of the stress response and immune/inflammatory reaction. *J. Clin. Invest.* 92, 1896–1902.

Viau, V. and Meany, M.J. (1991) Variations in the hypothalamic-pituitary-adrenal responses to stress during the estrous cycle in the rat. *Endocrinology* 129, 2503–2511.

Wang, R. and Millam, J.R. (1999) Corticotropin-releasing hormone-immunopositive nerve elements in apposition to chicken gonadotropin-releasing hormone I-containing perikarya in Japanese quail (*Coturnix coturnix japonica*). *Cell Tissue Res.* 297, 223–228.

11   Behaviour, learning and memory

General

Becker, J.B., Breedlove, S.M. and Crews, D. (1992) *Behavioral Endocrinology*, MIT Press, Cambridge, 574 pages.

Kandel, E.R., Schwartz, J.H. and Jessell, T.M. (1995) *Essentials of Neural Science and Behavior*, Prentice-Hall International, Norwalk, Connecticut, 743 pages.

Schulkin, J. (1999) *Neuroendocrine Regulation of Behavior*, Cambridge University Press, Cambridge, 323 pages.

Sexual behaviour

Argiolas, A. (1999). Neuropeptides and sexual behaviour. *Neurosci. Biobehav. Rev.* 23(8), 1127–1142.

Benelli, A., Bertolini, A., Zoli, M., Leo, G., Filaferro, M., Saltini, S. and Genedani, S. (2002) Pharmacological manipulation of brain galaninergic system and sexual behavior in male mice. *Psychopharmacology (Berl)* 160(3), 325–330.

Gimpl, G. and Fahrenholz, F. (2001) The oxytocin receptor system: Structure, function and regulation. *Physiol. Rev.* 81, 629–683.

Memory

Bartus, R.T., Dean, R.L.D., Beer, B., Lippa, A.S. (1982) The cholinergic hypothesis of geriatric memory dysfunction. *Science* 217, 408–414.

Chan-Palay, V. (1988) Galanin hyperinnervates surviving neurons of the human basal nucleus of Meynert in dementias of Alzheimer's and Parkinson's disease: A hypothesis for the role of galanin in accentuating cholinergic dysfunction in dementia. *J. Comp. Neurol.* 273, 543–557.

Chepurnov, S.A., Chepurnova, N.E. and Berdiev, R.K. (1998) Galanin controls excitability of the brain. *Ann. N.Y. Acad. Sci.* 865, 547–550.

Crawley, J.N. (1993) Functional interactions of galanin and acetylcholine: Relevance to memory and Alzheimer's disease (Review). *Beh. Brain Res.* 57, 133–141.

Crawley, J.N. (1996) Galanin-acetylcholine interactions: Relevance to memory and Alzheimer's disease. *Life Sci.* 58, 2185–2199.

Mazarati, A.M., Hohmann, J.G., Bacon, A., Liu, H., Sankar, R., Steiner, R.A., Wynick, D., Wasterlain, C.G. (2000) Modulation of hippocampal excitability and seizures by galanin. *J Neurosci.* 20(16), 6276–6281.

Pare, D. (2003) Role of the basolateral amygdala in memory consolidation. *Prog. Neurobiol.* 70, 409–420.

Fear and reward

Baxter, M.G. and Murray, E.A. (2002) The amygdala and reward. *Nature Rev. Neurosci.* 3, 563–573.

Fanselow, F.S. and Gale, G.D. (2003) The amygdala, fear and memory. *Ann. N.Y. Acad. Sci.* 985, 125–134.

Sanders, M.J., Wiltgen, B.J. and Fanselow, M.S. (2003) The place of the hippocampus in fear conditioning. *European Journal of Pharmacology* 463, 217–223.

Mazarati, A.M., Langel, U. and Bartfai, T. (2001). An endogenous anticonvulsant? *Neuroscientist* 7, 506–517.

Mazarati, A. and Wasterlain, C.G. (2002) Anticonvulsant effects of four neuropeptides in the rat hippocampus during self-sustaining status epilepticus. *Neurosci. Lett.* 331(2), 123–127.

Melander, T., Staines, W.A. and Rokaeus, A. (1986) Galanin-like immunoreactivity in hippocampal afferents in the rat, with special reference to cholinergic and noradrenergic inputs. *Neuroscience* 19, 223–240.

Mesulam, M.M., Mufson, E.J., Levey, A.I. and Wainer, B.H. (1983) Cholinergic innervation of cortex by the basal forebrain: Cytochemistry and cortical connections of the septal area, diagonal band nuclei, nucleus basalis (substantia innominata) and hypothalamus in the rhesus monkey. *J. Comp. Neurol.* 214, 170–197

Rada, P., Mark, G., Hoebel, B.G. (1998) Galanin in the hypothalamus raises dopamine and lowers acetylcholine release in the nucleus accumbens: a possible mechanism for hypothalamic initiation of feeding behavior. *Brain Res.* 798, 1–6.

Steiner, R.A., Hohmann, J.G., Holmes, A., Wrenn, C.C., Cadd, G., Jureus, A., Clifton, D.K., Luo, M., Gutshall, M., Ma, S.Y., Mufson, E.J., Crawley, J.N. (2001) Galanin transgenic mice display cognitive and neurochemical deficits characteristic of Alzheimer's disease. *Proc. Natl. Acad. Sci. USA* 98(7), 4184–4189.

Wasterlain, C.G., Mazarati, A.M., Naylor, D., Niquet, J., Liu, H., Suchomelova, L., Baldwin, R., Katsumori, H., Shirasaka, Y., Shin, D. and Sankar, R. (2002) Short-term plasticity of hippocampal neuropeptides and neuronal circuitry in experimental status epilepticus. *Epilepsia* 43 (Suppl. 5), 20–29.

Wilcock, G.K., Esiri, M.M., Bowen, D.M. and Smith, C.C. (1982) Alzheimer's disease: Correlation of cortical choline acetyltransferase activity with the severity of dementia and histological abnormalities. *J. Neurol. Sci.* 57, 407–417.

Xu, Z.D., Shi, T.S., Hokfelt, T. (1998) Galanin/GMAP- and NPY-like immunoreactivities in locus coeruleus and noradrenergic nerve terminals in the hippocampal formation and cortex with notes on the galanin-R1 and -R2 receptors. *J. Comp. Neurol.* 392, 227–251.

12 Pheromones and chemo-attractants

Pheromones in invertebrates

Christensen, T.A. and Hildebrand, J.G. (2002) Pheromonal and host odor processing in the insect antennal lobe: How different? *Curr. Opin. Neurobiol.* 12, 393–399.

Leinders-Zufall, T., Lane, A.P., Pusche, A.C., Ma, W., Novotny, M.V., Shipley, M.T. and Zufall, F. (2000) *Nature* 405, 792–796.

Monnin, T., Ratnieks, F.L., Jones, G.R. and Beard, R. (2002) Pretender punishment induced by chemical signalling in a queenless ant. *Nature* 419, 61–65.

Seybold, S.J. and Tittiger, C. (2003) Biochemistry and molecular biology of the de novo isoprenoid pheromone production in the Scolytidae. *Ann. Rev. Entomol.* 48, 425–453.

Pheromones in vertebrates

Devriot, J.H. (1984) Functional anatomy of the peripheral olfactory system of the African lungfish *Protopterus annectens* Owen: Macroscopic, microscopic and morphometric aspects. *Am. J. Anat.* 169, 177–192.

Dulka, J.G. (1993) Sex pheromone systems in goldfish: Comparisons to vomeronasal systems in tetrapods. *Brain Behav. Evol.* 42, 265–280.

Eisthen, H.L. (2000) Presence of the vomeronasal system in aquatic salamanders. *Philos. Trans. R. Soc. Lond. B Biol. Sci.* 355, 1209–1213.

Ichkawa, M. (2003) Synaptic mechanisms underlying pheromonal memory in the vomeronasal system. *Zoolog. Sci.* 20, 687–695.

Kolattukudy, P.E. and Rogers, L. (1987) Biosynthesis of 3-hydroxy fatty acids, the pheromone components of female mallard ducks, by cell-free preparations from the uropygial gland. *Arch. Biochem. Biophys.* 252, 121–129.

Novotny, M.V. (2003) Pheromones, binding proteins and receptor responses in rodents. *Biochem. Soc. Trans.* 31, 117–122.

Oikawa, T., Suzuki, K., Saito, T.R., Takahashi, K.W. and Tanigushi, K. (1998) Fine structure of three types of olfactory organs in *Xenopus laevis. Anat. Rec.* 252, 301–310.

Rasmussen, L.E., Lazar, J. and Greenwood, D.R. (2003) Olfactory adventures of elephantine pheromones. *Biochem. Soc. Trans.* 31, 137–141.

Stacey, N.E., Cardwell, J.R., Liley, N.R., Scott, A.P. and Sorenson, P.W. (1994) Hormones as sex pheromones in fish. *Perspect. Comp. Endocrinol.,* pp. 438–448.

Webb, D.M., Cortes-Ortiz, L. and Zhang, J. (2004) Genetic evidence for the coexistence of pheromone perception and full trichromatice vision in Howler monkeys. *Mol. Biol. Evol.* 21, 697–704.

Zufall, F., Kelliher, K.R. and Lenders-Zufall, T. (2002) Pheromone detection by mammalian vomeronasal neurons. *Microsc. Res. Tech.* 58, 251–260.

13   Xenobiotics and hormone mimics

General

Dewick, P.M. (2002) *Medicinal Natural Products: A Biosynthetic Approach*, 2nd Edition, John Wiley & Sons, Ltd, Chichester, UK, 506 pages.

Figuier, L. (1888) *The Ocean World*, Cassell and Company Ltd, London, 656 pages.

Hansen, H.A. (1978) *The Witches Garden*, Unity Press, Santa Cruz, CA, 128 pages.

Krimsky, S. (2000) *Hormonal Chaos*, Johns Hopkins University Press, Baltimore, 284 pages.

Mann, J. (1994) *Murder Magic and Medicine*, Oxford University Press, Oxford, 232 pages.

McLachlan, J.A. (2001) Environmental signaling: What embroyos and evolution teach us about endocrine disrupting chemicals. *Endocr. Rev.* 22, 319–341.

Spinella, M. (2001) *The Psychopharmacology of Herbal Medicine*, MIT Press, Cambridge, Massachusetts, 578 pages.

Ion channel agonists and antagonists

Brown, R.I., Haley, T.L., West, K.A. and Crabb, J.W. (1999) Pseudechetoxin: A peptide blocker of cyclic nucleotide-gated ion channels. *Proc. Natl. Acad. Sci. USA* 96, 754–759.

Corona, M., Coronas, F.V., Merino, E., Becerril, B., Gutierrez, R., Rebolledo-Antunez, S., Garcia, D.E. and Possani, L.D. (2003) A novel class of peptide found in scorpion venom with neuro-depressant effects in peripheral and central nervous system of the rat. *Biochim. Biophys. Acta* 1649, 58–67.

Church, J.E. and Hodgson, W.C. (2002) Adrenergic and cholinergic activity contributes to the cardiovascular effects of lionfish (*Pterois volitans*) venom. *Toxicon* 40, 787–796.

Church, J.E. and Hodgson, W.C. (2002) The pharmacological activity of fish venoms. *Toxicon* 40, 1083–1093.

Dai, Q., Liu, F., Zhou, Y., Lu, B., Yu, F. and Huang, P. (2003) The synthesis of SO-3, a conopeptide with high analgesic activity derived from *Conus striatus*. *J. Nat. Prod.* 66, 1276–1279.

Datta, G. and Tu, A.T. (1997) Structure and other chemical characterizations of gila toxin, a lethal toxin from lizard venom. *J. Pept. Res.* 50, 443–450.

Floresca, C.Z. (2003) A comparison of the mu-conotoxins by [3H] saxitoxin binding assays in neuronal and skeletal muscle sodium channel. *Toxicol. Appl. Pharmacol.* 190, 95–101.

Heading, C.E. (2002) Conus peptides and neuroprotection. *Curr. Opin. Investig. Drugs* 3, 915–920.

Hu, J.F., Schetz, J.A., Kelly, M., Peng, J.N., Ang, K.K., Flotow, H., Leong, C.Y., Ng, S.B., Buss, A.D., Wilkins, S.P. and Hamann, M.T. (2002) New antiinfective and human 5-HT2 receptor binding natural and semisynthetic compounds from the Jamaican sponge *Smenospongia aurea*. *J. Nat. Prod.* 65, 476–480.

Kinoshita, E., Maeijima, H., Yamaoka, K., Konno, K., Kawai, N., Shimizu, E., Yokote, S., Nakayama, H. and Seyama, I. (2001) Novel wasp toxin discriminates between neuronal and cardiac sodium channels. *Mol. Pharmacol.* 59, 1457–1463.

Jimenez, E.C., Shetty, R.P., Lirazan, M., Rivier, J., Walker, C., Abogadie, F.C., Yoshikami, D., Cruz, L.J. and Olivera, B.M. (2003) Novel excitatory *Conus* peptides define a new conotoxin superfamily. *J. Neurochem.* 85, 610–621.

Le, M.T., Vanderheyden, P.M., Fierens, F.K., Vauquelin, G. (2003) Molecular characterization of the high affinity [3H] neuropeptide Y-binding component from the venom of *Conus anenome*. *Fundam Clin. Pharmacol.* 17, 457–462.

Li, D., Xiao, Y., Hu, W., Xie, J., Bosmans, F., Tytgat, J. and Liang, S. (2003) Function and solution structure of haninantoxin-I, a novel insect sodium channel inhibitor from the Chinese bird spider Selenocosmia hainana. *FEBS Lett.* 555, 616–622.

Miyawaki, T., Tsubokawa, H., Yokota, H., Oguro, K., Konno, K., Masuzawa, T. and Kawai, N. (2002) Differential effects of novel wasp toxin on rat hippocampal interneurons. *Neurosci. Lett.* 328, 25–28.

Nobile, M., Noceti, F., Prestipino, G. and Possani, L.D. (1996) Helothermine, a lizard venom toxin, inhibits calcium current in cerebellar granules. *Exp. Brain Res.* 110, 15–20.

Oberdorster, E. and McClellan-Green, P. (2002) Mechanisms of imposex in the mud snail, *Ilyanassa obsolete*: TBT as a neurotoxin and aromatase inhibitor. *Mar. Environ. Res.* 54, 715–718.

Shiau, Y.S., Huang, P.T., Liou, H.H., Liaw, Y.C., Shiau, Y.Y. and Lou, K.L. (2003) Structural basis of binding and inhibition of novel tarantula toxins in mammalian voltage-dependent potassium channels. *Chem. Res. Toxicol.* 16, 1217–1225.

Tytgat, J., Vandenberghe, I., Ulens, C. and Van Beemen, J. (2001) New polypeptide components purified from mamba venom. *FEBS Lett.* 491, 217–221.

Vassas, A., Bourdy, G., Paillard, J.J., Lavayre, J., Pais, M., Quirion, J.C. and Debitus, C. (1996) Naturally occurring somatostatin and vasoactive intestinal peptide inhibitors. Isolation of alkaloids from two marine sponges. *Planta Med.* 62, 28–30.

Zhang, M., Fishman, Y., Sher, D. and Zlotkin, E. (2003) Hydralysin, a novel animal group-selective paralytic and cytolytic protein from a noncnidocystic origin in hydra. *Biochemistry* 42, 8939–8944.

Index

α-amino-3-hydroxy-5-methyl-
   4-isoxazoleproprionate
   (AMPA) receptor   129, 144, 357
   see also Glutamate, receptors

Abdominal gland   340
Abu Sina   10
Acetylcholine   100, 130, 143, 234,
   311, 348
   muscarinic receptors   130, 314
   nicotinic receptors   130
Acetylcholinesterase   352
Acheta domesticus   278
Acoelomorpha   86, 89, 92, 99
Acromegaly   197
Acropora millepora   79
ACTH, *see* Adrenocorticotropic hormone
Actinopterygii   101, 103, 108, 112, 153, 193,
   254, 311
Activin   135
Adenohypophysis   108, 109
Adenoma   197
Adenosine   124
Adenosine triphosphate   124
Adenylyl cyclase   128, 253
ADH, *see* Vasopressin
Adipose   190
Adrenal cortex, *see* Adrenal gland
Adrenal gland   250
   adrenal cortex   255
   adrenal medulla   126, 167, 250
   adrenalectomy   263
Adrenal medulla, *see* Adrenal gland
Adrenaline, *see* Epinephrine
Adrenergic receptors   99, 168, 314, 320

Adrenocorticotropic hormone   108, 134, 155,
   201, 247
Adrenomedullin   102
African catfish   293
African green monkey   288
Ageing   208, 302, 315
Agnathans   153
Agonist   145
Agouti-related protein   181, 261
al-Razi   10, 12, 13, 23
Alcmaeon   6
Aldosterone   151, 153
Alexandria   9
Alexandria Medical School   9
Alkaloids   348, 349, 358
Allatostatins   170
Allatotropins   171
   profile   183
Alleochemicals   346
Allomones   346
Alzheimer's disease   324
L-aromatic amino acid decarboxylase   127
Amazon   358
Ambystoma mexicanum   259
Amphibia   113, 226, 293, 340,
   348, 351
Amphioxus   97, 103, 170
Amphiuma tridactylum   338
Amplitude modulation   290
Amygdala   172, 255, 311
   basolateral   312, 315
   central nucleus   155, 268, 303, 304, 313
   medial nucleus   160, 174, 317
Amylin   102
Anaesthetics   11

Anandamide   125
   receptors   125
Anas platyrhynchos   340
Anaximander   8
Androgen-binding protein   280
Androgens   125, 205, 277, 341, 362
Androstenedione   280, 342
Androvandi, Ulisse   17
Anemone   80
   see also Anthozoa; Cnidaria
Angel dust   129
Angiotensin-converting enzyme   152
Angiotensin-I   152
Angiotensin-II   151, 153, 154, 263
Angiotensin receptors   153, 263
Angiotensinogen   152
Anguilla anguilla   259
Annelida   88, 94
Anoles   324
Anorexia nervosa   302
ANP, *see* Atrial natriuretic peptide
Antagonist   145
Antarctica   38
Anterioventral tip of the third ventricle
   (AV3V)   154
Anthozoa   357
Anthropogenic activity   364
Antidiuretic peptide, *see* Vasopressin
Anti-Mullerian hormone (AMH)   141
Antioxidant   230
Ants   335, 349, 356
Anura   113
Aplysia   171, 232, 308
Apoptosis   248
Appetite   161
Apteronotus leptorhynchus   259, 321
Arabic science   10, 11
Arachidonic acid   73, 93, 125
Arachnids   354
Archistriatum, robust nucleus of   320
Arcuate nucleus   107, 174, 263, 288, 303
Area postrema   104, 105, 175
Area X   320
Arginine   123
Arginine-vasopressin, *see* Vasopressin
Aristotle   3, 9
Aromatase   206, 362
Arrestin   139
Arthropoda   88, 102, 127, 354
Aryl hydrocarbon receptor   362
Arylalkylamine *N*-acetyltransferase
   (AANAT)   231
Asexual species   276
   see also Parthenogenic species
Aspilia   359

Astrocytes   207, 268
Atomism   7, 23
Atrial natriuretic peptide   159,
   160, 161
Atropa belladonna   358
Australia   52
Autism   320
Autocatalytic reactions   43, 48
Autocrine   57, 79
Autonomic nervous system   99, 244
Aves   113
Ayurvedic writings   3

Babylon   3
Bacon, Roger   12
Barbaro, Ermolao   17
Barbiturates   130
Bargmann   32
Bark beetle   342
Barreswill   30
Basal lamina   281
Basement membrane   281
Batidae   348
Batrachordiformes   349
Batrachotoxin   349
Bed nucleus of the stria terminalis   154, 172,
   268, 303, 322
Behaviour   154
   affiliative   319
   aggressive   318, 342
   brooding   322
   courtship   235, 317
   ingestive   158, 166, 179, 207
   locomotion   323
   maternal   199, 322
   motivational   207
   pair-bonding   319
   parental   321
   paternal   322
   reproductive   205, 317
   reward   308, 311
   scent marking   318
   sexual   205
   singing in birds   205, 317
   stress   154
Belgium   14
Belon, Pierre   18
Benzodiazepine   130, 219, 271
Bernard, Claude   22, 29
Bilateral organisms   86, 87
Biological clocks   216
Bipolar disorder   165
Birds   266, 299, 317, 340
Bisphenol A   362
Black goby   341

Blood–brain barrier 100, 101, 103, 105, 154, 314, 351
Blood–testes barrier 280
BNP, *see* Atrial natriuretic peptide
BNST, *see* Bed nucleus of the stria terminalis
Bombesin 179, 351
Bombyx mori 182, 337
Bone morphogenic protein (BMP) 74, 75, 141
Bougery 25
Boyle, Robert 22
Bracciolini, Poggio 12
Brachiostoma californiensis 196
Brachiostoma lanceolatum 233
Bradykinesia 210
Bradykinin 153
Brainstem 173, 179, 255
Branchiostoma californiensis 196
Breast-feeding 264
Brevicomin 342
Bromocriptine 268
Brown-Sequard 31
Bunodosoma granulifera 357
Burgess shale 95
Byzantine Empire 10–12

Caenorhabditus elegans 92, 209, 230
Caerulein 351
Caffeine 359
Calcitonin 102, 165
Calcitonin-gene–related peptide 102, 165, 271
Calcitonin receptor 165
Calcium 57, 122, 123, 163, 164, 191, 253, 357
Cambrian Period 64
Cambridge University 32
Camellia sinensis 359
Canada 64
Candida albicans 330
Cannabinoids 93, 125, 326, 360
Cannabis sativa 360
Cannon, Walter 32
Carassius auratus 258
Carbohydrates 50, 51, 251
Carbon monoxide 123, 124
Carboniferous Period 113, 352
Carp 323, 325
CART, *see* Cocaine and amphetamine regulated transcript (CART)
Cartilaginous fish, *see* Chondrichthyes
Catalase 210
Catecholamines 126, 249
Catostomus commersoni 251
Caudate putamen 319
Caulepa taxifola 358
CCK, *see* Cholecystokinin
Cell theory 26

Cellular dehydration 150
Celsus 12
Central grey 173, 322
Centruroides limpidus limpidus 354
Cephalochordate 97
Cerebrospinal fluid 103, 132, 165
Cetaceans 338, 342
c-fos expression 219
CG 289
Chasmagnathus granulatus 162
Chelonia 113
Chelonia mydas 233
Chelyosoma productum 196
Chicken 198, 266
Chimpanzee 288, 359
Chin gland 340
China 11, 12
Chipmunks 223
Chloride channels 130, 144, 145
Cholecystokinin 133, 173, 179, 270
Cholesterol 56, 93, 125
Choline acetyltransferase 130
Cholinergic projections 91
Chondrichthyes 105, 110, 196, 273
 see also Elasmobranchii; Holocephali
Chondrostei 114
Chordata 86, 87
Chorionic gonadotrophin, *see* Gonadotropin
Choroid plexus 170
Christian pilgrimages 11
Chromaffin cells 249
Chrysolorus, Manuel 12
Cilia 53, 63, 81
Ciona intestinalis 108, 270
Circadian rhythms 204, 216
 profile 240
Circumventricular organ 102, 104, 302
 see also Area postrema; Median eminence; Organum vasculosum of the lateral terminalis (OVLT); Subfornical organ
Clock genes 224, 225
Clover 361
Cnemidophorus inoratus 317
Cnidaria 67, 70, 72, 79, 80, 87, 357
CNP, *see* Natriuretic peptides
Cocaine 311, 360
Cocaine and amphetamine regulated transcript (CART) 181
Coccinellines 349
Cockroach 94, 170
Codeine 359
Coelacanth 112, 151, 289
Coelenterata 79, 81

Coffee   359
Coffee arabica   359
Cola nitida   359
Colonial organisms   63
Columbus livia   259
Columbus, Realdus   13
Conopeptides   158
Conotoxins   354
Constantinople   11
Conus   354
   Conus anemome   354
   Conus geographus   156
   Conus striatus   156
Corpora allata   93, 170
Corpus cardiacum   32, 93, 162
Corpus luteum   296
Corticosterone   153
Corticotrophin-releasing factor   102, 134, 147,
   163, 222, 236, 247, 254
   binding protein   259
   profile   213
   receptors   259
Cortisol   106, 233, 246
Coturnix japonica   318
Coumestrol   361
Cranial nerves
   IX   171
   X   171
Crayfish   102
CRF, *see* Corticotrophin-releasing factor
CRH, *see* Corticotrophin-releasing factor
Cricket   170, 279
Croaker   301
Crocodilia   105, 113, 338
Crocuta crocuta   318
Crustacea   204
Crustacean hyperglycaemic hormone   204
Cryptochrome   227
Ctenophora   67, 70, 79
Cubozoa   357
Curare   358
Cuvier   25
Cyanobacteria   54, 55
Cyclosporin A   267
Cyprinus carpio   323
Cysteine   55
Cytochrome P   450
   cholesterol side cleavage enzyme   125
Cytokines   134, 140, 179
Cytoskeleton   53, 58, 163

da Verona, Guarino   12
Dalton, John Call   30
Darwin, Charles   21, 25
Darwin, Erasmus   25

Dasyatis sabina   106
Decahydraquinolines   349
Decidua   195
Dehydration   150, 158
Deiodinase   169, 198
Deltorphin, *see* Opioids
Democritus   7
Dendroaspis augusticeps   352
Dendrobatidae   349
Dentate gyrus   315
Depression   165, 220, 246, 302
Dermorphin, *see* Opioids
Descartes, Rene   23
Deuterostomes   86, 91, 95
Diagonal band of Broca   324
Diapause   209
Diencephalons   256
Dihydroxytestosterone   280
Dinoponera quadriceps   335
Dinosaur   113
Diploblastic organisms   72, 133
Diploptera punctata   163
Dipnoi   105, 112
Distal convoluted tubule   151
Diuresis   156
Diuretic hormone (DH)   163, 171
DNA   51, 52, 217
Dogs   197
Dolichol   335
DOPA   101, 126, 249
Dopamine   91, 107, 210, 249, 252, 298, 313,
   318, 336, 360
Dopamine β hydroxylase   127, 249
Dopamine receptors   127, 210
Dorsal medial complex   173
Dorsal vagal complex (DVC)   174
Drosophila melanogaster   76, 79, 130, 209,
   230, 270
Du Vigneaud, Vincent   32
Dugesia japonica   91

Ecdysozoa   86, 91–3, 99, 102, 103, 115, 141,
   256, 353
Ecdysteroids   142, 203, 277
   ecdysone   277
   20 hydroxy ecdysone   277
Echinodermata   80, 86, 87, 95
Eclosion hormone (EH)   203
Ediacaran organisms   60, 64–7, 80, 82, 357
Edinger-Westphal nucleus   256
Egypt   3
Eicosanoids   125
Elapidae   352
Elasmobranchii   110, 114, 153
Electroencephalogram (EEG)   325

Electrolytes   194
Elephants   342
Empedocles   3, 6
Encephalization   89
Encephalomyelitis   268
Endoplasmic reticulum   56, 125
Endozepines   271
Energy   167, 263
Enkephalin   133
   met-   102
Entorhinal cortex   315
Epicurus   3
Epididymis   297
Epinephrine   126, 167, 250, 314, 360
Eptatretus stouti   105–6
Erpetoichthyes   105
Erythropoietin   140
Erythroxylon coca   360
Esox lucius   227
Estienne, Charles   13
Eustachio, Bartolomeo   14
Exercise   167
Exo-brevicomin, *see* Brevicomin
Exocrine   52, 57, 350
Extracellular matrix   68, 132

Facial nerve   181
Faeces   337
Fallipio, Gabriele   14
Fatty acids   245, 250
Fear   312
Fernel, Jean   20
Fertility   302
FGF, *see* Fibroblast growth factor
Fibroblast growth factor   91
Fibronectin   141
Fight or flight   245
Flagella   53, 63
FMRFamide   91, 92, 133
Follicle-stimulating hormone (FSH)   110, 135, 280
Foraging   167
Forebrain   97, 314
Formaldehyde   38, 44
Franco–Prussian war   26
Frequency modulation   290
Freshwater   151
Fritsch   27
FSH, *see* Follicle-stimulating hormone (FSH)
β-Funaltrexamine   269
Furin   71

Galanin   174, 268, 297, 300, 323
Galen   9, 12, 13, 360
Gallus domesticus   259

Galvani   25
Gametes   71, 276
γ-amino butyric acid (GABA)   69, 130, 143, 252, 286
   receptors   69, 130, 143, 144, 325
Gaskell   31
Gastrin   173
Gastrin-releasing peptide (GRP)   226, 270
Gastropod   362
General adaptation syndrome   32, 245
   alarm reaction   32
   countershock phase   32
   shock phase   32
Genome expansion   116
Geodia cydonium   69
Germany   26
Gesner, Conrad   17
GH, *see* Growth hormone (GH)
GHRH, *see* Growth hormone-releasing hormone (GHRH)
Gill-withdrawal reflex   309
Gillichthys mirabilis   262
Gills   155, 158, 161, 165
Glia   102
   see also Astrocytes; Schwann cells
Glisson   25
Glossopharyngeal nerve   181
GLP-1, *see* Glucagon-like peptide
Glucagon-like peptide   1, 176
Glucocorticoid receptor   237, 315
   Type I   263
   Type II   263
Glucocorticoids   201, 248, 263, 314, 315
   responsive elements   316
   synthesis   126
Gluconeogenesis   248
Glutamate   69
   receptors   137, 143
Glutamate decarboxylase   130
Glutathione   231
Glutathione peroxidase   54
Glycera convolute   354
Glycera dibranchiate   354
Glycine   143
Glycogen   245
Glycogenesis   248
Glycogenolysis   248
Glycolysis   167, 248
Glycoprotein   105, 110, 129, 135, 165, 266, 289, 293
   see also CG; FSH; LH; TSH
Gnathonemus   115
GnRH, *see* Gonadotropin-releasing hormone
Gobius jozo   341

Goldfish   258
Golgi, Camillo   27
Gonad-inhibiting hormone (GIH)   204
Gonadotropin   233
   -I   288
   -II   288, 295
   chorionic   289
Gonadotropin-releasing hormone   108, 121,
   133, 209, 235, 282
   evolution   283
   expression   284
   function   288
   migration   285
   structure   135
Gonadotropin-releasing hormone II   287, 325
GPCR, *see* G-protein-coupled receptor
G-protein-coupled receptor   53, 72, 73, 76,
   123, 137–9
Granulosa cells   281
Greece   3, 34
Green, John   33
Greenland   40
GRF, *see* Growth hormone-releasing hormone
   (GHRH)
Ground squirrels   223
Growth hormone (GH)   110, 134, 190, 209, 265
Growth hormone-releasing hormone
   (GHRH)   107, 134, 190
Guanylyl cyclase   124
Guillemin, Roger   34
Guppy   362
Gymnophiona   113

Habituation   308
Haemoglobin   30
Haemolymph   94
Hagfish   103, 107, 110, 153
   see also Myxini
Haller   25
Hamster   217
   Djungarian   223, 224
   Siberian   223
   Syrian   232, 233
Harderian gland   232
Harris, Geoffrey   32
Harvey, William   13, 23
Hatschek's Pit   108
Heat shock proteins   143
Heavy metals   246
Hedgehog   76, 133
Helix aspera maxima   232
Heloderma horridum horridum   353
Hemichordata   86
Heraclitus   3
Heterochrony   199

Heterodontus japonicus   106
Hibernation   223
High vocal center   320
Hindbrain   97
Hindu culture   3
Hippocampus   311, 315, 316, 322
Hippocrates   3–5
Histone   52
Hitzig   27
5-HT, *see* 5-hydroxytryptamine
Holocephali   110
   see also Chondrichthyes
Holostean fishes   114
Holy Land   11
Homeobox-containing genes   79
   hox   79
   Pax   79
Homeostasis   3, 30, 45, 55, 71, 243
Honeybee   355
Hoppe Seyler   30
Hot vents   40
Hox genes, *see* Homeobox-containing genes
Hydra   67, 70–5, 79–81, 86
Hydra vulgaris   71
Hydractinia   76
Hydrazoa   357
Hydrin   158
Hydrolagus colliei   106
Hydroxide radical   54, 55
11-β-Hydroxyandrostenedione   294, 295
Hydroxyindole-*O*-methyltransferase
   (HIOMT)   128, 228
11-Hydroxysteroid dehydrogenase   315, 316
5-Hydroxytryptamine (HT; serotonin)   73,
   127, 128, 209, 228, 229, 234, 239
   receptors   127, 128, 209
5-Hydroxytryptophan   127
Hyena   318
Hyla caerulea   270
Hyla cinerea   321
Hylidae   350
Hyoscyamine   358
Hypophyseal portal system   110–13
Hypophysis, *see* Pituitary gland
Hypothalamus   110–13, 152–5, 173–5, 206–8,
   225–6, 234–8, 247, 248, 254, 263–9, 277, 302
Hypothalamus–pituitary systems
   adrenal   247
   gonadal   277
   thyroid   168, 198
Hypoxia   251

Ibn al-Nafs   11
Ibn al Quff   11
Ibn Baytar   11

Ibn Sina   23
I.C.V., *see* Intracerebroventicular injection
IGF-II receptor   193
Iguana iguana   227
Ilex paraguariensis   359
Imposex   362
India   11–12
Indoleamine hormones, *see* Melatonin;
   Serotonin
Inferior lobes   173
Infradian rhythms   216, 220
Infundibulum   108
Inhibin   135, 141, 280
Insects   92, 332, 356
Insulin   135, 179, 181, 209, 263
Insulin-like growth factor   103, 191, 209
   binding proteins   192
   IGF-I   192
   IGF-II   192
   receptors   192
Insulin receptor   140
Intergeniculate leaflet   219, 234
Interleukin   102, 179, 190
Intermediate filaments   286
Intracerebroventicular injection   325
Intracrine   52, 57
Iodine   128
Ischaemia   166
Islam   10, 11
Islets of Langerhans   181
Isoflavonoids   361
Isomer   44
Isoprenoid   56
Isoproterenol   127
Izidines   349

JAK, *see* Janus kinase
Janus kinase   76, 140
Jellyfish   357
Jerusalem   11
Jet lag   237
Juvenile hormone (JH)   170, 203, 209, 277,
   336, 361
Juxtaglomerular cells   151

K$^+$, *see* Potassium ion
Kainate receptors   325, 357
Kairomones   346
Kaliuretic peptides
   BNP   159
Ketones
   methyl (garter snakes)   340
11-Ketotestosterone   294, 295
Kidney   152
   head   250

Killifish   362
Kinases   141–2
   casein   218
Kindling   325
King snake, *see* Snakes
Kola   359

Lactotrophs   298
Lagomorpha   322
Lamarck   25
Lamna cornubica   270
Lamprey   110, 153, 201, 226
Lateral hypothalamus   269
Lateral tuberal nucleus   251
Latipinna poecilia   259
Laudanum   22
Leech   161
Leibniz   23
Leptin   134, 175, 180, 263
Leptin receptor   181
Leucophaea maderae   196
Leucophora maderae   270
Leukotrienes   125
Leydig cells   281
LH, *see* Luteinizing hormone (LH)
Libido   300
Limbic system   268, 344
Lingulodinium   230
Linnaeus, Carolus   21
Lionfish   348
Lipids   47, 49, 50, 56, 298, 333
   see also Fatty acids
Lipolysis   250
Lipotropin   261
Lissemys punctata punctata   237
Liver   248, 280
lizards   113, 226, 227, 317, 352, 353
Llyanassa obsoleta   362
Locus coeruleus   173, 259, 269, 313
Locust   162, 332
Locusta migratoria   157, 277
Locustomyotropin   162
Long-term potentiation   309
Lophotrochozoa   86, 91, 92, 99, 115,
   141, 353
Lordosis   207, 325
Low density lipid (LDL) receptors   133
Lucretius   7, 8
Lungfish   105, 153
Luteinizing hormone (LH)   110, 135, 280
   see also Gonadotropin
Luteinizing hormone–releasing hormone,
      see Gonadotropin-releasing hormone
Lymnaea stagnalis   156
Lyonet   21

Macaque   265
Macroglomerular complex   333
Macrophage colony–stimulating factor   190
Magendie, Francois   29
Magnesium   122
Magnus, Albertus   19
Major histocompatibility complex   344
Malpighi, Marcello   21
Malpighian tubules   163
Mammary glands   297
Mammosomatotrophs   195
Manduca sexta   196
Mannose-6-phosphate receptor   193
   see also IGF-II receptor
MAP kinase   301
Marmosets   288
Mars   38
Median eminence   104
Mediobasal hypothalamus   235
Mediterranean Sea   358
Meiosis   276, 281
Melanin-concentrating hormone (MCH)
      102, 173, 253
   profile   185
Melanocortin receptors   181, 261
Melanocyte-stimulating hormone (MSH)   113
Melanophore   253
Melanostatin   252
Melanotrope   252
Melatonin   54, 218, 359
   biosynthesis   127, 230
   evolution   229
   functions of   230
   hypothesis   226
   patterns   232
   receptors   234
Memory   307, 310
Mendel, Gregor   25
Menstrual cycle   221
Mesocorticolimbic projections   311
Mesocricetus auratus   268
Metallothioneins   210
Metamorphosis   3, 198
   Anura   3, 202
   insects   3, 202
   lamprey   170, 202
   salmonids   202
Metazoa   75, 78
Meteorite   40, 51
5-Methoxytrypophol (5-ML)   232
Methyl farnesoate (MF)   203
   see also Juvenile hormone (JH)
Mexican beaded lizard   353
Mexico   64
Microtus montanus   322

Microtus ochrogaster   223, 268, 322
Midbrain   97, 225, 311
Miller, Stanley   40
Millipedes   349
Mineralcorticoid receptor, *see* Glucocorticoids
      receptor, type I
Mineralocorticoids   263
Molluscs   86, 94, 157
Mongolia   11
Monoamine   71
   see also catecholamines; Indoleamine
      hormones
Monosiga brevicollis   76
Monro   25
Mood disorder   314
Morphine   262, 359
Moth   279
Motivated behaviour   207
Moult-inhibiting hormone (MIH)   204
Moulting   202, 203, 277
Mudpuppies   338
Mushroom bodies   279
Mustelus   105
Myokinins   163
Mytilus edulis   262
Myxine glutinosa   233
Myxini   105, 233
   see also Hagfish

Na$^+$, *see* Sodium
Naja naja   353
Naloxone   269
Nasal embryonic LHRH factor (NELF)   286
Nasal epithelium   285
Natriuretic peptides   159
NCAM, *see* Neural cell-adhesion molecule
      (NCAM)
Necturus maculosus   338
NELF, *see* Nasal embryonic LHRH factor
      (NELF)
Nematoda   91
Neocortex   312
Nephron   151
Nereis diversicolor   161
Nerve net   97, 99
Neural cell-adhesion molecule (NCAM)   286
Neural ridge   285
Neurexin   102
Neurodegeneration   325
Neurohypophysis   155
   see also Pituitary gland
Neurokinin A   271
Neuropeptide F   91
Neuropeptide Y   91, 134, 173, 174, 219, 291
Newt   264, 318, 323, 340

Newton, Issac   24
Nicotiana tabacum   360
Nicotine   311
Nigrostriatal pathway   210, 311
Nissl, Frans   27
Nitric oxide   123, 153, 292
Nitrogen   191
N-methyl D-aspartate (NMDA) receptor   129, 145, 225, 354
   see also Glutamate, receptors
Nodes of Ranvier   102
Non-photic input   219
Norepinephrine   99, 126, 168, 180, 291, 305, 311, 360
Noscapine   359
Notch   76
NPY, *see* Neuropeptide Y
NTS: nucleus of the solitary tract   172, 174, 175, 181
Nuclear receptors   143
   see also Orphan receptors; Retinoids; Steroids; Thyroid hormone
Nucleus accumbens   175, 311
Nucleus basalis   315
Nucleus of medial longitudinal fasciculus (nMLF)   256, 287, 323
Nucleus of the solitary tract (NTS)   160, 171, 322
Nudibranch   308
   see also Molluscs
Nutrients   357

Obesity   166
Ocelli   97
Octopus vulgaris   94, 157
Oestradiol   295, 319, 356
Oestrogens   125, 205, 223, 277
   receptors   143
Oestrous cycle   221
Olfactory bulb   199, 285, 338
   accessory   338
   main   338
   projections   338
Olfactory epithelium   199
Olfactory lobe   173
Olfactory placode   284
Oligochaete, *see* Leech
Oncorhynchus kisutch   266
Oncorhynchus nerka   256
Oncorynchus mykiss   248, 270, 323, 362
Oocytes   281
Oogonia   281
Opioids   261, 304, 311
   deltorphins   262, 351
   dermorphins   262, 351

dynorphins   261
endorphins   261, 304
enkephalins   261, 304
morphine   262
orphinins   261
Optic gland   95
Optic lobe   173
Optic tectum   233
Orexin   173
Organum vasculosum of the lateral terminalis (OVLT)   105, 154, 291
Orinoco   358
Orphan receptors   146
Orthology   120
Oryzia postica   279
Osmolality   150, 159
Osmoreceptors   154
Osmoregulation   87, 113
Osteoglossum   105, 115
Ovary   341
Ovary-maturing peptide (OMP)   277
OVLT, *see* Organum vasculosum of the lateral terminalis (OVLT)
Oxford University   12
Oxygen   54–6, 169, 216, 250
Oxytocin   32, 133, 156, 179, 234, 247, 317, 321
   receptors   158
Ozone   216

Pacemaker   225
Paleologus, Manuel   12
Pallium   234
Pancreas   153
   see also Islets of Langerhans
Papaver somnoferum   359
Papaverine   359
Parabranchial nucleus   174, 181
Paracelsus   19, 20
Paracrine   57, 79
Paralogy   120
Paralysins   205
Paramecium   230
Parapineal organ   227
Paraponera clavata   356
Parasympathetic nervous system   99, 249
Parathyroid gland   164
Parathyroid hormone   164
Parathyroid hormone–related peptide   165
Paraventricular nucleus   107, 173, 234, 257, 268, 288, 313
Paraventricular organ, *see* Circumventricular organs
Parietal eye   227
Paris   12

Parkinsons disease   210
Parr   202
Pars distalis   114
    see also Pituitary gland
Pars intercerebralis   277
Pars intermedia   114
    see also Pituitary gland
Pars nervosa   110, 111, 113
    see also Pituitary gland
Pars neurointermedia   110
    see also Pituitary gland
Pars tuberalis   235
Parthenogenic species   276, 317
Passer domesticus   227
Pax genes, see Homeobox-containing genes
Pedunculo-pontine nuclei   360
Pelage   235
Pepsin   173
Pepsinogen   173
Peptidase   132
Peptides   131
Periaqueductal central grey   185
Periodicity   216
Peripherin   286
Peromyscus maniculatus   268
Peroxide   54
Persia   10
Petramyzontiformes   105
    see also Lamprey
Petromyzon marinus   106, 193
Phase-shifting   219
Phencyclidines   129
Phenylethanolamine-O-methyltransferase
    (PNMT)   127
Pheromone   57, 138, 330
    aggregation   334
    alarm   335
    courtship   334
    dispersion   335
    exocrine glands   335
    sex attractants   335
    trail marking   335
Pheromone biosynthesis–activating peptide
    (PBAN)   336
Phosphate   166, 191
Photoperiod   220, 264, 300
Phyllobates terribilis   349
Phyllomedusa sauvagei   352
Phyllomedusinae   258, 351
Phytoecdysteroids   361
Phytoestrogens   361
Pigeons   259
Pimpla hypochrondriaca   356
Pineal gland   104, 233
    function of   226

locus of the soul   23
    melatonin secretion   227
    neuroendocrine regulation   225
Pinealectomy   227, 300
Piso, William   18
Pit-1   298
Pituitary adenylate cyclase activating
    peptide (PACAP)   190
    profile   211
Pituitary gland   32
    anterior lobe   108
    buccal lobe   110
    evolution of   110
    hormones of   107
    intermediate lobe   108
    neural lobe   104, 107, 110
    neurointermediate lobe   110, 114
    ontogeny of   109
    portal system   33, 112
    teleost   114
    ventral lobe   110
Placenta   199
Placental lactogen   194
Placozoa   67, 68, 78, 80, 81
Planaria   89
Plants   357
Plasma membrane   27, 49
Plato   4, 6, 9
Platyhelminthes   86, 89
Plethon, Gemistos   12
Pleurodeles waltii   259
Pliny the Elder   9, 17
Poikilothermy   194
Poison-arrow frogs   349
Polychaete
    fanged bloodworm   354
Polychlorinated biphenyls   362
Polypterus   105
POMC, see Proopiomelanocortin (POMC)
Pompilidotoxin   355
Poneratoxin   356
Porifera   67–70, 78, 80, 81, 357
Post-translational modifications   135
    acetylation   135
    amidation   135
    endoproteolytic cleavage   135
    exoproteolytic cleavage   135
    glycosylation   135
    sulphation   135
Potamotrygon   105
Potassium   101, 129
    channel   309
    channel toxins   357
Precambrian explosion   64, 82, 91, 95, 115
Prefrontal cortex   322

Preoptic area   154, 206, 303
Primates   342
Primordial follicle   281
PRL, *see* Prolactin
Prodynorphin   261
Proenkephalin   261
Progesterone   205, 281, 317
Prohormone   135–7
Prohormone convertase   71, 136
Prokaryotes   52, 53
Prolactin   108, 110, 202, 223, 321
   functions of   161, 295
   receptor   194
   role in lactation   296
   role in osmoregulation   161
   role in stress   265
   structure   134
Proliferin   194
Proliferin-related protein   194
Proopiomelanocortin (POMC)   108, 110,
   181, 261
   brain   273
   evolution   261, 273
   processing   261
   profile   272
Proorphinin   261
Prostacyclins   125
Prostaglandins   125, 340
Prostate gland   280
Protein kinase   146
Prothoracic gland   171
Prothoracicotropic peptide (PTTH)   203
Protocell   42, 46, 48–50
Proximal convoluted tubule   164–5
Psychotropic agents   346
Puberty   281, 293, 342
   in fish   293
   in mammals   281, 293
Purines   124
PVN, *see* Paraventricular nucleus
Pyriform cortex   315
Pyrophosphate   41

Quail   318
Quiescence   218

Radiata   73, 87, 95
Raja binoculata   106
Raja erinacea   233, 282
Ramon y Cajal, Santiago   27
Rana catesbeiana   202
Rana dybowskii   222
Rana esculenta   201, 234, 293
Rana pipiens   362
Rana ridibunda   252, 259, 271

Rana sphenocephala   321
Rana temporaria   222
Rana tigrina   259
Ranakinin   271
Raphe nuclei   173, 322
RAS, *see* Renin-angiotensin system
Ras oncogene   140
Rathke's pouch   108, 109
Ray-finned fishes, *see* Actinopterygii
Ray, John   21
Reactive oxygen species (ROS)   230
Receptor kinase   75, 135
Red deer   223, 301
Reissner's Fibre   105
Relaxin   135
Renaissance   12, 20
Renilla kollikeri   232
Renin   152
Renin-angiotensin system   151–3, 159
Reproductive cycles   279
Reptiles   105, 113, 226, 340
Resveratrol   230
Reticular formation   325
Retina   225, 227
Retinohypothalamic tract (RHT)   226, 241
Retinoic acid   75, 130, 147
   receptors   130, 142, 203
Retinoids   130
Retrochiasmatic nucleus   236
Reward   308, 311
Rhodnius prolixus   163
Rhodopsin   137
Rhynchocephalians   113
Ring doves   322–3
Rivier, Jean   34
RNA   43, 51, 52
   polymerase   52
Roman Empire   9, 10
Roman medicine   9
Rome   9
Russia   64

Saccharomyces cerevisiae   232, 330
St Augustine   11
St Johns wort   359
St Thomas Aquinas   11
Salamander   340
Saliva   337
Salmonids   202, 287
Salt gland   151
   nasal   151
   rectal   151
Saltwater   151, 159
Santorio   23
Sarcopterygii   103, 106, 112, 114, 193, 254, 311

Sauvagine   258, 351
Scaphiopus hammondii   202
Schally, Andrew   34
Scharrer, Berta   31, 32
Scharrer, Ernst   31, 32
Schleiden, Mattias   27
Schwann cells   102
Schwann, Theodor   27
SCN, *see* Suprachiasmatic nucleus
Scopolamine   326
Scorpaeniformes   348
Scorpion   354
Scyliorhinus canicula   254, 262
Scyphozoa   357
Sea bream   284
Seaweed   358
Sebaceous gland   337
Secretin   6, 31, 137, 173
Secretory granules   135
Segmental ganglia   161
Segmentation   88
Selenocosmia hainana   354
Selye, Hans   32, 34, 244, 301
Seminal vesicles   280
Seminiferous tubules   280
Semiochemicals   346
Sensilla   333
Sensitization   308
Sepia   102, 103
Septum   179
Serotonergic pathways   91
Serotonin, *see* 5-Hydroxytryptamine (HT;
    serotonin)
Sertoli cells   280
Servetus, Michael   13
Sexual receptivity   322
Sexually dimorphic nuclei   206
Shift work   237
Shrew   287
Silkworm   337
Siren intermedia   338
Skate   31, 233, 282
Sleep   237
SMAD   74, 141, 142
Smenospongia aurea   357
Smolt   202
Smoltification   202
Snake
    asp   353
    cobra   353
    garter   340
    green mamba   352
    king brown   353
    pit vipers   352
Snowshoe hares   246

Sodium   129, 151, 263
    channels   356, 360
Soldierfish   348
Somatolactin   134, 193, 195
Somatostatin   107, 133, 190
Somatotropin, *see* Growth hormone (GH)
SON, *see* Supraoptic nucleus
Song nuclei   320
South America   349
Spain   14
Spermatogenesis   281, 293
Spiders   354
Spinal cord   97, 129, 269
Spiropyrrolizines   349
Sprague-Dawley rats   175
Squalus acanthias   106, 270, 285
Squamata   352
    see also Snake; lizards
Squid   94
Squirrel   246
SS, *see* Somatostatin
STAT (signal transducers and activators
    transcription)   140, 181,
    296, 316
Steroids   71, 76, 93, 294
Stomatogastric nervous system   99
Stonefish   348
Stress   154
Stress syndrome, *see* General adaptation
    syndrome
Striatum   311
Sturgeons   114
Sturnus vulgaris   320
Subcommissural organ   104
    see also Circumventricular organ
Subfornical organ   104, 105, 155
    see also Circumventricular organ
Suboesophageal ganglion   157, 336
Substance P   153, 269, 271, 318
Substantia innominata   310, 315
Substantia nigra   311
Subtilisin family of enzymes   136
Superoxide dismutase   210
Superoxide radical   54, 55
Suprachiasmatic nucleus   173, 217, 225, 234,
    252, 322
Supraoptic nucleus   154, 173, 288
Swammerdam   21
Sydenham, Thomas   20, 22
Symmetry   79
Sympathetic nervous system   93, 99,
    245, 249
Synaptic transmission   349
Synomones   346
Syria   10

T3, *see* Thyroid hormone
T4, *see* Thyroid hormone
Tachykinin   153, 271
Tamias amoenus   223
Tanycytes   103
Taricha granulosa   323
Tau   217
Tau mutant   217
   profile   239
T-cells   267
Teleostei   113, 114
Teneurin C-terminal associated peptide
      (TCAP)   256
Termites   333
Testis   281
Testosterone   205, 223, 246, 295, 342,
      356, 362
   see also Steroids
Tetraodontiformes   349
Thalamus   179
Theca externa   281
Theca interna   281
Thermogenesis   169
Theromyzon tessulatum   161
Thirst   161
Thoracic ganglia   162
Thromboxanes   125
Thurniesser, Leaonary   22
Thyroglobulin   129
Thyroid hormone   71, 128, 142, 147, 266
   T3   169, 198, 222
   T4   169, 198, 222
   receptors   143
Thyrotropin, *see* Thyroxine stimulating
      hormone (TSH)
Thyroxine, *see* Thyroid hormone
Thyroxine stimulating hormone (TSH)
      110, 113, 135
Ticks   336, 354
Tilapia   193, 292
Toadfish   349
Tobacco hornworm, *see Manduca sexta*
Torpor   223
Toxins, *see* Xenobiotics
Transcription element binding protein
      (BTEB)   201
Transforming growth factor (TGF)
      74–6, 141, 209
Transgenic   79, 202
Transthyretins   170
Tree frogs, *see* Hylidae
TRH, *see* TSH-releasing hormone
Tributyl tin   362
Trichoplax adherens   67
Triglycerides   245

Triploblastic organisms   72, 82, 86–8, 150
Triturus carniflex   234
Trypsin   352
Tryptophan   127
Tryptophan hydroxylase   128
TSH, *see* Thyroxine stimulating
      hormone (TSH)
TSH-releasing hormone   107, 166, 168
Tuatara   113
Tubero-infundibular region   299
Tunicates   108
Tupaia glis belangeri   287
Turkey   9, 322
Turtles
   Green   233
   soft-shelled   237
Typhlonectes   105
Tyrannosaurus rex   121
Tyrosine hydroxylase   126, 318
Tyrosine kinase   73, 140, 253
   receptor   191

Ubiqinone   335
Ultradian rhythms   216
Ungulates   288, 322
   artiodactyls ruminants   147, 196
   cetartiodactyls   196
   perissodactyl   255
United Kingdom   64
Urey, Harold   40
Urinary bladder   155
Urochordate   97, 196
Urocortin   155, 256, 304
   -II   176, 256
   -III   176, 256
Urodela   113, 340
Urophysis   105, 155
Uropigial gland   340
Urotensin-I   105, 155, 251, 304
   see also Sauvagine; Urocortin
Urotensin-II   105, 133, 155
   profile   187

Vagus nerve   99, 173, 179
   dorsal motor complex   179
Vale, Wylie   34
Van Helmont   22
Van Leeuwenhoek   21
Vasoactive intestinal peptide (VIP)
      202, 226, 299
Vasoconstriction   151
Vasopressin   32, 133, 155, 234, 247, 257, 319
   receptors   158, 319
Vasotocin   71, 133, 155, 234, 321
Venom   348

Ventral tegmental area   311, 360
Ventromedial hypothalamus   179, 183,
    206, 207, 223, 263, 317, 322,
    338, 344
Ventromedial nucleus   173, 206
Vesalius, Andreas   13, 14
Vitamin A, *see* Retinoic acid
Vitamin C   54
Vitamin D   125
Vitamin E   54, 230
Vitellogenin   209, 277
Vitronectin   193
VMH, *see* Ventromedial hypothalamus
Voles   319
Vomeromodulin   343
Vomeronasal organ   286, 338
    evolution   338
    neural projections   339
    structure   339

Wallaby   301
Wallace, Alfred Russell   21, 25

Wasp   333, 355
Wharton, Thomas   24
Willis, Thomas   24
Wingless-related   76, 133
    receptor (frizzled)   76, 146
Wistar rats   269
Wnt, *see* Wingless-related

Xenobiotics   345
Xenopus laevis   108, 158, 202, 234, 252,
    259, 321, 338, 362
Xenoturbella bocki   95
Xestospongia   357
Xth cranial nerve, *see* Vagus nerve

Yalow, Rosalyn   34
Yohimbine   269

Zebrafish   193
Zinc-finger   142
Zona glomerulosa cells   153
Zucker rats   175